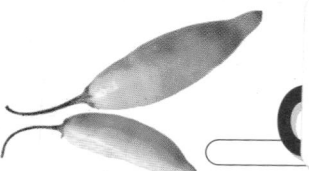

Page ▽

Calorie, Fat & Carbohydrate Counter:

Weight Control Tips

✅ Eat Sensibly
- Avoid fad diets. Eat 3 sensible meals daily.
- Limit fats and fatty foods, sugar, soda and alcohol.

(Sample Diet Plan, Page 9)

✅ Exercise Daily
- Get active and exercise every day!
- Include muscle-strengthening exercises. You'll lose more fat and keep it off. You'll also feel and look better, and you can eat a little more food. *(Exercise Guide, Page 10)*

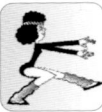

✅ Reshape Eating Behaviors
- Be aware of eating and shopping behaviors that lead to overeating.
- Also focus on social and emotional situations that make you snack compulsively.

(Extra notes - Page 12

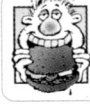

✅ Keep a Food & Exercise Diary
- A diary helps you see exactly what you eat and drink, and how much you really exercise.
- An excellent motivator.
- Keeps you honest! *(Page 13)*

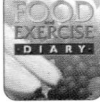

✅ Arrange Moral Support
Gain the support of family and friends. Get extra professional help if required, from your doctor, dietitian, psychologist, exercise trainer, or slimming group. Beware of family saboteurs who discourage you from adopting a healthier lifestyle!

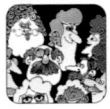

DOCTOR CHECK-UP
Ask your doctor to check you for high blood pressure, diabetes, and high blood cholesterol.

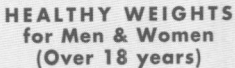

HEALTHY WEIGHTS for Men & Women (Over 18 years)

Based on weights with least risk of disease or death from heart disease, diabetes, stroke and cancer.

Based on Body Mass Index - range 20-25.

BMI calculated as: $\dfrac{\text{Weight (kg)}}{\text{Height (m)}^2}$

Height (No Shoes)	Healthy Weight Range
Ft Ins	Pounds
4'7"	86-108
4'8"	88-110
4'9"	92-114
4'10"	97-121
4'11"	99-123
5'0"	101-127
5'1"	105-132
5'2"	110-136
5'3"	112-140
5'4"	114-145
5'5"	119-149
5'6"	123-156
5'7"	127-158
5'8"	129-162
5'9"	134-167
5'10"	138-173
5'11"	143-178
6'0"	145-182
6'1"	149-187
6"2"	156-193
6'3"	158-198
6'4"	162-202
6'5'	170-211
6'6"	172-215
6'7"	175-220

Body Fat Distribution & Health

Fat above the hips carries a far greater health risk than fat on or below the hips - better to be a **'pear-shape'** than an **'apple-shape'**.

Abdominal obesity greatly increases the risk of developing diabetes, heart disease, high blood fats, hypertension, stroke and some cancers. So-called **'cellulite'** carries no extra health risk.

Waist Measurement (High Health Risk)

Men: Over 39 inches **Women:** Over 34 inches

Women who become obsessed with dieting away their thighs and buttocks on an otherwise lean body, are fighting mother nature and may well be inviting health problems.

If you are within a healthy weight range, it is better to exercise regularly to maintain body shape, rather than to be constantly dieting and lacking in energy. Accept your body shape and focus on other pursuits and enjoying life!

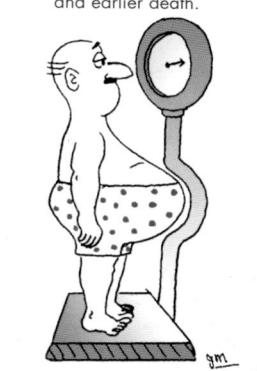

Abdominal obesity greatly increases the risk of ill-health and earlier death.

Estimating Body Fat Percentage

Body fat percentage is a better indicator of health than total weight.

Bioelectric impedance analysis (BIA) is gaining support as a practical and economical method for estimating body fat in both clinical and home settings.

BIA measures the resistance of a weak electrical current that is passed through the body. A computer within the body fat analyzer calculates the amount of body water, fat and muscle.

More Information: www.calorieking.com

BODY FAT & OBESITY

Men: Above 25% body fat
Women: Above 32% body fat

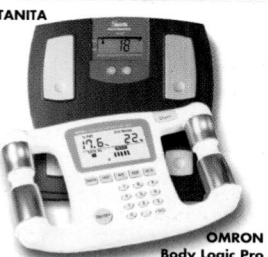

OMRON
Body Logic Pro

Easy-to-use
body fat monitors for home
and professional use.

HEALTHY BODY FAT RANGES

Men:	Under 30 years	~	14 - 20%
	Over 30 years	~	17 - 23%
Women:	Under 30 years	~	17 - 24%
	Over 30 years	~	20 - 27%

Note: Less than 13% body fat in women can be unhealthy.

Calories in Food

Calories in food are derived from protein, fat and carbohydrate. Alcohol also provides calories. Vitamins, minerals and water provide no calories.

Calorie Values Per Gram

Fat/Oil	~	9 Calories
Carbohydrate	~	4 Calories
Protein	~	4 Calories
Alcohol	~	7 Calories

Note that fats have over double the calories of protein and carbohydrate. The higher the fat content of food, the higher the calories.

Sample Calculation

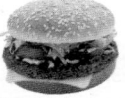

QUARTER POUNDER® WITH CHEESE has 534 calories derived from:

30g Fat (x 9 cals/gram)	=	270
38g Carbohyd.(x 4 cals/gram)	=	152
28g Protein (x 4 cals/gram)	=	112
Total Calories	**=**	**534**

Calorie Levels for Weight Loss

Commence with a calorie-controlled diet that allows a moderate weight loss of $1/2$ - 1 pound per week. Weight loss is usually much larger in the first few weeks due to extra fluid losses.

Note: It is better to increase exercise rather than lessen food calories too drastically.

Suggested Calories for Weight Loss

Women:	Non-active	1000 - 1200
	Active	1200 - 1500
Men:	Non-active	1200 - 1500
	Active	1500 - 1800
Teenagers:		1200 - 1800

Food Guide Pyramid

Fats Sweets — ◄ Use Sparingly

2-3 Servings ► Milk Soy / Meat Beans Nuts ◄ 2-3 Serving

Vegetables 3-5 Servings / Fruit 2-4 Servings

Bread, Cereals, Rice, Pasta
6-11 Servings
(4-6 Servings For Weight Loss)

The **Food Guide Pyramid** emphasizes eating a wide variety of foods from the 5 major food groups. For weight loss, make lowfat choices and eat the lower number of servings.

Examples of Serving Size

Bread & Cereal Group:
- 1 slice bread
- $1/2$ bun, bagel or English muffin
- 4 small crackers or 1 tortilla
- 1 oz ready-to-eat cereal
- $1/2$ cup cooked cereal, rice, pasta

Fruit Group:
- 1 medium apple, orange, banana
- $1/2$ cup canned fruit
- $1/4$ cup dried fruit
- $3/4$ cup fruit juice
- $1/4$ medium avocado

Vegetable Group:
- 1 cup raw leafy vegetables
- $1^1/2$ oz raw chopped vegetables
- $1/2$ cup cooked vegetables
- $1/2$ - $3/4$ cup vegetable juice

Meat & Alternatives Group:
- 2-3oz (cooked) lean meat/poultry/fish
- 2 eggs **or** 7oz tofu **or** $1/2$ cup nuts
- 1 cup (cooked) dried beans or chickpeas
- 4 Tbsp peanut butter

Milk & Alternatives Group:
- 1 cup (8 fl.oz) milk, soy drink, yogurt
- $1^1/2$ oz cheese or $1/2$ cup cottage cheese

Recommended Fat Intake

Americans consume too much fat with many having over 40% of total calories from fat - either as fat or oil, or as fat in foods and drinks. A range of 20-30% is healthier.

Fat Intake – Healthy Ranges

Children	30-60g
Teenagers (Active)	40-80g
Women	30-60g
Men: Active	40-80g
Heavy Activity/Athlete	80-120g

The chart below recommends maximum fat intake for different calorie levels.

MAXIMUM DESIRABLE FAT INTAKE (Daily)

Calories	Fat	% Fat Cals
1200 cals	30g fat	23%
1500 cals	40g fat	24%
1800 cals	50g fat	25%
2000 cals	60g fat	27%
2200 cals	70g fat	28%
2500 cals	80g fat	29%
2800 cals	90g fat	29%
3000 cals	100g fat	30%
3500 cals	117g fat	30%
4000 cals	135g fat	30%

Infants Fat Intake

Infants and toddlers under 3 years should not be restricted in their fat intake because much larger volumes of food would be required to guarantee adequate calorie intake and growth. Whole milk should be used rather than light milk (1%) or nonfat milk. Similarly, a high fiber diet is also not suitable for infants.

Calories Versus Fats

For successful weight control it is important to be aware of both fats and calories in foods. It widens your choices at the supermarket and when eating out.

While choosing more lowfat foods is wise, it does not guarantee that total calories will be reduced, particularly if portion size is not limited.

It is a mistake to think that eating lowfat or fat-free foods allows you to eat double the quantity.

Be aware that lowfat and fat-free cakes, cookies and ice cream are **not calorie-free.** Nor are soda drinks, fruit juices, beer, alcoholic spirits, sugar and sugar candy which are also fat-free. Bread, rice and pasta also have negligble fat.

Carbohydrate Calories Count

It is also a fallacy that carbohydrate calories don't count. Carbohydrates in excess of body needs can still be converted to and stored as body fat - particularly in women in their child-bearing years.

Total Calories Count!

Ultimately, **it is food portion size and total calories that count** whether from fat, carbohydrate or protein. Remember, cows get fat on grass!

FOOD LABEL MEANINGS
FDA Nutrition Claim Definitions
(All are on a Per Serving Basis.)

Low Calorie: 40 calories or less
Light or Lite: One third fewer calories or, 50% or less fat than regular product
Fat-Free: Less than half a gram of fat
Low-Fat: 3 grams or less of fat
Reduced-Fat: 25% less fat than regular product
Fewer or Less Calories: At least 25% fewer calories than regular product

Hints to Reduce Fat

Meats & Poultry

- **Choose lean cuts** of meat with little marbling. Choose the white meat of chicken and turkey, and extra lean ground beef.

- **Trim all visible fat** from meat and remove the skin from poultry. Removal of fat after cooking is okay (to prevent dryness).

- **Eat modest portions** (3-4 oz cooked weight) of meat, poultry or fish. **Add extra** beans, lentils, tofu, tempeh, vegetables, potatoes, rice, pasta, bread, or tortillas.

- **Avoid high-fat meat products** such as salami, bacon, sausage and franks. Choose lowfat and fat-free brands. Choose lean luncheon meats (90% or more fat-free).

- **Broil or bake. Avoid frying.** Allow casseroles to cool and skim off surface fat.

Fish & Seafood

- **Choose fresh or frozen fillets,** and canned fish (in water pack).

- **Avoid fried fish,** frozen fish in batter, canned fish in oil.

Fats & Oils

- **Use minimal amounts** of all types of fat and oil. All are high in calories.

- **Choose** 'light' and 'reduced fat' spreads but still use sparingly. Check the Fats and Spreads section of this book for lower fat brands.

- Use minimal amounts of oil when stir-frying. Use no-stick sprays like *Pam*.

Salad Dressings & Sauces

- **Avoid regular mayonnaise and oil dressings.** Choose 'light', 'reduced fat' or 'fat-free' brands (Check salad dressings section of this book).

- **Choose** lowfat or fat-free sauces. Most tomato-based pasta sauces are lowfat but avoid 'pesto', 'alfredo', cheese and 'creamy' sauces.

Milk, Dairy, Soy Drinks

- **Choose** lowfat or skim milks and yogurt. Avoid full-cream milk, cream, *Half & Ha* coffee creamers.

- **Soy Drinks:** Choose lowfat brands.

- **Cheese:** Choose fat-free, lowfat and fa reduced (e.g. cottage, part-skim ricotta Cheese substitutes can still be high in fat.

- **Icecream:** Choose lowfat and fat-fr brands, frozen yogurt, sorbet, sherbet an ices. Limit regular icecream to a small servin Avoid rich high-fat icecreams.

Frozen Meals & Entrees

- **Choose** lowfat varieties such *Lean Cuisine, Healthy Choice* and *Weig Watchers.* Add extra vegetables.

Soups

- **Choose lowfat brands.** Avoid high-f ramen noodle blocks/soup.

FRYING ADDS FAT!

The greater the surface area of potato exposed to fat or oil, the higher the fat content.

Whole Potato (3 oz)
Nil Fat, 65 Cals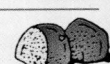

Roast Potato (3 oz)
5g Fat, 155 Cals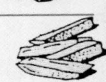

Fries (Large, 3 oz)
12g Fat, 220 Cals

Fries (Small, 3 oz)
15g Fat, 265 Cals

Potato Chips (3 oz)
30g Fat, 450 Cals

Bread, Bagels, Crackers

All breads are suitable as well as pita, bagels, English muffins and rice cakes. Avoid croissants, sweet rolls, danish pastry and doughnuts. **Avoid** fat-soaked toast and garlic bread.

Choose lowfat crackers such as graham, saltines, matzo, bread sticks, crispbreads. Avoid regular cheese or butter crackers.

Cereals, Pasta, Noodles, Rice

Most cold and hot cereals are low in fat and nil in cholesterol. Avoid granola made with hydrogenated oils.

Choose plain pasta or rice. Avoid dishes made with cream, butter or cheese sauces. **Avoid** high-fat ramen noodle blocks/soups.

Fruits & Vegetables

Choose all types. (Note: Avocados contain no cholesterol. Their fat and fiber can help lower blood cholesterol). Use mashed avocado on bread in place of fat.

Choose dried beans, lentils, chick peas, baked beans.

Avoid french-fried potatoes and regular potato salad. Avoid vegetables made in butter, cream or sauce.

Avoid deli-style salads made with high fat dressings. Choose lowfat brands. Use lowfat and fat-free salad dressings.

Snacks, Cookies, Candy

Avoid high-fat snacks such as potato chips, corn/tortilla chips, cheesy balls, buttered popcorn, chocolate and carob bars.

Choose fat-free potato chips and tortilla chips made with *olestra* (such as *Wow!* brand) but still limit quantity.

Choose plain popcorn, lowfat cookies and muffins, hard candy, jelly beans, fruit rolls and frozen fruit bars and popsicles.

Choose fresh and dried fruits, vegetables. Limit nuts and seeds if overweight.

Desserts/Sweets

- **Avoid high-fat desserts**, such as fruit pies, pastries, cheesecake, cheese board.
- **Choose** fresh fruits, fresh fruit salad, lowfat custard and lowfat yogurt. Use yogurt in place of cream or ice cream.
- **Avoid** regular icecream. *Choose* lowfat brands but still limit quantity.
- **Choose** sugar-free gelatin desserts such as *Jell-O* (sugar-free package).

Fast-Foods & Take-Out

Check the Fast-Foods Section of this book for actual fat counts and wise selections.

- **Delis:** Choose sandwiches/bread rolls, pitas with lowfat fillings and plain salad. Limit meat/cheese to small portions. Request half quantities.
- **Avoid** high-fat deli salads. Choose plain salads and add your own lowfat dressing. Eat more fruit.
- **Chicken & Fish:** Avoid deep-fried chicken or fish, BBQ chicken with fat or skin, chicken nuggets. Choose broiled or baked chicken breast without fat or skin.
- **Hamburgers:** Choose medium size, lower fat burgers. Avoid bacon. Have a side salad (without dressing).
- **Pizzas:** Avoid sausage/pepperoni. Choose vegetarian topping and modest quantity of cheese. Eat a moderate serving. Eat extra salad and fruit.
- **Desserts:** Avoid apple pie, danish, choc chip cookies. Choose lowfat muffins (e.g. *McDonald's*), fresh fruit or fruit salad.
- **Avoid** regular shakes and sundaes. Choose lowfat milk, lower fat shakes (such as *McDonald's*), and orange juice, but choose smaller sizes.

• While reducing the amount of fat is an important dietary focus for weight control, sugar intake also needs to be watched.

• Many overweight, inactive persons consume over 500 calories of refined sugars per day (equivalent to over 30 level teaspoons) - a significant amount in weight control terms. Halving this amount would be reasonable and worthwhile.

Note: Naturally occurring sugars in fruits, vegetables and milk are fine when consumed in normal recommended amounts.

• Most sugar in our diet is 'hidden' in processed foods such as soft drinks, fruit drinks, candy, cookies, cake, jam, sauces, icecream, desserts, canned foods, and breakfast cereals.

Certainly enjoy moderate quantities of these foods, but for serious weight control, look for 'low calorie', 'diet' or sugar-free alternatives. Be careful not to substitute sugar-rich foods with high-fat foods which might boost calories even more!

• Sweeteners such as *Equal, NutraSweet, Splenda, Sweet'n Low* and *Stevia* make it easy to reduce sugar in drinks and recipes. (Most recipes can be adapted to contain less sugar with little effect on taste or quality.)

• The body can obtain sufficient sugar for its needs from carbohydrate-rich foods such as bread, rice, spaghetti and other pasta, potatoes, corn, fruit, vegetables, beans, nuts, seeds and lactose in milk.

These foods are also rich in other nutrients. Refined sugar is referred to as 'empty calorie' because it supplies calories but negligible nutrients and no fiber.

DIFFERENT FORMS OF SUGAR

Be aware that sugar comes in different forms. Check the label.

- Sugar
- Brown Sugar
- Dextrose
- Fructose
- Corn Syrup
- Honey
- Maple Syrup
- Sucrose
- Confectioners' Sugar
- Glucose
- Malt, Maltose
- High-Fructose Corn Syrup
- Molasses
- Turbinado Sugar

SUGAR CONTENT OF SOME COMMON FOODS

	Teaspoons of Sugar
Coca Cola or *Pepsi*, 12 oz	10
20 oz size	17
Iced tea, sweetened, 12 oz	8
Choc malted Milk, 12 oz	4.5
Honey Smacks Cereal, 1 oz	4
Popcorn, caramel, 1 cup	3.5
Chocolate Bar, 1.5 oz	6
M&M's, 1.7 oz pkg	7
Cake, sponge, jam-filled	8
Choc Chip Cookie, 1 oz	2
Donut, iced	6
Apple Pie, 1 piece	7
Jell-O, 1/2 cup	4.5
Jam, 1 Tbsp, 20g	2.5
Syrup, maple, 1 Tbsp	3

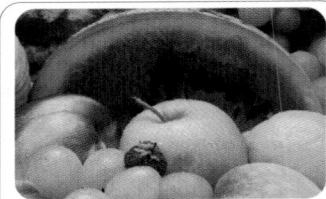

Reach for fresh fruit when you want to snack instead of candy or snack products rich in sugar and fat.

Sample Diet Plan - 1200 Calories

For Overweight Persons. Please Check With Your Doctor.
(Menu contains approximately 30-35 Grams Fat)

 Breakfast (approx. 250 cal)
1 Small Fruit or $^1/_2$ oz Dried Fruit

Plus   Cereal: $1^1/_2$ oz Dry (high fiber)
or 1 cup cooked Oatmeal

Plus   Milk (from daily allowance)

Milk Allowance (160 calories)
2 cups Skim Milk or $1^1/_2$ cups LowFat Milk
or equivalent Soy Drink, Yogurt, Cheese, Tofu

Fat Allowance (140 calories; 15g Fat)
4 tsp Fat or 6-8 tsp Diet Margarine or 3 tsp Oil
or $1^1/_2$ Tbsp Mayonnaise or $^1/_2$ medium Avocado
or $1^1/_2$ Tbsp Peanut Butter or 30g Nuts/Seeds

Breakfast ~ Choice 2
1 Small Fruit

Plus 1 Toast (no added fat)

or $^3/_4$ oz Cheese
or 2 oz Cottage Cheese
or $^1/_4$ cup Baked Beans

Plus 1 Toast or $^1/_2$ Muffin (English)

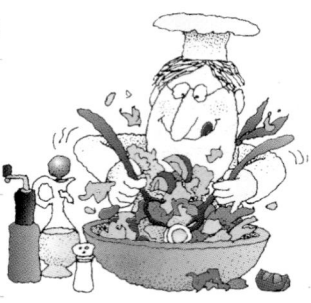

 Lunch (approx. 440 calories)
2 slices Bread (2 oz) or 1 medium Roll or Bagel
or 4 Crispbreads/Crackers or 6" Pita

Plus   2 oz lean Meat, Chicken or Turkey
or $3^1/_2$ oz Tuna (in water) or $2^1/_2$ oz Salmon
or 1 oz Cheese or 3 oz Cottage Cheese
or $2^1/_2$ oz Ricotta Cheese
or $^1/_2$ cup, 4 oz Fruit Yogurt (lowfat)
or $^1/_2$ cup (4 oz) Baked Beans or Bean Salad

Plus   Large Salad (Oil-free dressing)
Plus   1 small Fruit or $^1/_2$ oz Dried Fruit

 Dinner (approx. 360 Calories)
Soup (fat-free)

Plus   3 oz lean Meat (cooked weight)
or 4 oz Chicken Breast (no skin)
or 3 oz Chicken Thigh/Leg (no skin)
or 5 oz Fish (grilled, no fat)
or $^3/_4$ cup (6 oz) Beans (Soy, Baked, Haricot etc)/Lentils
or LowFat Recipe Dish (e.g. Lean Cuisine)

Plus   1 small Potato or $^1/_2$ cup Rice/Pasta or 1 slice Bread
Plus   2-3 servings Vegetables/Salad
Plus   1 small Fruit + Diet Gelatin Dessert

 Between Meals: Water, Coffee, Tea, Diet drinks,
Fruit from main meals; Raw vegetable pieces, Milk from Allowance
Note: Take a multivitamin/mineral supplement daily while dieting.

- Persons who exercise regularly **lose more weight** and keep it off longer than non-exercisers.

- Exercise also improves general health and well-being. **Mood, confidence and self-esteem** are enhanced by a sense of control and accomplishment.

- **Exercise increases the metabolic rate** of the body even for hours after exercise - a good way to 'wake up' a sluggish metabolism and burn extra fat.

   Exercise compensates for any decrease in metabolic rate with increasing age and also in some heavy smokers who stop smoking.

- **Strength training** further builds muscle and aids body reshaping. You can also eat more food!

Note: It is muscle which burns fat. Each extra pound of muscle burns an extra 100 calories daily ~ even while you sleep! Weight from exercised muscles is okay. It is surplus fat that is potentially harmful.

- **Avoid injury** by beginning with walking, low impact aerobics, or weight-supported exercise (e.g. swimming, cycling). Avoid competitive sports.

- **How Much?** Start with 10 - 20 minutes/day and progress to 30-45minutes/day - even if broken into 5-10 minute lots. It all adds up! **Aim to achieve 250-500 calories of exercise daily.**

   Also walk up stairs instead of using lifts. Take a brisk walk at lunch. Use an exercise bike, treadmill or stair machine while watching TV.

- **How Often?** While aerobic fitness requires only 3 - 4 sessions weekly, **weight control is a daily event which requires daily exercise.**

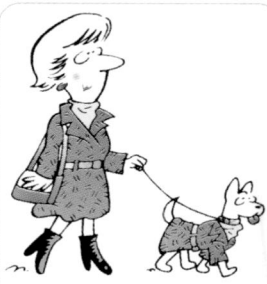

Brisk walking each day is a safe and effective way to keep trim and fit. Try it - you'll like it!"

Strength-training with light weights helps to retain or rebuild muscle tissue and enhances weight control.

TV CAN BE FATTENING!

Many adults and children watch over 20 hours of television per week and indulge in high-fat snacks at the same time - potent contributors to obesity.

Are you a TV couch potato? Limit your TV hours and plan healthy physical activities. At least use an exercise bike or treadmill while watching TV!

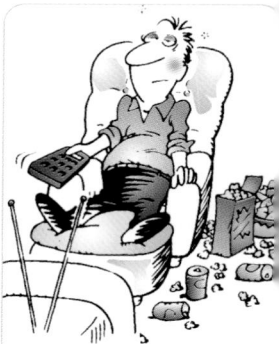

Middle-age spread has little to do with getting older. Too little exercise is the main culprit.

Daily exercise and sensible eating can minimize middle-age spread.

Calories Used in Exercise

LIGHT
4 Calories/Minute

Walking, slow
Cycling, light
Gardening light
Golf, social
Tennis, doubles
Housework, cleaning
Callisthenics, Yoga
Ten Pin Bowls
Ping-pong, social
Ice Skating
Aquarobics
Skate Boarding
Line/Square Dancing

MODERATE
7 Calories/Minute

Walking, brisk
Cycling, moderate
Swimming, crawl
Weight-training, light
Tennis, singles
Racquetball, beginners
Aerobics, light
Football, Grid Iron
Basketball, Baseball
Walking Downstairs
Snow Skiing (downhill)
Shoveling snow
Dancing (vigorous)

HEAVY
10 Calories/Minute

Walking (power), Jogging
Cycling (vigorous), Spinning
Swimming, strenuous
Weight-training, heavy
Wrestling/Judo, advanced
Racquetball, advanced
Tae Bo, Kick Boxing
Football, training
Basketball (Pro)
Climbing Stairs, Skipping
Skiing (cross country)
Aquarobics, advanced
Dancing (strenuous)

Note: Only those sports or activities that are sustained over a period of time (e.g running) qualify for heavy exercise. Stop-start sports such as tennis are considered 'moderate'.

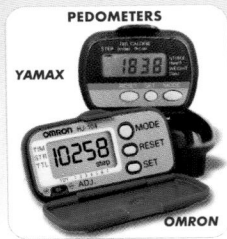

PEDOMETERS
YAMAX
OMRON

10,000 STEPS PER DAY

A pedometer can motivate you to be more active every day.

Different models count steps, miles and even calories used. It clips to your belt or waist band and registers each step.

Aim for 8,000 - 10,000 steps per day, instead of an average of only 3,000 - 4,000 steps.

Extra information: www.CalorieKing.com
Ordering Details ~ Page 287

WALKING PROGRAM

Weeks		Distance To Walk	Time Taken	Calories Used (140lb Person)
Weeks 1-2	▶	1 mile	20 mins	140 calories
Weeks 3-5	▶	1.5 miles	28 mins	200 calories
Weeks 6-8	▶	2 miles	35 mins	250 calories
Weeks 9-10	▶	2.5 miles	45 mins	310 calories
Weeks 11+	▶	3.5 miles	60 mins	420 calories

- Eating is a behavior that is largely controlled by people with whom we live or socialize, places in which we carry out our lives, and our emotions. Become aware of those situations that commonly lead to extra food being eaten.

- We may also be unaware of 'bad' eating habits that can lead to excess calorie intake; e.g. eating quickly, large mouthful, eating when tense or bored, finishing a large serving of food when not hungry.

Hints to help uncover and correct those 'bad' eating habits include:

- **Don't eat while engaged in other activities;** e.g. watching TV, reading. Eat only at the table, not at the fridge or while standing.

- **Don't eat quickly.** Chewing slowly allows time to register a feeling of fullness. Don't use fingers, only utensils. Cut food into smaller pieces. Don't load your fork until the previous mouthful is finished.

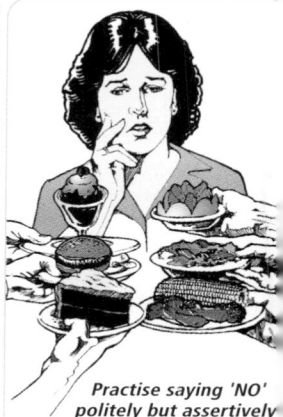

Practise saying 'NO' politely but assertively

- **Don't purchase problem high calorie foods.** Shop from a set list to prevent impulse buying. Avoid shopping with children.

- **Buy snack foods** in the smallest package. The larger the serving size or package, the more you are likely to eat or drink.

- **Plan meals in advance. Stick to a set menu.**

- **Plan a strategy to avoid uncontrolled eating** and drinking at social events, or when your emotions urge you to binge.

  Rehearse repeatedly in your mind exactly what you will do in such situations. Remind yourself several times each day that you are in charge of your actions and that you can be strong-willed. Seek counseling or coaching on various strategies.

- **Promise yourself** that when you feel the urge to snack, you will engage in some activity that will distract you away from food (e.g. go for a walk, brush your teeth, phone a friend.)

  If you eat out of boredom, find some new hobby or interest that gets you out of the house. Even enrol in an adult education class.

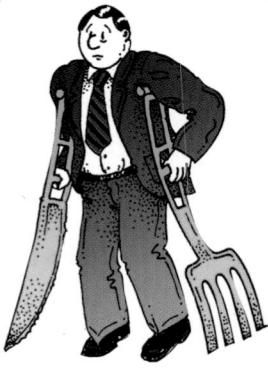

Do you use food as an emotiona[l] crutch? If so, professional counseling may be helpful.

The food diary is the most powerful proven aid for dieters. Persons who keep a food and exercise diary not only lose more weight they also keep it off. Here are some of the reasons:

- Recording your eating and exercise habits jolts you into realizing just what you do eat and drink each day; and also whether you exercise sufficiently.

- **Helps you identify problem foods** and drinks with excessive calories and fat.

- **Helps identify moods**, situations and events that lead to excessive eating of unwanted calories. You can then plan to overcome or avoid them.

- **Prevents 'calorie amnesia'**, the forgetfulness that leads to rebound weight gain after successful weight loss. Recording puts you back on the right track.

- **Helps you develop greater self-discipline.** You will think twice about over indulging if you have to record it - especially if someone checks your diary regularly. It certainly keeps you honest!

- **Motivates you** to carefully plan your meals and to exercise each day.

- **Serves as a check system** for your doctor, dietitian or counselor to assess your progress and make recommendations.

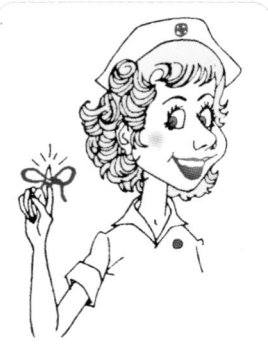

"Keeping a diary gives me feedback on exactly what I eat each day.
It helps prevent 'calorie amnesia' and reminds me to exercise each day.
It's a must for successful weight control!"

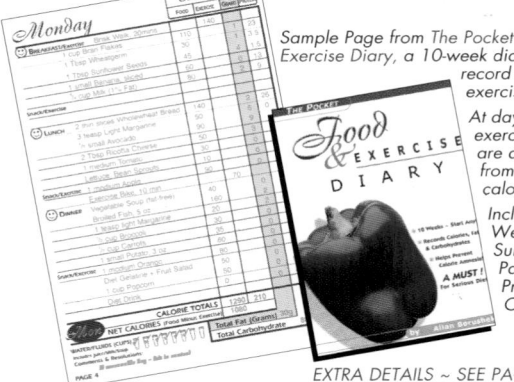

Sample Page from The Pocket Food & Exercise Diary, a 10-week diary to record food and exercise.

At day's end, exercise calories are deducted from food calories.

Includes Weekly Summary Page & Progress Checklist.

EXTRA DETAILS ~ SEE PAGE 288

What is Diabetes?

Diabetes is a disorder in which the body cannot make proper use of carbohydrates (sugar and starches).

- After digestion, sugar and starches are changed into **glucose** - the simplest form of sugar that is vital to body cells for energy and growth.

- **Insulin** is the hormone which acts like a key that opens the door to body cells and allows glucose to enter.

- **Without sufficient insulin**, unused glucose builds up in the blood and passes into the urine. This produces symptoms of frequent urination, continual thirst and tiredness.

- **Untreated diabetes** increases the risk of damage to nerves and blood vessels. This, in turn, increases the risk of heart disease, stroke, blindness, kidney damage, foot ulcers and gangrene, impotence and other complications.

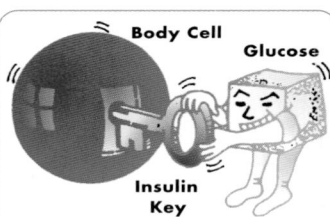

*Insulin acts like a key.
It opens the door to body cells
and allows glucose to enter.*

Some persons with diabetes (Type 1) have too few or no keys and require insulin injections.

Others (Type 2) have ample keys but 'mis-shapen' key holes (insulin resistant) - particularly if obese and inactive.

TYPE-1 DIABETES

Insulin-Dependent Diabetes

- Occurs in 10% of diabetes cases.

- Usually children and young adults.

- Pancreas gland produces little or no insulin. Daily insulin injections are necessary, plus:

- Regular meals with even carbohydrate distribution to match insulin dosage. Regular exercise and weight control are also important.

WARNING SIGNALS

- Frequent urination
- Continual thirst
- Rapid weight loss
- Unusual hunger
- Extreme weakness/fatigue
- Nausea, vomiting, irritability

TYPE-2 DIABETES

Non-Insulin Dependent

- Occurs in 90% of diabetes cases.

- Occurs mainly in adults - particularly in overweight and inactive persons.

- Insulin is produced but body cells resist its action and glucose cannot enter cells.

- Usually treated with diet and exercise. Sometimes requires medication (pills or insulin injections).

WARNING SIGNALS

- Any Type-1 symptom
- Blurred vision
- Excessive itching
- Skin infections with slow healing
- Tingling/numbness in feet

Importance of Weight Control

- **Type-2 diabetes** occurs 2-3 times more often in overweight persons - particularly if inactive.

- Such persons do not usually lack insulin. Rather, their insulin is less effective. As obesity develops, muscle and other body cells may resist insulin in varying degrees. The resultant build-up of blood glucose may lead to diabetic symptoms.

- **Weight loss alone** often corrects this condition in Type-2 diabetes. If overweight, try a moderate diet of 1200-1500 calories **plus daily exercise**.

  Within several weeks, body cells can lose their resistance and become sensitive once again to the effects of insulin. Insulin and blood glucose levels may normalise, and symptoms may disappear.

  Further, the need for oral antidiabetic drugs might be prevented or much lessened in dosage. **So, give diet and exercise a fair go** - and maintain them to keep symptoms under control.

Managing Diabetes

Don't battle diabetes alone. Establish a partnership with your doctor, dietitian, nurse educator and pharmacist. For extra support, contact the *American Diabetes Association* 1-800-342-2383.

Hints to keep blood glucose within safe limits:

- **Control your diet.** Know what and when you will eat. Seek referral to a dietitian for expert advice.

- **Exercise regularly.** It assists weight control and can improve sensitivity of body cells to insulin. Plan exercise into your daily routine.

- **Monitor your blood glucose** at home and work - ideally with a portable blood glucose meter. It will help you become familiar with your blood glucose patterns, and the effects of diet, exercise and medication. **Insulin pumps** can also help control blood glucose levels around the clock.

- **Don't skip prescribed insulin or oral medication.** If on insulin, know what action to take if hypoglycaemia (low blood glucose) occurs. Also educate family and friends.

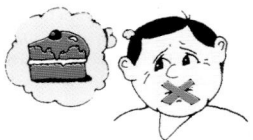

Modest weight loss and daily exercise can greatly improve control of Type-2 diabetes.

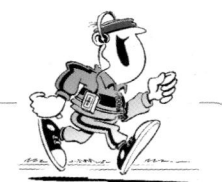

Get Moving! Everyday, do at least 30 minutes of moderate intensity exercise. It's the key to improving insulin sensitivity.

Add strength-training 3-4 times a week to double the benefits.

Blood glucose meters, insulin pumps and pens can greatly improve control of diabetes and lifestyle choices.

Diabetes ~ Diet Hints

Guidelines for choosing a healthy diet apply equally to persons with or without diabetes. Eating a wide variety of foods with the emphasis on low-fat, high fiber and low in refined sugars, is recommended.

However, actual food quantities, as well as when you eat, will also influence control of blood glucose. Your dietitian will individualize a diet plan to suit your food preferences, lifestyle and medical status. Here are a few hints:

- **Maintain a healthy weight.** If overweight, even a modest weight loss plus daily exercise can help to normalise blood glucose in Type-2 diabetes.

- **Don't skip meals.** If you take insulin or an oral hypoglycemic agent, regular meals are important.

- **If on insulin**, eat meals at the same time each day. Eat a similar amount of food at each meal. An even distribution of carbohydrate over the day will make best use of the available insulin and prevent wide fluctuations in blood glucose levels. Leave an interval of about 30 minutes between insulin injection and breakfast.

- **Avoid sugars and foods high in added sugar** particularly if overweight. Small amounts of sugar as part of a meal may occasionally be okay. Check with your dietitian. Use *Equal, Splenda* and *NutraSweet*-sweetened foods and drinks.

- **Choose wholegrain breads, cereals and pasta.** Eat fresh fruits, vegetables and legumes. These foods contain more fiber and slow the release of glucose into your blood after a meal.

- **Limit foods high in saturated fat and cholesterol.** Enjoy fish, soy foods, and other foods rich in omega-3 fats. *(See Fats & Cholesterol Guide, Pages 246-252)*

- **Foods (and supplements) rich in antioxidant vitamins C, E and beta-carotene**, as well as omega-3 fats, magnesium, zinc and chromium may help prevent long-term complications of diabetes (such as damage to small blood vessels and nerves). Be sure to check with your doctor.

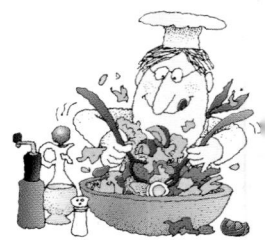

Eat a well-balanced diet, high in fiber-containing foods and low in fat.

NEW BLOOD SUGAR LEVEL FOR DIAGNOSING DIABETES
(Adopted by American Diabetes Assoc.)

Blood Sugar Levels
Previously: 140 mg/dL
New: 126 mg/dL

Everyone 45 and older should have a blood test every 3 years.

Excess Alcohol contributes to obesity, diabetes, and high blood pressure.

The risk of hypoglycemia (low blood sugar) and drug interactions with alcohol is also increased.

Carbohydrates & Diabetes

Carbohydrate foods in their more natural forms are an important part of a healthy diet. They provide energy, fiber, vitamins, minerals, protein and water.

Carbohydrates are found mainly in cereal grains, fruit, vegetables and milk. Animal flesh foods contain negligible amounts. A healthy diet of at least 2000 calories is based around carbohydrate foods and should provide over 50% of total calories - whether or not we have diabetes. Lower calorie diets for weight control will have as little as 40% carbohydrate calories.

Carbohydrates include sugars, starches and fibers. Sugars and starch provide energy to body cells. Even though fiber is not digested, it benefits the body - more so in diabetes. (See Fiber Guide ~ Page 262)

The **various forms of carbohydrate** affect blood glucose levels in different ways; and it is difficult to predict the effect of particular foods, sugars or meals, simply by their actual carbohydrate content. Thus, the **same amount** of carbohydrate from different foods may affect blood sugar differently. It depends on many factors.

For example, fiber can slow digestion and absorption of sugars by acting as a physical barrier or by forming a gel. Both fiber and fat also slow the emptying rate of the stomach into the intestines where further digestion and absorption takes place. The physical form of food (solid, puree, liquid) also matters - the more natural the better.

Generally, raw foods rather than cooked foods, and whole-foods rather than ground-up foods, are more slowly absorbed.

- **Sugar: Small amounts** eaten as part of a meal, may not adversely affect blood glucose in persons with good blood glucose control. Nevertheless, minimal amounts of sugar are encouraged for nutritional and weight control reasons.

Glycemic Index

- Glycemic index (GI) indicates how fast a carbohydrate containing food is digested and how much it causes blood glucose to rise (glycemic response).

LOWER GLYCEMIC FOODS

Slower Acting Carbohydrates

These foods are more slowly digested and absorbed. They help maintain more even blood glucose levels. Use these foods regularly. Examples:

- Dried beans, peas, lentils
- Nuts and seeds
- Wholegrain breads, pita
- Bran cereals, oats
- Barley, buckwheat, bulgur
- Spaghetti, pasta, Basmati Rice
- Fresh fruit: apples, avocados, bananas (firm), cherries, grapefruit, grapes, olives, oranges, peaches, pears, plums
- Vegetables: sweet corn, yam
- Milk, yogurt, soy drinks

HIGHER GLYCEMIC FOODS

Quicker Acting Carbohydrates

These foods more rapidly raise blood glucose levels. Eat in moderation.

- White bread, rice cakes, bagels, croissants, doughnuts
- Low fiber cereals: Cornflakes, *Rice Krispies, Froot Loops*
- White potato, white rice
- Watermelon, ripe bananas, cantaloupe, pineapple
- Glucose drinks and candy

(See Carbohydrate Distribution next page)

17

- **For people with diabetes,** regular meals with even distribution of carbohydrate over the day are important for good control of blood sugar levels.
- **Smaller amounts of food** eaten more frequently result in steadier, more even blood glucose levels. (Be sure to control your weight.)

Recommended daily eating patterns for good blood glucose control:

1. **Three Meals & Three Snacks ~**
   Best for persons on insulin (Type-1 diabetes) with normal blood glucose variations.

2. **Three Meals ~**
   Best for Type-2 diabetes (especially if overweight).

Note: If blood sugar levels show excessive variations see doctor and dietitian.

- **Your doctor or dietitian** will select the lev of calories and carbohydrate mo appropriate to your weight, medication ar activity. (Regular blood glucose checks w provide feedback on the level of control.

- **Amounts of carbohydrate** in the guid below provide an average of 50% of tot calories. **A rough rule of thumb** 13 grams of carbohydrate per 100 calorie

At calorie levels above 2000, carbohydrat approach 50-60% of total calories.

At lower calorie levels used for weight lo (1200-1500 calories), carbohydrates accour for as little as 40% of total calories. This because protein has nutritional priority.

These carbohydrate quantities (an percentages) apply equally to persons wit or without diabetes.

IDEAL CARBOHYDRATE DISTRIBUTION
For Type-1 Diabetes (Insulin Dependent)

3 MEALS & 3 SNACKS
Balanced Blood Sugar Levels

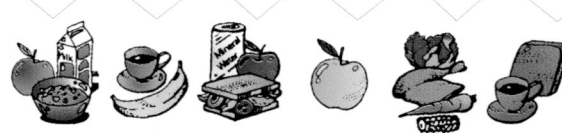

GUIDE TO CARBOHYDRATE DISTRIBUTION

Daily Total Calories		Daily Total Carbohyd.	Percent Carbohyd. Cals	Each Main Meal (3)	Between Meals (3)
1200 Cals	~	120g	40%	30g	10g
1500 Cals	~	170g	45%	40g	15g
2000 Cals	~	250g	50%	60g	25g
2500 Cals	~	345g	55%	70g	45g
3000 Cals	~	450g	60%	90g	60g

Fat Percentages Explained

Percent Fat Calories
(Percentage of Calories from Fat)

While health authorities recommend that not more than 30% of our total food calories should come from fat, it is not implied nor even recommended that you eat only those foods with less than 30% calories from fat.

Our normal diet is made up of foods that are either well above or below 30%. Only on average should the total diet be less than 30% calories from fat.

Some higher fat foods such as avocados, nuts and seeds, are highly nutritious and favor lower blood cholesterol levels. **Moderation is the aim . . . not elimination.**

Nevertheless, knowing the percentage of calories from fat can be useful in spotting high-fat foods and drinks.

> ### FORMULA FOR CALCULATING PERCENTAGE CALORIES FROM FAT
>
> $$\frac{\text{Grams of Fat/Serve} \times 9}{\text{Total Calories/Serve}} \times \frac{100}{1}$$
>
> **EXAMPLE:**
>
> Mars Bar (11g fat, 240 cals)
>
> Percentage Calories from Fat
> $$= \frac{11 \times 9}{265} \times \frac{100}{1} = 37\%$$

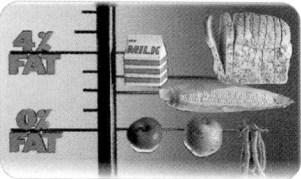

Fat Percentage Content
(Percentage of Fat in Food)

Don't be fooled by promotion of foods claiming to have a low percentage of fat. It's **serving size and total grams of fat that count.**

For example, whole milk with 3.5% fat sounds low (3.5g fat/100ml) but an 8fl.oz cup contains 8g fat (and 2 cups contain 16g fat).

Icecream with 10% fat seems high, yet a large scoop (3fl.oz) has only 5g fat. (Low-fat icecream has less than 2g fat/serve.)

❖   ❖   ❖

Also note that the percentage of fat in a food is not the same as the percentage of calories derived from fat.

Foods with a low percentage of fat can still have a high percentage of calories derived from fat - as shown below.

For example, around 50% of total calories in whole milk comes from fat - yet whole milk has less than 4% fat. Low fat/light milk with less than 1% fat has only 18% of total calories from fat - a much better choice.

FAT CONTENT & PERCENTAGES OF MILK

	Whole Milk	Reduced Fat	Low-Fat (light)	Non-Fat Skim
Percentage Fat	3.5%	2%	1%	0%
Fat (Grams) in 8 fl.oz Cup	8g	5g	2g	0g
Calories	150	120	100	95
Percent Calories From Fat	48%	38%	18%	0%

Notes, Abbreviations, Measures

- Calorie and fat values have been rounded off.
  Calories - to the nearest 5 or 10 calories.
  Fat - to the nearest half gram.
  Note: Trace amounts of fat (less than 0.3 grams per serving) have been treated as zero.

- Because manufacturer's figures on labels are rounded off, figures in this book may differ slightly from the label. Serving sizes may also vary.

- Food product formulations change from time to time, and hence the need to regularly update this type of publication. Many products also come and go. Check the food label for any changes.

- **Seek Professional Advice:** This book is intended for educational purposes only. It is not a substitute for professional advice.

- **Feedback Welcome:** Please contact the author directly with your queries, and suggestions for foods to be included in future editions.

  Write to: Allan Borushek (Dietitian)
  PO Box 1616, Costa Mesa CA 92628
  Email: allan@calorieking.com

- **Free Information Service:** Check the author's website for new food product updates.

  www.calorieking.com

C ~ Calories
F ~ Fat (grams)
Cb ~ Carbohydrate (grams)

Abbreviations

tsp	=	teaspoon
Tbsp	=	Tablespoon
oz	=	ounce(s)
c	=	cup
fl.oz	=	fluid ounce(s)
g	=	gram(s)
<1	=	less than 1

Volume Measures

3 tsp	=	1 Tbsp
2 Tbsp	=	1 fl.oz
1/2 cup	=	4 fl.oz
1 cup	=	8 fl.oz
		or 16 Tbsp
2 cups	=	1 Pint
2 Pints	=	1 Quart

(All measures are level)

Note: 8 oz weight is not the same as 8 fl.oz volume (space occupied). Dense foods weigh more per set volume. Examples:
1 cup popcorn weighs 1/2 oz
1 cup milk weighs 8 1/2 oz
1 cup pudding weighs 10 oz

Metric Conversion

1/2 oz	=	14 grams
1 oz	=	28.4 grams
2 oz	=	57 grams
3 1/2 oz	=	100 grams
1 fl.oz	=	30 mls
1 cup (8 fl.oz)	=	240 mls
33 fl.oz	=	1 liter (volume)

SOURCES OF INFORMATION

- U.S. Dept. of Agriculture
- Food Manufacturers
- Food Industry Boards & Councils
- Independent laboratory analysis
- Scientific publications
- Overseas food composition tables
- Author extrapolations

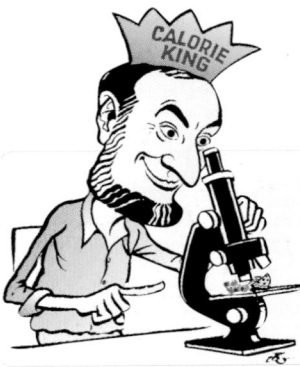

CALORIE KING

20

Quick Guide

	C	**F**	**Cb**

Cow Milk
Average All Brands

Whole (3.5% fat):

	C	F	Cb
2 Tbsp, 1 fl.oz	20	1	1.5
1 Glass, 6 fl.oz	110	6	8.5
1 Cup, 8 fl.oz	150	8	12
1 Pint, 16 fl.oz	300	16	23
1 Quart, 946 ml	600	32	46

Reduced-fat (2% fat):

	C	F	Cb
2 Tbsp, 1 fl.oz	15	0.5	1.5
1 Glass, 6 fl.oz	90	4	8.5
1 Cup, 8 fl.oz	130	5	13
1 Pint, 16 fl.oz	260	10	26
1 Quart, 946 ml	520	20	52

Light/Lowfat (1% fat):

	C	F	Cb
2 Tbsp, 1 fl.oz	12	0.3	1.5
1 Glass, 6 fl.oz	75	2	8.5
1 Cup, 8 fl.oz	120	2.5	14
1 Pint, 16 fl.oz	240	5	28
1 Quart, 946 ml	480	10	56

Fat Free/Skim:

	C	F	Cb
2 Tbsp, 1 fl.oz	10	0	1.5
1 Cup, 8 fl.oz	90	0.5	13
1 Pint, 16 fl.oz	180	1	26
w. Replace (Oatrim Fiber): 1 cup	85	0	12

Protein-Fortified:

	C	F	Cb
2% fat, 1 cup	140	5	14
1% fat, 1 cup	120	3	14
Skim, 1 cup	100	0.5	14

Acidophilus: Average All Brands

	C	F	Cb
Reduced Fat (2%), 1 cup	130	5	13
Lowfat (1%), 1 cup	100	2	13

Buttermilk: Average All Brands

	C	F	Cb
Reduced Fat (2%), 1 cup	120	5	10
Low Fat (1%), 1 cup	100	2.5	12
Oak Farms (1%), 1 cup	100	2.5	12

Lactose-Reduced:

	C	F	Cb
Reduced Fat: Lactaid, 1 cup	130	5	12
Dairy Ease 100, 1 cup	130	5	12
Lowfat, Lactaid, 1 cup	110	2.5	13
Fat Free Lactaid/Lucerne, 1 cup	80	0	13

Soy & Non-Dairy Drinks
~ See Page 23 ~

Goat & Sheep Milk

	C	**F**	**Cb**
Goat's Milk (Meyenberg):			
Whole, 1 cup, 8 fl.oz	140	7	11
Light/Lowfat (1%), 8 fl.oz	90	2.5	9
Evaporated, reconst., 8 fl.oz	145	8	11
Kefir: Alta Dena, 1 cup	240	4.5	41
Steve's Kefir Peach, 1 cup	220	9	25
Sheep's Milk: Whole, 1 cup	265	17	13

Canned & Dried Milk

	C	F	Cb
Condensed: Reg. 2 Tbsp, 1 fl.oz	130	3	22
Lowfat (Eagle), 2 Tbsp	120	1.5	23
Fat Free (Eagle), 2 Tbsp	110	0	24
Evaporated: Whole, 2 Tbsp	40	3	3
Whole, 1/2 cup	170	10	13
Lowfat (Carnation), 2 Tbsp	25	1	3
1/2 cup	110	3	12
Light/Skim, 1/2 cup	100	0.5	14
Dried: Whole, 1/4 cup, 1 oz	150	8	11
Skim/Nonfat, 1/3 cup	80	0	12
Made-up, 1 cup, 8 fl.oz	80	0	12
Buttermilk, sweetcream, 1 oz	110	2	3
Nonfat, 1 Tbsp	25	0	3

Whey Drink

	C	F	Cb
Acid: Dry, 1 Tbsp, 3g	10	0	2
Fluid, 1 cup, 8 fl.oz	60	0	13
Sweet: Dry, 1 Tbsp, 8g	25	0	6
Fluid, 1 cup, 8 fl.oz	65	1	13
Nutri Mil: Orig./Low Fat 8 fl.oz	80	3	11
Chocolate, 8 fl.oz	110	3	19
Fat Free (Calcium Enriched)	60	0	11

Flavored Milk Drinks

Quick Guide   C F Cb

Chocolate Milk

Average All Brands: Per Cup, 8 fl.oz

	C	F	Cb
Whole Milk (3.3%): 1 cup	225	9	26
1 Pint	450	18	52
Reduced Fat (2%), 1 cup	190	5	26
Lowfat (1%), 1 cup	160	3	26

Brands ~ Chocolate Milk

Ready-To-Drink: Per 8 fl.oz Cup

Albertson's, lowfat	170	2.5	30
Bodywise, nonfat	180	0	35
Borden: Dutch Choc., 1 cup	220	8	28
Bosco	230	8	33
Brown Cow Farm, 1 cup	250	8	39
Deans 'Chug': Regular	220	9	26
Lowfat, 1 cup	160	2.5	27
Dominick's Lowfat, 1 cup	170	2.5	28
Golden Guernsey, 1 cup	130	2.5	15
Grocers Pride Choc D'Lite, 1 cup	120	3	22
Hershey's: Lowfat (2%) Choc Milk	190	5	25
Whole Milk, 1 cup, 240ml	230	9	28
Hood, Lowfat (1%)	150	2	27
Horizon Organic	160	2.5	27
Knudsen	200	3	32
Kroger (3.25% milk)	220	9	28
Lactaid (1%)	160	3	28
Land O'Lakes, lowfat (0.5%)	150	1.5	35
Meadow Gold (3.5%)	210	8	25
Nesquik: 1 cup	230	8	31
Fat Free, 1 cup	160	0	31
Oak Farms, 1 cup	210	8	26
Parmalat (2%)	180	5	28
Quik: (Nestle) Chocolate Milk	230	8	30
Strawberry Milk	220	9	31
Ralph's	240	3	34
Sobe Love Bus Chocolate, 8 fl.oz	140	1	28
Yoo Hoo Choc Drink, 9 fl.oz	150	1	33

Bottled Chocolate (Chilled)

Ready-To-Drink: Per Bottle

Blue Luna: Cafe Latte 12½ fl.oz	195	3	36
Lite Cafe Mocha, 12½ fl.oz	114	3	15
Main St Cafe:			
French Van. Ice Latte, 12 fl.oz	190	33	31
Nescafe: Caffe Latte	140	3.5	23
Mocha	140	3	26
Starbucks: Coffee; Mocha	190	3	40

Shakes & Smoothies

Smoothies   C F Cb

Made Up Ready-To-Drink

(8 fl. oz Milk/Soy + Fruit): Per 12 fl.oz

Average all types: w. Whole Milk	300	8	50
+ Icecream, 1 scoop	400	13	62
with Nonfat Milk	240	0	50
Langers: 8 fl.oz, all flavors	135	0	34

Shakes

Regular: Chocolate, 10 fl.oz	360	11	58
Vanilla/Strawberrry, 10 fl.oz	320	9	53
McDonald's Reduced Fat,			
Small (14 fl.oz), all flavors	360	9	59
Burger King: Vanilla, medium	430	9	73
Chocolate w. Syrup, medium	560	10	105
Killer Shake (14oz): Choc./Van., 1 c.	210	5	36

Cocoa-Chocolate Mixes

Add extra cals/fat/carbohydrate for milk

Alba '66 Milk Choc, 1 pkt	60	0	14
Carnation Cocoa Mixes:			
Chocolate Rich, 3 Tbsp/1 pkt	110	1	24
Milk Chocolate, 3 Tbsp	110	1	24
w.mini Marshmallows, 1 oz pkt	110	1	24
Malted Milk Original, 3 Tbsp	90	2	15
70 Calorie Cocoa Mix, 3 tsp	70	0.5	15
Fat-Free, 2 Tbsp/1 pkt	25	0	4
No Sugar, 1 pkt	50	0.5	8
Land O' Lakes: Per 1¼ oz pkt			
Choc.Mint/Raspb./Supreme	160	5	25
Nestle Hot Cocoa Mix, 1 oz	110	1	23
w. Marshmallows, 1 oz	120	1	23
French Vanilla	120	3	22
Ghirardelli: Per 2 heaping tsp			
Choc. Mocha/Hazelnut/Dble Choc	80	1.5	21
Pralines & Creme, 2 Tbsp	90	0	23
Ovaltine Cocoa Mixes, 4 tsp	80	0	20
Swiss Miss Cocoa Mixes:			
Milk Chocolate, 1 oz pkt	110	1.5	22
w. Marshmallows, 1.2 oz pkt	140	3	27
Choc. Sensation, 1.25 oz pkt	150	4	27
Lite, 1 pkt	70	0	18
Diet Cocoa Mix, 1 pkt	20	0	4
Sugar Free	60	0	10
Fat Free, 0.53 oz	50	0	9
Vending Machine, 1.34 oz pkt	145	2	24
Weight Watchers: Hot Cocoa Mix	70	0	10

Soy & Non-Dairy Drinks

Soy ~ Ready-To-Drink

Per 1 Cup Serving (8 fl.oz)

	C	F	Cb
Advantage \10 Fruit Smoothies, average all flavors, 11 oz pkg	225	2.5	47
Balanced:			
Chocolate; Strawberry	230	3	37
Vanilla, 1 cup	230	3	35
Eden Blend: 1 cup	120	3	18
Edensoy: Original, 1 cup	130	5	13
Vanilla	150	3	23
Carob	170	4	27
Light: Original, 1 cup	95	2	14
Vanilla	120	2	21
8th Continent: Chocolate, 8 fl.oz	140	3	23
Original	80	3	8
Vanilla	90	3	11
Hain Soy Supreme: Original	80	3	9
Vanilla, 1 cup	100	3	12
Harmony Farms: Regular, 1 cup	80	3	10
Enriched; Vanilla, 1 cup	100	3	14
Health Source: All flavors	150	1.5	23
Health Source Plus	160	1	17
Soy Protein Shake	100	1	4
Health Valley: Soy Moo	110	0	21
It's Soy Delicious: Vanilla	110	1	22
Awesome; Chocolate	120	2	22
Lifeway:			
Soy Treat, Apple; Caramel	160	4	23
Pacific:			
Original unsweetened	100	5	5
Enriched (Soy Isoflavin): Plain	90	2.5	14
Vanilla, 1 cup	110	2.5	16
Fat Free: Plain	70	0	14
Vanilla	90	0	17
Select (Soy Isoflavin), Plain	100	2.5	13
Ultra: Plain/Vanilla	150	5	20
PowerDream: Soy Energy,			
Java Jolt, Chai, Vanilla Blast	250	5	42
Mango Passion	320	5	65
X-treme Chocolate	260	5	48
Silk (White Wave): Plain	100	4	8
Chai, Mocha	140	3	20
Chocolate	145	3.5	23
Vanilla	100	3.5	10
Silk Creamer, 1Tbsp	15	1	1
SoyDream: Orig./Enriched 8 fl.oz	130	4	17
Carob/Chocolate Enriched	210	4	37
Vanilla; Vanilla Enriched	150	4	22
Soy Fusion: Berry, 1cup	120	1.5	24
Matcha Green Tea, 1cup	110	2	19
Soy Nice: Natural, 8 fl.oz	70	3.5	2
Original	80	3	6
Chocolate, 1 cup	110	3	17
Vanilla	100	3	11
SunSoy: Chocolate, 1 cup	140	3	23
Creamy Original	80	3	8
Ulltra Slim-Fast: Juice based			
With Soy, all flavors, 11 oz can	220	1	46
Vitasoy:			
Refrigerated: Creamy Original	110	4	12
Rich Chocolate	160	4	24
Low Fat Vanilla Delite	90	2	13
Long Life: Creamy Original	110	5	9
Creamy Unsweetened	80	4	5
Carob Supreme	150	4.5	20
Rich Cocoa	150	4.5	21
Vanilla Delite	120	4	14
Light: Original	60	2	7
Cocoa	110	2.5	18
Vanilla	90	2	14
Enriched: Original	90	4	9
Light Original	60	2	7
Vanilla	110	4	14
Light Vanilla	90	2	13
WestSoy: *Per 1 Cup, 8 fl. oz*			
Plus: Plain	130	4	18
Vanilla	140	3.5	19
100% Organic: Original (2% fat)	140	5	18
Unsweetened, Plain	90	4.5	4
Unsweetened, Vanilla	100	4.5	5
Nonfat: Plain	80	0	16
Vanilla	90	0	17
Lite: Plain, 1 cup	100	2	15
Cocoa	120	2.5	28
Vanilla	120	2.5	21
Lowfat: Plain	90	1.5	14
Vanilla	110	1.5	20
Café: Coffee; Mocha; Fr. Vanilla	130	2.5	24
Chai: Orig./Green Tea	140	3	26
Smoothies, all flavors	140	1.5	28
Soy Shakes: Choc; Vanilla	180	3.5	30
Vigor Aid: French Vanilla	260	6	44
Choc Mocha, Creamy Choc,	240	6	38
Juice Bar, average all flavors	120	1.5	24

Soy Powder Mix   **C** **F** **Cb**

(1 oz (¹/₄ cup) mix makes 1 cup, 8 fl.oz)

	C	F	Cb
Better Than Milk: Original, 1 oz	100	2.5	16
Light, 1 oz	80	0.5	13
Joy Soy: Extra (Carob/Van.), 2 T.	80	3	11
Revival Soy: Plain, 1 oz pkt	110	1.5	2
Vanilla w/Fructose, 2 oz pkt	220	2	31
Unsweetened/Aspartame, 35g	120	2	6
Soyagen: Reg./No Sugar, 1 oz dry	130	6	12
Carob, 1 oz dry	130	6	13
Soy Protein Isolate, 1 oz dry	95	1	0
Soy Quik *(Ener-g),* 1 oz dry	100	4.5	8

Rice & Cereal Drinks

Per 1 Cup, 8 fl. oz

	C	F	Cb
Almond Breeze: Original, 8 fl.oz	60	3	8
Vanilla, 8 fl.oz	90	3	16
Amazake: Almond Light, 8 fl.oz	110	2	16
Don José Horchata, 8 fl.oz	140	4	25
Eden Blend: Rice & Soy, 1 cup	120	3	18
Eden Rice: 1 cup, 8 fl.oz	110	3	21
Hain Rice Supreme: Lowfat Orig.	100	3	16
Lowfat Cinnamon	130	3	22
Pacific Foods: Multigrain, 8 fl.oz	150	2	31
Naturally Oat: Original, 1 cup	110	1.5	21
Vanilla, 1 cup	130	1.5	24
Naturally Almond: Original, 1 cup	70	2.5	10
Vanilla, 1 cup	90	2.5	15
Pacific Rice: Lowfat, Plain, 1 cup	90	2	18
Fat Free: Plain	80	0	18
Cocoa	100	0	21
Vanilla	110	0	24
Rice Dream: Carob, 1 cup	150	2.5	32
Chocolate; Enriched, 1 cup	170	3	36
Vanilla/Vanilla Enriched, 1 cup	130	2	28
Original/Original Enriched,	120	2	25
Westbrae: Oat Plus, 1 cup	150	3	26
Original Vanilla, 1 cup	150	3	20
Rice: Plain, 1 cup	100	2.5	18
Vanilla, 1 cup	120	2.5	22

Rice/Nut Drink Mixes

	C	F	Cb
Better Than Milk: Light, 19g	70	0.5	14
Original, 23g	100	2.5	16
Nut Quik, 2 Tbsp powder, 18g	110	9	3
Rice Moo, 2 Tbsp powder, 19g	72	0	17
Solait, 3 tbsp powder, 22g	80	1.5	13
Sun's Up, 2 scoops, 40g powder	160	2	36

Quick Guide   **C** **F** **Cb**

Yogurt

Average All Brands: Per 8 oz Cup

	C	F	Cb
Plain Yogurt: Whole, 8 oz	180	7	11
Lowfat	140	4	16
Nonfat	110	0	18
Fruit Flavored: Whole, 8 oz	250	6	38
Lowfat	230	3	32
Nonfat, regular	150	0	32
Nonfat, no sugar added	120	0	32
Goat's Milk Yogurt-Same as Regular Yogurt			

Yogurt ~ Brands

	C	F	Cb
Alex Rod: Fat Free, all flav., 8 oz	70	0	12
Albertson's: Plain, lowfat, 8 oz	140	2.5	17
Fruit on the Bottom (lowfat):			
Average all flavors, 8 oz	220	2	42
Swiss (Nonfat), average, 6 oz	90	0	14
Indulgents (Lowfat), 6 oz	180	2	35
Alta Dena: Lowfat: Plain, 8 oz	170	4.5	20
Vanilla, 8 oz	260	3.5	44
Nonfat: Plain, 8 oz	110	0	17
Flavors, average	190	0	39
America's Choice: Swiss Style	210	2.5	41
Fruit on the Bottom: Cherry Van.	270	2.5	55
Other flavors, average	220	2.5	40
Nonfat, all flavors, 8 oz	100	0	15
Berkeley Farms (8 oz Cup)			
Lowfat: Boysenberry/Cherry	230	2.5	46
Raspberry	220	2.5	43
Strawberry, Lemon, Vanilla	270	2.5	42
Nonfat: Average all flavors	100	0	16
Breyers: Light n' Lively	125g	130	1	25
Lowfat: 1% fat, all flavors, 8 oz	250	2.5	48
1.5% fat, plain	130	3	15
Flavors, average	220	3	38
Smooth & Creamy: 125g	130	1	25
Brown Cow Farm (Fat Free): Plain	80	0	11
Cappuccino/Maple Alm./Vanilla	170	0	33
Cherry Vanilla/Strawberry, 8 oz	190	0	39
Chocolate, 8 oz	220	0	45
Whole Milk, 8 oz	210	8	30
Plain, 8 oz	170	10	12

Yogurt ~ Brands (Cont)

	C	F	Cb
Cabot			
Plain, 8 oz	140	4	16
Flavors, 8 oz	220	3	42
Cascade Fresh			
Lowfat, 6 oz	140	2	23
Fat Free, all flavors, 6 oz	110	0	20
Colombo			
Light, all flavors, 8 oz	100	0	17
Classic (Fruit on the Bottom), 8 oz	200	4	43
Non Fat: Plain, 8 oz	110	0	17
Continental: Nonfat, 8 oz	200	0	38
Nonfat Fruit on the Bottom:			
average all flavors, 8 oz	190	0	38
Dannon			
Plain (Natural), 8 oz	170	8	14
Light: All flavors, 8 oz	100	0	16
w. Crunchy Toppings, aver. 8 oz	170	0	33
Nonfat: Snackpack, 4 oz	60	0	11
Light 'n Fit: All flavors, 8 oz	120	0	22
Fruit on the Bottom (99% FF):8 oz	230	2.5	40
Minipack, 4 oz	110	1	20
Nonfat: Plain, 8 oz	130	0	19
Blended, 4 oz	100	0	21
Chunky Fruit (Nonfat), aver., 6 oz	160	0	32
Low Fat: All types, 8 oz	220	3.5	36
Double Delights Lowfat:			
w. Fruit Topping, aver., 6 oz	170	1	34
w. Choc. Topping, 6 oz	220	1	46
Light Duets: w. fruit topping, 6 oz	90	0	34
Danimals (lowfat), 4 oz	120	1.5	20
Sprinkl'ins: All types, 4 oz	125	1	23
Dominick's			
Lowfat, 8 oz	230	2	40
Fruit on the Bottom, aver., 8 oz	230	2	40
Fat Free 80 Calories, 8 oz	80	0	13
Plain: Lowfat, 8 oz	130	2.5	15
Nonfat, 8 oz	120	0	17
Friendship			
Fruit Flavors, 6 oz	190	5	31
Grocer's Pride			
Lowfat, 4.4 oz	140	1.5	28

	C	F	Cb
Horizon Organic			
Nonfat: Cherry, 6 oz	140	0	28
Other fruit flavors, aver., 6 oz	130	0	26
Plain: 1 cup, 8 oz	170	0	32
Fat Free, 6 oz	80	0	11
Vanilla, 1 cup, 8 oz	110	0	15
Hood			
Fat Free, Plain, 8 oz	130	0	18
Average all flavors, 8 oz	190	0	40
Imperial Supreme			
Lowfat, 6 oz	140	1.5	26
Jerseymaid (Vons)			
Fruit on the Bottom, 8 oz	240	2.5	46
Prestirred (lowfat), average	240	2.5	46
Plain, lowfat, 8 oz	140	3.5	18
Jell-O			
Kid Pack, all flav., 125g	130	1	25
Jewel: **Lowfat**, average, 8 oz	250	2.5	48
Knudsen			
70 Calories, 6 oz	70	0	11
Free, average, 6 oz	170	0	33
Cottage Doubles, 5.5 oz	140	2.5	18
Kroger			
Lite, aver. all flav., 8 oz	100	0	14
Lowfat, average all flavors, 8 oz	210	1.5	40
Health Indulgence (Nonfat):			
Fruit on the Bottom, aver.	170	0	35
Fat Free: Plain, 8 oz	120	0	18
Vanilla, 8 oz	190	0	36
98% Fat Free: Plain, 8 oz	140	4	16
Vanilla, 8 oz	240	4	42
Lactaid: **Lowfat Vanilla**, 8 oz	240	2.5	45
La Yogurt			
Fruit Flavors, average, 6 oz	170	2	32
Light, average all flavors, 6 oz	70	0	12
Fruit La More, average, 6 oz	160	0	32
Light n'Lively			
Free 50 Calories, 4 oz	50	0	8
Free 70 Calories, 6 oz	70	0	11
Free (Regular) 6 oz: Vanilla	160	0	32
Strawb. Fruit/Peach/Lem./Berry	170	0	34
Strawberry/Raspberry	180	0	36
Kidpack/Multipack, aver. 4.4 oz	140	1	28

	C	F	Cb
Lucernes			
Light, Pre-Stirred, 8 oz	90	0	17
Fat Free, Pre-Stirred, 8 oz	180	0	33
Meadow Gold			
Plain, 8 oz	160	5	16
Flavors, average, 8 oz	250	4	42
Mountain High			
Original: Plain, 8 oz	190	8	18
Fat Free Plain, 8 oz	120	0	20
Fat Free: all flavors, 8 oz	170	0	33
Mystic Lake Dairy (Goat Milk Yogurt)			
Plain, 1 cup, 8 oz	120	6	9
Pavel's: Original Russian, 8 oz	140	8	10
Lowfat Vanilla, 8 oz	120	4	12
Nonfat Russian, 8 oz	110	0	15
Private Selection (Ralph's)			
Lowfat, average all flavors, 8 oz	220	2	43
Fat Free: Coconut Cream Pie, 6 oz	130	0	23
Other flavors, average, 6 oz	100	0	16
Mountain Dairy, 6 oz	150	1.5	27
Publix			
Light, average, 8 oz	130	0	21
Fruit on the Bottom, aver., 8 oz	250	2.5	43
Fat Free: Plain, 8 oz	140	0	23
Swiss Style (lowfat), 8 oz	240	2.5	41
Redwood Hill Farm (Goat Milk Yogurt)			
Fruit flavors, average, 8 oz	180	5	28
Vanilla, 8 oz	190	6	28
Plain, 8 oz	120	6	9
Snackwell's: Nonfat, 6 oz	160	0	36
Stonyfield Farm			
Lowfat, 8 oz	120	1.5	22
Nonfat, aver. all flavors, 8 oz	160	0	31
Frozen: Nonfat, 1/2 cup, 11.4 oz			
Vanilla; Decaf Coffee	90	0	19
Chocolate; Raspberry	100	0	21
Vanilla Fudge Swirl	110	0	23
Lowfat: 1/2 cup, 11.4 oz			
Choc Mint; Mocha Almond	130	3	22
"TCBY" Fat Free (Fantasies):			
Banana Creme Pie, 6 oz	110	0	18
White Chocolate, 6 oz	90	0	12

	C	F	Cb
Trader Joe's			
Nonfat, 8 oz	190	0	40
Lowfat, average, 8 oz	230	2.5	44
Yofarm			
All flavors, aver., 8 oz	220	6	37
Yo Crunch: Lowfat w. Toppings, 6.5 oz			
Oreo Cookies & Cream	190	4	35
Peach/Strawberry w. Granola	220	2	46
Strawberry w. Nestlés Crunch	270	6	46
Vanilla w. Choc Crunch	240	7	39
Yoplait			
Light: All flavors, 6 oz	90	0	16
Original Lowfat: C'nut Creme, 6oz	200	3	35
99% Fat Free, all flavors, 6 oz	180	1.5	34
Multipack, 4 oz	120	1	22
Exprèsse: all flavors, 2.25 oz tube	70	1.5	11
Go-Gurt: 64g tube	80	2	12
Custard Style: All flavors, 6 oz	190	3.5	32
Trix: Multipack, 4 oz	130	1.5	24
Yumsters, 4 oz	120	2	21

Soy/Non-Dairy Yogurt

	C	F	Cb
Health Source: Soy Nonfat, 6 oz	150	0	32
Nancy's Soy: Aver. all flav., 8 oz	210	4	37
Soy Nonfat, 6 oz	150	0	32
Silk (White Wave) Cultured Soy:			
6 oz Cup: Black Cherry	160	2	30
Vanilla	170	2	27
Average other flavors	170	2	34
32 oz Pkg: Plain, 1 cup, 8 oz	150	3.5	24
Vanilla, 1 cup, 8 oz	190	3.5	35

Yogurt Drinks

	C	F	Cb
Alta Dena: Drinkables, 1 cup	220	0	46
Dannon: Danimals, 6 oz	180	3	32
Glen Oaks: All flav., aver., 1 cup	250	4	46
Yonique, 6 fl.oz: Pina Colada	190	4	30
Peach; Banana; Guava	170	2	30
Yo Soy, 8 fl.oz	80	4	4

Frozen Yogurt

See Page 27

Quick Guide — C F Cb

Icecream

Vanilla: Average All Brands
Other flavors ~ See Brand Listings.

Regular Icecream (10% fat):
(Examples: *Borden/Hood*)

	C	F	Cb
3 fl.oz scoop	100	5	12
1/2 cup, 4 fl.oz	130	7	16
1 Pint, 16 fl.oz	520	28	62
1/2 Gallon (4 Pints)	2100	112	248

Rich (16% fat):

	C	F	Cb
3 fl.oz scoop	130	8	12
1/2 cup, 4 fl.oz	170	10	17
1 Pint	690	40	68

Super-Rich (20% fat): (*Haagen-Dazs/Ben & Jerry's*)

	C	F	Cb
3 fl.oz scoop	200	14	16
1/2 cup, 4 fl.oz	270	18	21
1 Pint	1100	72	84

Reduced Fat/Light (6% fat):
(*Breyer's Light/Hood Light*)

	C	F	Cb
3 fl.oz scoop	100	3	14
1/2 cup, 4 fl.oz	140	4	18
1 Pint	560	16	72

Low Fat (less than 4% fat):
(*Healthy Choice/Weight Watchers/Snackwell's*)

	C	F	Cb
3 fl.oz scoop	90	2	17
1/2 cup, 4 fl.oz	120	2.5	22
1 Pint	480	10	88

Fat Free: (*Baskin-Robbins FF/Borden FF/*
Breyers FF/Dreyers FF/Hood FF))

	C	F	Cb
3 fl.oz scoop	75	0	17
1/2 cup, 4 fl.oz	100	0	22
1 Pint	400	0	88

Soft Serve:

	C	F	Cb
Regular, 1/2 cup	140	5	20
1 cup	280	10	40
Nonfat, 1/2 cup	90	0	23
1 cup	180	0	46

Quick Guide — C F Cb

Frozen Yogurt

Average All Brands

		C	F	Cb
Hard:	Lowfat, 1/2 cup	140	3	26
	Nonfat, 1/2 cup	110	0	29
Soft:	Lowfat, 1/2 cup	120	2.5	28
	Nonfat, 1/2 cup	100	0	30

Brands ~ See Icecream & Ices Section

Quick Guide — C F Cb

Gelato/Ices

	C	F	Cb
Gelato: *Per 1/2 Cup*			
Milk base: Vanilla	200	15	18
Choc. Hazelnut	370	29	26
Water base: 1/2 cup	100	0	25
Ice (Milk base): Average all flavors			
Hard (4% fat), 1/2 cup	100	3	15
Soft Serve (3% fat), 1/2 cup	110	2	19
Shaved Ice: Average, 12 fl. oz	160	0	40
Sherbet: Average, 1/2 cup	120	2	28
Sorbet: Fruit (no fat), 1/2 cup	120	0	30
Fruit Ice Pops	80	0	20
Tofu Frozen Desserts ~ Page 30			

Sundaes

	C	F	Cb
Denny's Sundaes:			
Single Scoop, no topping	190	14	14
Double Scoop, no topping	375	27	29
Banana Split	895	43	112
Butterfinger® Hot Fudge	780	38	106
Toppings:			
Blueberry, 2 oz	70	0	17
Chocolate, 2 oz	320	25	27
Fudge, 2 oz	200	10	30
Strawberry, 2 oz	80	1	17
McDonald's Sundaes:			
Hot Fudge Sundae, 6.3 oz	340	12	52
Oreo® Cookie McFlurry™	570	20	82
Toppings: Nut/Sundae, 1/4 oz	40	3.5	2

~ Full Analysis: See Fast-Foods Section ~

Icecream Bars & Pops

See Pages 32-34

Icecream Cones & Cups

	C	F	Cb
Wafer Cone/Cup, average	20	0	4
Sugar Cone, average	40	0	9
Waffle Cone:			
Small	60	0	11
Large	100	1	22
Brands:			
Oreo Chocolate Cone	50	1	10
Comet Sugar Cone	50	0	11
Keebler Sugar Cone	45	0	11

Icecream & Ices

Brands

	C	F	Cb
Alta Dena: Per 1/2 Cup			
Honey Chocolate	160	9	19
Golden Honey Vanilla	160	10	17
Baskin-Robbins: See Page 173 (Fast-Foods)			
Ben & Jerry's: Per 1/2 Cup			
Aloha Macadamia	330	21	30
Butter Pecan	330	25	22
Bovinity Divinity	160	18	30
Cherry Garcia; Vanilla	260	16	23
Choc. Chip Cookie Dough	300	17	34
Choc. Fudge Brownie	280	15	32
Chubby Hubby	350	21	33
Chunky Monkey; Coffee Heath	310	19	32
Concession Obsession	310	19	32
Dilbert's World Totally Nuts	310	21	27
Jerry's Jubilee	260	14	29
Kaberry Kaboom	240	13	27
Mint Choc. Cookie	280	17	28
New York Super Fudge Chunk	320	21	28
Nutty Waffle Cone	310	19	32
Peanut Butter Cup	380	25	32
Peanut Turtles	320	19	33
Phish Food	300	14	41
2 Twisted: Half Baked	280	15	33
Everything But The . . .	320	19	30
From Russia With Buzz	270	17	26
Monkey Wrench	310	20	29
S.N.A.F.U.	250	14	28
This Is Nuts!	300	20	26
Vanilla Caramel Fudge	300	17	33
Vanilla Heath Bar Crunch	310	19	30
Wavy Gravy	340	20	32
Lowfat: Coconut Cream Pie	160	2.5	29
Blondies	200	2	38
S'mores	190	2	35
Frozen Yogurt:			
Vanilla Heath	210	6	34
Choc. Cherry/Chip	190	4	35
Choc. Fudge Brownie	190	2.5	36
Cherry Garcia	170	3	32
Sorbet: Devil's Food Chocolate	170	2.5	36
Average other flavors	130	0	30
Pops: See Page 32			

Bon Bon's	C	F	Cb
Vanilla w. choc. coating, 5 pieces	200	14	17
8 pieces	330	23	27
Bresler's: Per 1/2 Cup			
All Flavors Icecream: average	230	12	23
Royal Cremes, average	260	16	24
Royal Lites, average	220	0	49
Breyers: Per 1/2 Cup			
Dulche de Leche	160	7	21
Homemade: Double Choc Fudge	180	9	23
Butter Pecan; Van.; Neopolitan	150	8	16
Fat Free: Average	110	0	24
Reduced Fat: Average	160	6	19
All Natural: Butter Pecan	180	12	15
Cherry Vanilla; Coffee	150	7	17
Chocolate; French Vanilla	160	10	15
Choc. Chip; Mint Choc. Chip	170	10	18
Cookies 'n Cream	170	9	19
Peach; Strawberry	130	6	18
Vanilla; Van./Choc./Strawberry	150	8	16
Van. & Choc.; Van. Fudge Twirl	160	8	18
Light: Average all flav., 1/2 cup	140	4	19
Icecream Parlor: Chips Ahoy	160	8	18
Candy Bar Sundae	170	8	21
Double Choc Malt	160	7	21
English Toffee	180	8	23
Heath Toffee	180	9	21
Hershey's Choc. w. Almonds	170	8	21
Icecream Sandwich	160	7	21
Mint w/Oreos	160	7	22
Oreo	160	8	19
Reese's P'nut Butter Cup	180	9	22
Vienetta: All flavors, 1 slice	190	11	17
No Sugar Added: Vanilla	80	4	11
Vanilla Fudge Twirl	90	3.5	14
Vanilla Chocolate Strawberry	90	4	11
Mint Chocolate Chip	100	5	11
Frozen Yogurt: Average, 1/2 cup	140	3	25
Carvel Icecream			
See Fast-Foods Section ~ Page 179			
Colombo: Per 1/2 Cup			
Frozen, Soft Serve: Nonfat var.	100	0	22
Slender Sensations varieties	65	0	11
Lowfat: Old Worlde; P'nut Butter	120	2.5	20
Vanilla varieties	110	1.5	21

28

Brands (Cont) C F Cb

Dairy Queen/Brazier
See Fast-Foods Section ~ Page 186

Dannon Frozen Yogurt: Per 1/2 Cup (4 fl.oz)
	C	F	Cb
Light Soft, all flavors, average	90	1	21
Light 'N Crunchy, all flavors, aver.	110	1	23
Pure Indulgence, all flavors, aver.	150	3	25

Dolewhip (Soft Serve): Per 4 fl.oz, 1/2 Cup
Chocolate; Vanilla	100	3	18
Fruit flavors, average	80	0.5	16

Dreyers: Per 1/2 Cup
No Sugar Added: Aver. all flavors	90	3	12
Fat Free: Average all flavors	110	0	25
No Sugar Added	95	0	20
Candy Bar: Twix	190	9	23
Snickers; M&M's Vanilla	180	9	22
M&M's Chocolate	170	8	22
Milky Way; 3 Musketeers	160	7	22
Grand: Cracker Jack	170	9	20
Scooby Doo!	160	8	16
Dexter's Lab.; Amazing Creation	160	7	21
Grand Light: Vanilla	100	3	15
Cookie Dough; P'nut Butter Cup	130	5	17
Other varieties, average	120	4	18
Homemade: Butter Pecan, 71g	160	9	16
Banana Crunch; Strawb. & Crm	130	6	17
Chocolate Peanut Butter, 71g	200	12	18
Cracker Jack; Scooby Snack	170	9	20
Orbit City Swirl	160	8	19
Peaches & Cream, 65g	120	5	16
Vanilla, 1/2 cup, 71g	140	7	16

"He misses the way you used to bend over and pat him."

Dreyers (Cont): Per 1/2 Cup C F Cb
	C	F	Cb
Dreamery: Banana Boogie	290	17	27
Black Raspberry Avalanche	250	14	27
Caramel Toffee Bar: Heaven	270	14	32
Vanilla	260	15	25
Cashew Praline Parfait	260	13	30
Choc P'nut Butter Chunk	310	18	29
Choc Truffle; Nuts About Malt	280	15	30
Cool Mint	280	14	34
Coney Island Waffle	300	18	31
Galactic Choc Swirl	280	12	37
Grandma's Cookie Jar	270	14	32
Harvest Peach; Strawb. Fields	220	11	25
New York Strawb. Cheesecake	250	13	27
Raspberry Brownie a la Mode	270	14	33
Frozen Yogurt: Vanilla	90	0	19
Chips Supreme, 1/2 cup	120	4	19
Fat Free, average all flavors	90	0	20
Starburst Sherbet: Aver. all flav.	150	2.5	30

Edys: Per 1/2 Cup
Banana Split; Choc. Fudge Mousse	160	8	19
Cherry Choc; Van./Choc.; Espresso	150	8	17
Choc. Fudge Sundae; Dble Fudge	170	9	19
Ice Cream Sandwich	140	8	14
Grand Light: Vanilla	100	3	15
Butter Pecan; Choc. Almond	120	5	16
Chiquita 'N Chocolate	110	5	13
Choc. Fudge Mousse	110	3	17
Cookie Dough; P'nut Butter Cups	130	5	18
Cookies 'n Cream; Rocky Road	110	4	16
French Silk	120	4	18
Fat Free: Average all flavors	115	0	25

Eskimo Pie: Per 1/2 Cup
Reduced Fat: Butter Pecan	140	7	16
Choc. Marshmallow	130	4	23
Neopolitan; Vanilla	110	4	18
Fudge Ripple	120	4	19
Bars ~ See Page 32			

Friendly's: Per 1/2 Cup
Icecream: Chocolate Almd Chip	170	10	18
Forbidden Chocolate	150	9	14
Fudge Nut Brownie	200	11	23
Vanilla Choc. Strawb.; Vanilla	150	8	16
Vienna Mocha Chunk	180	11	19
Frozen Yogurt: Lowfat flav., aver.	120	3	20
Regular flavors, average	150	4	24

Icecream & Ices (Cont)

Brands (Cont)

	C	F	Cb
Frostline (Soft Serve): Choc.	90	2	20
Vanilla, 1/2 Cup	90	3	18
Frusen Gladje: *Per 1/2 Cup*			
Butter Pecan	280	21	16
Chocolate	240	17	17
Chocolate Choc. Chip	270	18	21
Mocha Chip; Praline & Cream	280	18	22
Strawberry	230	15	20
Swiss Choc. Candy Almond	270	19	18
Vanilla	230	17	16
Vanilla Swiss Almond	270	19	18
Godiva: *Per 1/2 Cup*			
Belgian Dark Chocolate	280	17	26
Choc Hazelnut Truffle	350	23	31
Choc Raspberry Truffle	290	16	32
Classic Milk Chocolate	290	18	28
Pecan Caramel Truffle	320	19	32
White Choc. Raspberry	260	12	32
Good Humor: *Per 1/2 Cup*			
Light: Coffee	110	3	18
Choc. Chip, Toffee Bar Crunch	130	4	20
Cookies n' Crm; Praline Alm. Crnch	130	3	21
Vanilla, Vanilla Choc. Strawb.	110	3	19
Haagen-Dazs: *Per 1/2 Cup*			
Baileys Irish Cream	270	17	23
Butter Pecan	310	23	21
Cappuccino Commotion	310	21	25
Cherry Vanilla	240	15	23
Chocolate	270	18	22
Chocolate Brownie w. Walnuts	290	19	25
Chocolate Chocolate Chip	300	20	26
Chocolate Swiss Almond	300	20	24
Cinnamon	250	17	20
Coffee	270	18	21
Coffee Fudge Low Fat	170	2.5	32
Coffee Mocha Chip	290	19	25
Cookie Dough Chip	310	20	29
Cookies & Cream	270	17	23
Creme Caramel Pecan	320	20	29
Dulce De Leche	290	17	28
German Chocolate Cake	290	18	28
Macadamia Brittle	300	20	25
Mango	250	14	28
Mint Chip	300	19	26

Haagen-Dazs (Cont):	C	F	C
Per 1/2 Cup			
Pineapple Coconut	230	13	25
Pistachio	290	20	22
Rum Raisin	270	17	22
Strawberry	250	16	23
Toffee Creme	285	17	29
Vanilla	270	18	21
Vanilla Swiss Almond	300	20	24
Sorbet: Chocolate	120	0	28
Mango	120	0	31
Orange	120	0	30
Orchard Peach	130	0	33
Raspberry; Strawberry	120	0	30
Zesty Lemon	120	0	31
Gelato: Cappuccino	240	7	39
Chocolate	240	8	37
Coconut	240	8	38
Hazelnut	260	12	33
Honey Almond	250	10	34
Raspberry	240	7	40
Tiramisu	250	10	35
Frozen Yogurt: Choc. Choc. Chip	230	7	32
Coffee; Vanilla	200	4.5	31
Dulce De Leche	190	2.5	35
Strawberry Non Fat	140	0	31
Vanilla Fudge	220	4	37
Vanilla Raspberry Swirl	170	2.5	31
Bars ~ See Page 33			
Healthy Choice: *Per 1/2 Cup*			
Banana Split; Cookies 'N Cream	130	2	24
Cherry Choc. Chunk; Peanut Butter	110	2	19
Dulce de Leche; Vanilla Bean	110	2	21
Praline & Caramel/Cluster	130	2	25
Rocky Road	130	2	25
Coffee Almd Fudge; Turtle Fudge	110	2	20
Vanilla; Mint Choc Chip	100	2	18
Other flavors, average	120	2	22
Lowfat, No Sugar Added: Vanilla	90	2	16
No Sugar Add: Coffee Almd Fudge	110	2	20

30

Brands (Cont)

	C	F	Cb
...ood: Per 1/2 Cup			
...ght: Almond Praline	110	5	23
Carrib. Coffee	110	5	18
Vanilla; Van.Choc.Strawberry	110	4	18
Other Flavors, average	140	5	22
...hocolate	140	7	17
...hocolate Chip; Maple Walnut	160	9	18
...ookie Dough; Cookies 'n Cream	160	8	21
...rasshopper Pie	160	7	22
...eavenly Hash; Vanilla Fudge	140	6	21
...trawberry	130	7	16
...anilla; Van. Choc. Strawberry	140	7	16
...owfat: No Added Sugar, 1/2 cup	115	3	18
...at Free: Average all flavors	120	0	27
...ecream Bars ~ See Page 32			
...Can't Believe It's Yogurt: See Page 203			
...'s Soy Delicious: Per 1/2 Cup			
...hocolate; Vanilla	130	4	23
...erseymaid (Vons): Per 1/2 Cup			
...fter Dinner Mint; Cookies & Crm	170	9	19
...hoc Chip; Mint Choc Chip	160	9	17
...eavenly Hash; Nut Chunky Choc.	170	8	22
...locha Almd Fudge; Rocky Road	160	7	20
...eopolitan; Vanilla	140	7	16
...trawberry	140	6	18
...ilwin's: Per 1/2 Cup			
...lack Cherry; Caramel Revel	90	0	22
...utter Pecan	190	13	16
...utter Pecan Yogurt	130	6	17
...hocolate	170	10	17
...hocolate Chip Cookie Dough	190	10	22
...hocolate Ripple	100	0	23
...rench Silk; Mud	190	11	20
...emon/Raspberry Sorbetto	100	0	25
...ld Fashioned Vanilla	180	9	20
...opping: Caramel	160	4.5	31
Fudge	110	6	28
...uigi's Real Italian Ice			
...queeze-Up Tube: 8 fl.oz each	150	0	37
...ice Dream (Non Dairy): Per 1/2 Cup			
...anilla Carob/Choc/Cappuccino	150	6	23
...hocChip/Cookies/Carob Chip	170	8	26
...upreme: Average all flavors	170	8	26

	C	F	Cb
Sealtest: Per 1/2 Cup			
Butter Pecan	160	9	16
Choc. Chip Cookie Dough	160	8	20
Fudge Royal; Heavenly Hash	150	7	20
Vanilla/Choc. Strawberry	140	7	16
Snackwell's: Per 1/2 Cup			
Brownie; Rocky Road	130	2	26
Praline Caramel	140	2	28
Vanilla	100	2	18
Soy Dream (Non-Dairy): Per 1/2 Cup			
Butter Pecan	160	10	17
Chocolate Fudge Brownie	150	8	20
Mint Chocolate Chip	150	9	19
Average other flavors	140	6	20
Rocket Bars: Choc/Vanilla	220	12	29
Heavenly Pies: Mocha/Van	290	14	40
Starbucks: Per 1/2 Cup			
Biscotti Bliss	240	12	30
Brownies & Caramel; Van. Mocha	270	14	31
Chocolate Chocolate Fudge	290	17	28
Classic Coffee; Italian Roast	230	12	26
Coffee Almond Fudge	250	13	28
Espresso Swirl	220	10	29
Java Chip	250	13	29
Java Toffee	260	14	30
Mud Pie	240	11	32
Lowfat: Mocha Mambo; Latte	170	3	30
Bars ~ see Icecream Bars & Pops Section			
Stonyfield Farm: Per 1/2 Cup			
Chocolate; Raspberry; Vanilla	120	2	22

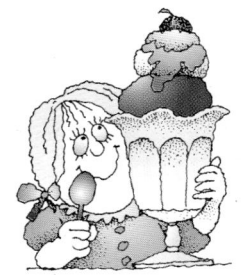

TCBY	C	F	Cb
Paradise Ice: Medium	430	0	110
Large	550	0	140
Froz. Yogurt Family Style: Peach	110	1	21
Dutch Choc:.Summertime Strawb	100	1.5	20
Other flavors, average	110	1.5	23
Hand-Dipped: Medium	310	6.5	57
Large	390	8.5	73
No Sugar Add. Non Fat: Med.	175	0	44
Large	225	0	56
Non Fat: Medium	240	0	51
Large	310	0	64
Regular, all flavors: Medium	285	6.5	51
Large	365	8.5	64
Hand-Dipped Icecream: Small	320	19	37
Medium	440	26	50
Large	560	34	64
Sorbet: Medium	220	0	53
Large	280	0	67
Tofutti Non-Dairy Dessert: Per 1/2 Cup			
Premium: Vanilla	190	11	20
Better Pecan; Alm. Bark	220	13	22
Choc. Cookie Crunch	210	11	26
Chocolate Supreme	180	11	18
Van. Fudge; Wildberry	190	9	24
Low Fat Supreme: Average	110	2	25
Cutie Pies: Average, 67g bar	250	19	28
Too Toos: Vanilla S'wich	215	10	28
Van. Choc. Swirl/Chip S'wich	230	11	30
Teddy Fudge: 52g bar	70	1	19
Turkey Hill: Per 1/2 Cup			
Black Cherry	140	7	18
Butter Pecan	170	11	16
Choco. Mint Chip, Cookies 'n Crm	160	10	17
Neapolitan, Vanilla & Choc.	150	8	18
Rocky Road	170	8	23
Vanilla, Vanilla Bean	140	8	16
Lite: Choco Mint Chip	140	5	19
Cookies 'n Cream	130	5	21
Vanilla & Choc., Van. Bean	110	3	18
Weight Watchers: Per 1/2 Cup			
Cookie Dough Craze	140	3.5	24
Oh! So Very Vanilla	120	2.5	20
Positively Praline Crunch	140	3	25
Reckless Rocky Road	140	3	23
Triple Chocolate Tornado	150	3.5	26
Bars ~ See Page 33			

Bars & Pops — Per Bar/Serving	C	F	C
Baby Ruth (Nestlé)	180	12	15
Baskin Robbins: Tiny Toons	140	17	20
Cappuccino Blast, average	120	4	20
Sundae Bar: Pralines 'n Cream	280	17	20
Ben & Jerry's: Vanilla Pop	330	22	29
Cookie Dough Pop	410	24	45
Totally Nuts	370	29	24
Big Bear: See Klondike	290	10	45
Big Ed's Super Saucer: 10 fl.oz	420	28	32
1/2 Sandwich, 5 fl.oz	210	14	16
Borden: Sundae Cone	210	10	27
Twin Pops	60	0	14
Bon Bons (Nestlé): Milk Choc., (8)	330	23	27
Dark Chocolate, 8 pces	310	21	26
Bounty: all varieties	70	5	7
Butterfinger Bar, 2.5 oz	190	13	16
Breyers: Vanilla Bar	250	17	21
w. chocolate coating	230	15	20
Sandwich (Vanilla)	250	11	32
Carnation: Orange Sherbet, 3 oz	90	1	19
Icecream Cup: Choc., 3 fl.oz	140	8	16
Strawb., Vanilla, 3 fl.oz	100	6	12
Choc./Vanilla Malt, 12 oz	270	6	48
Sundae Cup, all types, 5 oz	210	9	30
Chipwich Jr: Choc. Chip S'wich	240	10	35
Chiquita: Swirls, all flavors	80	3	12
Cool Creations: Mini Sandwich	110	5	16
Cookies & Cream Sandwich	240	11	34
Pops, all types, 2 oz	60	0	14
Mickey Mouse: 2.5 oz Bar	120	8	10
4 oz Bar	170	11	17
Creamsicle: Sugar-free pops	25	0	15
Orange, 2.8 fl.oz	110	3	20
Crunch (Nestlé): King, 4 oz	270	19	21
Reduced Fat, 2.5 oz	130	7	14
Regular Icecream Bar, 3 oz	200	14	16
Crystal Light: Cool 'n Creamy	50	2	7
Dole Bars: Coconut, 4 oz	210	7	33
Fruit Juice, reg., 1.75 oz	45	0	11
No Added Sugar, 1.75 oz	25	0	6
Fruit 'n Juice: Small, 2.5 oz	70	0	16
Pine-Coconut, 4 oz	150	4	27
Other flavors, 4 oz	120	0	28
Dove Bar: Almond	340	22	30
Bite Size, 5 pces, average	350	22	36
Caramel Pecan	350	35	35
Mocha Cashew	260	17	25

Per Bar/Serving	C	F	Cb
Dove Bar (Cont): Peppermint	390	17	31
Vanilla Dark Choc; Cookie	340	21	35
Single Vanilla Dark	200	12	24
Vanilla Milk Chocolate	350	24	35
Dreyers: Icecream Bars, average	250	17	22
Fruit Bars, 3 fl.oz	90	9	23
Smoothie Bars, average	95	0	21
Sundae Cone, 4 fl.oz	240	11	31
Whole Fruit Bars, 1.75 fl.oz	60	0	14
Drumstick *(Nestlé):* Chocolate	320	17	36
Choc. Dipped	320	16	40
Original Vanilla	340	19	35
Vanilla Caramel/Fudge	360	20	39
Eskimo Pie: Arctic Madness, 2.5 oz	230	15	23
Bars: Milk/Dark Choc, 50g	160	11	15
Fudge Bar, 55g	60	1	11
Reduced Fat varieties	120	8	13
Crispy Bar, 47g	130	8	13
Pecan, 51g	190	15	12
Big Bar, 99g	300	20	26
Icecream Sandwich, 65 g	160	4	27
Cones, 74g	210	12	24
No Sugar Added: Bar, 49g	120	8	13
Pudding Bar, 59g	90	1.5	16
Flintstones: Push Up Sherbet	100	2	20
Push Up Pebbles, 2.75 oz	120	6	15
Cool Cream, 2.75 oz	90	2	18
Frosty Dreams	100	2	19
Frosty Pops *(Nestlé)*	40	0	11
Froz-Fruit: Cherry	60	0	15
Strawberry	80	0	20
Fruit A Freeze: Coconut	130	5	20
Lime	65	0	16
Banana; Strawberry	90	1.5	19
Dark Choc-Dipped Strawberry	90	3.5	14
Fudge Bar *(Nestlé)*	110	1	23
Fudgesicle: Fudge Bar (1)	45	0.5	9
Fat Free (1)	60	0	13
Fudgetastics: Sticks Sundae	220	15	37
Good Humor: Candy Crunch	280	21	21
Chocolate Eclair; Colonel Crunch	170	9	21
Chocolate Taco	320	17	38
Classic Almond	210	12	21
Dinosaur	110	2	25
Giant Sandwich, 5 fl.oz	240	10	35
Icecream Sandwich	190	8	28
King Cone	300	14	38
Good Humor (Cont):			
Strawberry Shortcake, 3.75 fl.oz	210	9	29
Cups: Sundae Twist	160	3	33
Combo (6 fl.oz)	200	10	25
Reese's P'nut Butter, 1 bar	250	16	24
Haagen-Dazs: *Per Bar*			
Caramel & Almond Crunch	310	21	27
Chocolate & Almond	380	27	27
Chocolate & Dark Chocolate	350	24	28
Multipack, 3 fl.oz	290	20	23
Coffee & Almond Crunch	370	27	27
Multipack, 3 fl.oz	310	22	23
Cookies & Cream Crunch	370	26	30
Dulce De Leche (Caramel)	370	24	34
Multipack, 3 fl.oz	300	19	28
Raspberry & Vanilla	90	0	21
Sorbet & Cream, Orange & Vanilla	120	5	16
Tropical Coconut	340	24	25
Vanilla & Almonds	380	28	26
Multipack, 3 fl.oz	320	23	22
Vanilla & Dark Chocolate	350	24	27
Multipack, 3 fl.oz	280	20	22
Vanilla & Milk Chocolate	340	24	25
Multipack: Caramel & Alm. Crunch	310	21	27
Chocolate Sorbet	80	0	20
Sorbet & Yogurt, Raspb. & Vanilla	90	0	21
Hood: Chocolate Eclair, 1 bar	150	10	14
Cooler Cup, 2.1 oz	80	1	18
Crispy Bar	180	13	15
Fabukous Fudgies, 1 bar	100	3	19
Fabulous Fudge P'nut Butter	110	4	17
Fudge Bar	100	1	21
Hendrie's Cherry Choc. Dips	120	9	11
Hoodsie Cup Van./Choc.	100	5	12
Orange Cream Bar	90	2	18
Rockets, each	120	5	18
Vanilla Bar	160	12	11
Icecream Sandwich *(Nestle)*	170	6	26
Jell-O: Pop Bars	31	0	7
Jigglers, all varieties, 6 oz	215	1.5	50
Pudding Bars	80	2	13
Klondike: Almond Bar	310	21	26
Big Bear Van. Icecream S'wich	290	10	46
Choc Chip Cookie Sandwich	520	21	77
Gold Bar	340	23	30
Heath Toffee	300	20	27
Krunch	290	19	26

Per Bar/Serving	C	F	Cb
Klondike (Cont): Lite Bar	110	6	14
Original Vanilla; Choc.; The One	290	20	25
Sandwich: Chocolate	270	10	41
Lite	100	2	18
Vanilla	250	9	37
York Peppermint Patty	290	20	24
Kool-Aid Pops	40	0	10
Krispy Frostick:	150	10	13
Juice Flavored Sticks	50	0	13
M&Ms: Cookie Icecream S'wich	240	12	32
Mars Almond Bar	210	14	20
Matterhorn: Cone, 10 fl.oz	510	38	19
Milky Way: Choc, Reduced Fat	140	7	19
Caramel Swirl, 1 bar	180	10	21
Snack Bar, Vanilla/Chocolate	70	4	9
Minute Maid: Fruit Juice Pops	60	0	15
Nestlé Icescreamers: Push Up Pop	90	1.5	19
Shock Tarts, 1 pop	45	0	11
Tiger Tails, 1 pop	60	0	15
Oreo: Choc; Vanilla	160	9	19
Big Stuf, 1 sandwich	240	10	33
Cookies n' Cream, 1 bar, 59g	180	12	18
Pathmark: Vanilla w. choc. coat.	150	10	14
Polar Bar: Vanilla w. choc. coat.	240	18	15
Choc. Chip Cookie Dough	450	28	48
Pops (water/juice), average	60	0	14
Popsicles: Fudgesicle Fudge Pop	90	1.5	16
Scribblers Icecream: 2 pces	130	7	15
Juice Pops, 2 pces	60	0	16
Sprinklers Icecream, 1 bar	130	6	18
Pokémon Ice w. Candy, 1 pce	80	0	19
Rugrats Cookie S'wich, 1 pce	150	7	20
Wildlife Icecream, 1 piece	110	6	14
Ice Pops: Aver. of flavors, 1 pce	45	0	11
Sugar-Free, 1 pce	15	0	3
Reece's: Peanut Butter Icecream	160	11	22
Rice Dream: Pies, all flavors	320	18	40
Bars: Stawberry	250	13	31
Chocolate, Vanilla	270	15	32
Choc/Vanilla Nutty	270	18	23
Smart Ones *(Weight Watchers)*:			
Chocolate Mousse	40	1	9
Chocolate Treat	100	0.5	20
English Toffee Crunch	110	6	12
Mocha Java	80	1.5	9
Orange Vanilla Treat	40	0.5	10
Vanilla Sandwich	150	3	28

Per Bar/Serving	C	F	Cb
Snackwell: Icecream Sandwich	90	1.5	18
Yogurt Bars, 1 bar, 80g	120	2	22
Snickers: Pralines n' Creme	220	13	22
Icecream Bar	180	11	18
Snack, 4 bars	390	25	38
Soy Dream (Non-Diary):			
Dreamwich Vanilla	130	6	15
Heavenly Pies: Mocha; Vanilla	290	14	40
Lil' Dreamers: Choc; Vanilla	60	3	7
Rocket Bars: Choc; Vanilla	220	12	29
Starbuck's:			
Coffee & Almond Bars, 81g	280	18	26
Coffee Frappuccino Bar	110	2	21
Mocha Frappuccino Bar	120	2	21
Java Ice Cream Bar	270	16	29
Starburst: Juice Bars	20	0	5
Super Sundae Bar, 86g	310	20	26
3 Musketeers: 2 fl.oz bars	170	10	21
Snack Bars, regular	60	4	16
Tandem *(Nestlé):* Sandwich	380	21	39
Twin Pop *(Nestlé)*	60	0	14
Vitari: soft serve, 4 fl.oz, average	80	0	20
Welch's: Fruit Juice Bars, 92g	80	0	18
Tropical Coolers, 92g	45	0	11
No Sugar Added, 1 bar	25	0	6
Fruit Smoothie, 1 ctn	240	0	59

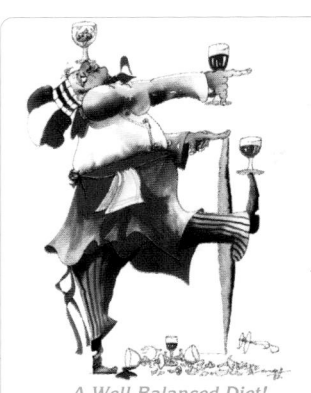

A Well-Balanced Diet!

Quick Guide

Cream

	C	**F**	**Cb**
Average All Brands			
Half & Half Cream: 1 Tbsp	20	2	0.5
2 Tbsp, 1 oz	40	4	1
Light, coffee/table (20% fat): 1 T.	30	3	0.5
2 Tbsp, 1 oz	60	6	1
Medium (25% fat), 1 Tbsp	40	4	0.5
Sour Cream:			
Regular, 1 Tbsp	30	3	0.5
1 cup	490	48	8
Lowfat/Light, 1 Tbsp	20	2	1.5
2 Tbsp, 1 oz	40	2.5	2
Half & Half, 1 Tbsp	20	2.5	0.5
Fat Free, 2 Tbsp	20	0	3
Fat Free: (*HeluvaGood*), 2 Tbsp	20	0	6
(*Kroger*), 2 Tbsp, 32g	25	0	5
(*Naturally Yours; Oak Farm*), 2 T.	20	0	3
(*Knudsen*), 2 Tbsp, 32g	35	0	6
Sour Cream Substitute:			
(*Albertsons/ IMO*), 2 T., 1 oz	50	5	1
(*Tofutti*) Sour Supreme, 1 oz	50	5	1
Whipping Cream:			
Heavy (37% fat):			
1 Tbsp fluid/2 T. whipped	50	5	1
1/4 cup whipped	100	11	2
1/2 cup fluid/1 c. whipped	400	44	8
Light (30% fat):			
1 Tbsp fluid/2 T. whipped	45	5	0.5
1/2 cup fluid/1 c. whipped	350	37	4

Coconut Cream/Milk

	C	**F**	**Cb**
Coconut Cream (Canned),			
Plain/unsweetened, 2 Tbsp, 1 oz	70	6	4
1/2 cup	280	24	16
Sweetened: *Coco Lopez*, 1 Tbsp	120	5	20
1/2 cup, 4 oz	480	20	80
Coconut Milk, can, 1/2 cup	225	24	3
Coconut Water (center), 1 cup	45	0.5	9

Whipped Toppings

	C	**F**	**Cb**
Average All Brands			
Cream (Pressurized): 1 Tbsp	10	1	0.5
1/4 cup	40	4	2
Cream Toppings: *Jewel*, Lite, 2 T.	20	1	2
Cool Whip: Extra Creamy, 2 T.	25	1.5	2
Lite, 2 Tbsp, 9g	20	1	2
Free, 2 Tbsp, 9g	15	0	3
Non Dairy, 2 Tbsp	22	2	2
Kraft: Whipped, 2 Tbsp	20	2	1
Real Cream, 2 Tbsp	20	2	1
Reddi-Wip: Original, 2 T., 8g	20	2	0
Original Light, 2 T.	15	1	2
Non-Dairy, 2 T., 8g	20	1.5	2
Extra Creamy, 2 Tbsp, 8g	30	3	0.5
1/4 cup/4 Tbsp	60	6	1
Fat Free, 2 Tbsp, 8g	10	0	2
Vetra: Light, sweetened, 2 T., 6g	15	1	1

Non-Dairy Coffee Creamers

	C	**F**	**Cb**
Powder *Coffee-Mate/Cremora/N-Rich:*			
Regular, 1 tsp	20	2	1
1 heaping tsp	25	2	2
Fat Free, 1 tsp	10	0	2
Lite, 1 tsp	10	0.5	2
Flavors: 1 1/3 Tbsp	60	3	9
Fat Free: Average, 1 1/3 Tbsp	50	0	11
Liquid/Refrigerated: *Per Tbsp*			
Coffee-Mate Non-Dairy Creamer:			
Plain: Regular/Plain, 1 Tbsp	20	1	2
Fat Free, 1 Tbsp	10	0	2
Lite, 1 Tbsp	10	0.5	1
Flavors: All flavors, 1 Tbsp	40	2	5
Fat Free, all flavors, 1 Tbsp	25	0	5
Hood (Non Dairy), 1 Tbsp	25	0	5
International Delight: 1 Tbsp	35	1.5	6
Fat Free flavors, 1 Tbsp	30	0	7
Mocha Mix: Original, 1 Tbsp	20	1.5	1
Fat Free, 1 Tbsp	10	0	1
Lite, 1 Tbsp	10	0.5	1
Morning Blend (Ralph's): 1 Tbsp	15	1.5	0
Fat Free, 1 Tbsp	5	0	2
Rich's Coffee Rich: Regular, 1 T.	25	1	2
Light	15	0.5	0.5
Rich's Farm Rich: Regular, 1 Tbsp	20	1	2
Light/Fat Free	10	0	0.5
Silk (White Wave) Creamer, 1Tbsp	15	1	1
French Vanilla, 1 Tbsp	20	1	3

Quick Guide   C F Cb

Butter & Margarine

Average All Brands

	C	F	Cb
Regular: 1 tsp (5g)	35	4	0
1 Pat (5g)	35	4	0
1 Tbsp, approx. 1/2 oz	100	11	0
2 Tbsp, 1 oz	205	23	0
1 Stick, 1/2 cup, 4 oz	810	92	0
1 Pound, 2 cups, 16 oz	3240	368	0
Light (Regular) 40% Fat:			
1 tsp, 5g	17	2	0
1 Tbsp, 1/2 oz	50	6	0
2 Tbsp, 1 oz	100	11	0
Whipped (Regular):			
1 tsp (4 g)	27	3	0
1 Tbsp (10g)	70	7.5	0
1 Stick, 1/2 cup, 2 2/3 oz	570	60	0
Light (Whipped) 40% Fat:			
1 tsp, 5g	10	1	0
1 Tbsp. 9g	35	3.5	0
2 Tbsp, 18g	70	7	0
Unsalted: Same as Regular			

Clarified Butter

	C	F	Cb
100% Fat: 1 Tbsp, 1/2 oz	130	15	0
2 Tbsp, 1 oz	260	30	0

Flavored Butter/Spread

Average All Brands

	C	F	Cb
Honey Butter (60% Fat):			
1 Tbsp, 1/2 oz	90	7	4
Downey's, 1 Tbsp, 1/2 oz	60	1	11
Garlic Butter (80% Fat):			
1 Tbsp, 1/2 oz	100	11	0
Sweet Cream Butter:			
Regular, 1 Tbsp	100	11	0
Stick (70% Fat), 1 Tbsp	90	10	0
Tub (60% Fat), 1 Tbsp	80	9	0

Other Spreads & Fats

	C	F	Cb
Copha, Dripping, Lard, Suet, Shortening:			
1 Tbsp, 1/2 oz	120	13	0
Chicken, Duck, Goose Fat:			
1 Tbsp, 1/2 oz	115	13	0

Light & Reduced Fat Spreads C F C

Per 1 Tbsp, 1/2 oz (Unless Stated)

	C	F	C
Benecol: Regular, single serve, 8g	45	5	
Light, single serve, 8g	30	3	
Blue Bonnet: Lowfat Margarine	45	4.5	
45% Veg. Oil Spread	70	7	
Breakstone's Whipped Butter	60	7	
Brummel & Brown: Spread	50	5	
Chiffon: Whipped, 1 Tbsp	70	7	
Country Crock: Regular	60	7	
Light	50	5	
Country's Delight (70% Veg.)	90	10	
Country Morning: Light	50	6	
Downey's Honey Butter	60	1	
Dutch Farms: 52% Veg. Spread	70	7	
Fleischmann's: Soft Spread	80	9	
Original	90	10	
Fat Free Spread	5	0	
'I Can't Believe It's Not Butter': Reg.	90	10	
Light; Sweet Cream	50	5	
Imperial: Diet, 1 Tbsp	50	6	
Jewel: Soft Spread	60	7	
Unbelievably Butter	90	9	
Kraft: 'Touch of Butter' (bowl)	50	6	
Land O'Lakes: Tub	80	8	
Honey Butter	90	7	
Light Whipped Butter	35	3.5	
Light Butter	50	6	
Mazola: Diet	50	6	
Mother's; Mrs Filbert's, 1 Tbsp	70	8	
Miracle: Soft	60	7	
Stick	70	7	
Nucoa: HeartBeat Margarine	25	3	
Olivio: Vegetable Spread	80	8	
Parkay: Squeeze, 1 Tbsp	80	9	
Stick, 1/3 Less Fat	70	7	
Tub, 1 Tbsp	60	7	
Tub, Light/Soft Diet	50	6	
Whipped	70	7	
Promise: Regular	90	10	
Extra Light	50	6	
Buttery Light	45	5	
Ultra, w. canola oil	35	4	
Smart Balance: Regular	80	9	
Light, 1 Tbsp	45	5	
Smart Beat: Fat Free	10	0	
Take Control: Regular Spread	50	6	
Light Spread	40	4.5	
Weight Watcher's: Light, all types	45	4	

Fats, Spreads & Oils (Cont)

Butter Substitutes

	C	F	Cb
Bake It Perfect (Fat Free Spread), 1 T.	5	0	0
Best O'Butter, 1/2 tsp	4	0	0
Butter Buds: 1 serving, 1/2 tsp	4	0	0
Butterlike Saute Butter, 1 Tbsp	35	2	0
Butter Sprinkles (Watkins): 1 tsp	5	0	0
Earth Balance, Non GMO, 1 tsp	35	3.5	0
Molly McButter: 1/2 tsp	5	0	0
Mrs Bateman's Baking Butter, 1 T.	35	1	0

Spreads Comparison

Mayonnaise: Regular, 1 Tbsp	100	11	0.5
Light, average, 1 Tbsp	50	5	1
Fat Free (e.g. *Wt. Watcher's*), 1 T.	12	0	3
Miracle Whip *(Kraft):*			
Regular, 1 Tbsp	70	7	2
Light, 1 Tbsp	40	3	3
Free, 1 Tbsp	15	0	3
SmartBeat Dressing: 1 Tbsp	12	0	2
Extra Listings for Mayonnaise & Dressings			
~ See Page 84 ~			
Peanut Butter, 1 Tbsp	100	8	3.5
Avocado, mashed, 1 Tbsp	25	2.5	2
Birdseye:			
No Fat Veggie Dip, 2 T., 1.1 oz	25	0	5

"I push myself away from the table but my wife's good cooking pulls me right back."

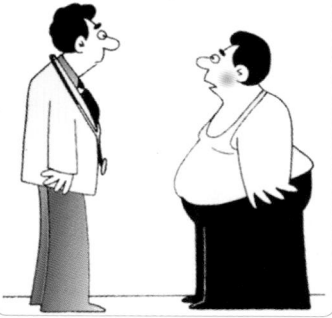

Animal Fats/Lards

Average All Types	C	F	Cb
Beef Tallow/Drippings, Lard (Pork),			
Chicken, Duck, Goose, Turkey.			
1 Tbsp (13g)	115	13	0
2 1/4 Tbsp, 1 oz	255	28	0
1 cup, 7 1/4 oz	1850	205	0
1/2 pound, 8 oz	2040	227	0
Ghee/Butter Oil: 1 Tbsp, 13g	110	13	0
2 1/4 Tbsp, 1 oz	250	28	0

Vegetable Shortening

Average All Types (example, *Crisco*)			
1 Tbsp	113	13	0
2 1/4 Tbsp, 1 oz	250	28	0
1 cup, 7 1/4 oz	1810	205	0

Vegetable Oils

Includes almond, avocado, canola, corn, coconut, flaxseed, grapeseed, linseed, mustard, olive, palm, peanut, rice-bran, safflower, sesame, sunflower, soybean, wheatgerm. Note: Oil is 100% fat.

1 tsp, 5g	45	5	0
1 Tbsp, 1/2 oz	120	14	0
2 Tbsp, 1 oz	250	28	0
1 cup, 7 3/4 oz	1930	205	0

Fish Oils

Average All Types (Includes cod liver, herring, salmon, sardine):			
1 Tbsp, 1/2 oz	125	14	0

Cooking Sprays

Cooking Sprays (*Pam, Mazola, Weight Watchers, Wesson*):			
Per serving	2	0	0
2-3 second spray	6	1	0
Parkay Buttery Spray	0	0	0

Olestra (Olean)

Olestra *(Olean)*	0	0	0

Olean is *Proctor & Gamble's* brand name for olestra - a no-calorie cooking oil that gives snacks (like potato chips, tortilla chips and crackers) taste and texture without adding fat or calories.

Cheese

Firm/Hard Cheeses
(American, Cheddar, Colby, Coon, Swiss)

Regular Cheese:	C	F	Cb
1 oz slice/piece	110	9	0.5
8 oz package	880	72	4
16 oz (1lb) package	1760	144	8
Cubes: 1" cube, 3/4 oz	55	5	0.5
1 1/4" cube, 1 oz slice	110	9	0.5
Diced: 1 cup, 4 1/2 oz	500	40	2
Grated: 1 Tbsp, 1/4 oz	27	2	0
Shredded:			
1/4 cup, 1 oz	110	9	0.5
1 cup, 4 oz	440	36	4
Sliced: 1 thin (3 1/2" sq.), 3/4 oz	85	7	0.5
Rectangular (7"x 4"x 1/8"), 1 1/2 oz	165	14	1
Round (3 1/4" diam. x 1/8"), 3/4 oz	85	7	0.5
Semi-circular, 1 1/4 oz			
(5 1/2" long, 3 1/2" radius, 1/8"thick)	140	11	0.5
Light: Average All Brands, oz	70	4.5	1
Fat Free: Average All Brands, 1 oz	50	0	2
Lowfat: Average All Brands, 1 oz	50	1.5	1

Cheese

Per 1 oz Unless Indicated

American:	C	F	Cb
Regular, 1 slice, 1 oz	110	9	1
Kraft Deluxe, 0.7 oz slice	70	6	0.5
Grated, 1 Tbsp, 1/4 oz	23	2	0
Light (*Borden*), 1 oz	70	4	0.5
Land O'Lakes, 1 oz	70	5	0.5
Smart Beat, 0.6 oz slice	35	2	1
Fat Free: Single, 0.75 oz	30	0	3
Alpine Lace, 1 oz	45	0	2
HealthyChoice, Singles, 0.7 oz	25	0	2
Weight Watchers, all types, 3/4 oz	30	0	3
Babybel (*Laughing Cow*), 1 oz	90	7	0
Crumbled, 1/2 cup, 2 1/2 oz	250	20	2
Dorman's Castello, 1 oz	135	12	1
Bonbel (*Laughing Cow*), 1 oz	100	8	0
Mini, 3/4 oz	75	6	0
Brick, 1 oz	100	8	0
Brie, 1 oz	95	8	1
Camembert, 1 oz	90	7	0
Caraway, 1 oz	105	8	1

Cheddar:	C	F	Cb
Regular, 1 oz	110	9	0.5
(Also see 'Quick Guide')			
Reduced Fat/Light, 1 oz	80	5	0.5
Weight Watchers, 1 oz	80	5	1
Fat Free: *Alpine Lace*, 1 oz	45	0	2
Weight Watchers, 1 sl., 3/4 oz	30	0	3
Cheese Balls (*Kaukauna*), 1 oz	100	7	0.5
Cheese Nut, Average, 1 oz	100	7	2
Cheese Logs, Average, 1 oz	100	7	0.5
Cheshire, 1 oz	110	9	1.5
Colby, Regular, 1 oz	110	9	0.5
Reduced Fat (*Alpine Lace*), 1 oz	80	5	1
Colby-Jack, 1 oz	110	9	0.5
Cottage Cheese: *Average All Brands*			
Creamed: 2 Tbsp, 1 oz	30	1	1
1/2 cup, 4 oz	120	5	4
w. fruit, 1/2 cup, 4 oz	130	4	15
Reduced Fat (2%), 2 T., 1 oz	25	<1	1
1/2 cup, 4 oz	100	2	4
Low Fat (1%), 2 Tbsp, 1 oz	20	<1	1
1/2 cup, 4 oz	80	1	3
NonFat, 2 Tbsp, 1 oz	20	0	1
1/2 cup, 4 oz	80	0	3
Borden Dry Curd (0.5%), 1/2 c., 4 oz	80	0	0
Friendship: Low Fat P'apple, 4 oz	120	1	17
NonFat Plus Peach, 1/2 c., 4 oz	110	0	15
Pot Style, 1/2 cup, 4 oz	90	3	3
w. Pineapple, 4 oz	140	4	16
Knudsen: 1.5% Fruit, 4 oz	110	2	12
Free, 1/2 cup, 4.3 oz	80	0	11
Cottage Dbles, 1 ctn, 5.5 oz	140	2.5	18
On the Go!, 1 cup, 4 oz	110	1.5	13
Light N' Lively: Garden Salad, 4 oz	90	2	5
Peach and Pineapple,			
1/2 cup, 4.3 oz	120	1	14
Chevre: See Goat's Milk Cheese			
Cream Cheese: See Page 41			
Edam: Regular, 1 oz	100	8	0
Farmer (*Friendship*), 2 Tbsp, 1 oz	50	3	0
Feta: Regular, *Frigo*, 1 oz	100	8	1
Crumbled, 1/2 cup, 2 1/2 oz	190	15	2.5
Reduced Fat (*Alpine Lace*),	60	4	1
Fontina (*Sargento/Classica*), 1 oz	110	9	0.5
Gjetost (Goat's Milk, fresh), 1 oz	85	7	0.5
Sargento, 1 oz	130	8	12
Goat's Milk: Soft: *Chevre*, 1 oz	70	6	0.5
Chavril, 3 Tbsp, 1 oz	60	4.5	0.5

	C	F	Cb
Goat's Milk Cheese (Cont)			
Semi-Soft: 1 oz	100	8.5	1
Hard: Sargento, 1 oz	130	10	0.5
Gorgonzola: 1 oz	110	9	0.5
Galbani Dolcelatte: 1 oz	95	8	1
Gouda: 1 oz	100	8	0.5
Gruyere, 1 oz	115	9	0
Havarti, 1 oz	120	11	0
Italian (*Classica Italiano*), 1 oz	110	10	1
Jarlsberg, 1 oz	100	7	1
Jarlsberg Lite shredded, 1 oz	70	4	1
Kefir, 2 Tbsp, 1 oz	60	4	1
Limburger, 1 oz	90	8	0
Mascarpone, 1 oz	130	13	1
Mexican (*Sargento* Recipe Blend),			
Shredded, 1/4 cup, 1 oz	110	9	0.5
Monterey, 1 oz	105	8.5	0
Monterey Jack: regular, 1 oz	110	9	0
Light Naturals (*Kraft*), 1 oz	80	5	0
Alpine Lace , Monti-Jack Lo, 1 oz	80	5	0
Weight Watchers, 1 oz	90	6	1
Mozzarella:			
Regular: *Kraft/Dorman's,* 1 oz	90	7	0.5
Land O'Lakes/Polly-O, 1 oz	80	6	0.5
Shredded, 1/4 cup, 1 oz	80	6	0.5
Light: *Polly-O Lite,* 1 oz	60	2.5	0.5
Kraft Light Naturals, 1 oz	80	5	0.5
Sorrento Lite, 1 oz	60	3	0.5
Part Skim (*Alpine Lace*), 1 oz	70	5	0.5
Polly-O, 1 oz	90	6	0.5
Fat Free: *Healthy Choice,* 1/4 c.,1oz	45	0	1
Polly-O, 1 oz	35	0	1
Kraft, shredded, 1/4 cup, 1 oz	50	0	2
Muenster: regular, 1 oz	110	9	0
Reduced Fat: *Dorman's,* 1 oz	80	5	0
Neufchatel: *Dominick's,* 1 oz	70	6	2
Philadelphia, 1 oz	70	6	1
Flavored: Fruit/Herbs	80	7	1
Chocolate (*Hickory Farms*), 1 oz	110	8	1
Parmesan: Fresh/Block, 1 oz	110	7	1
Shredded/Grated, 1 Tbsp	22	1.5	0
Grated (Packaged): 1 Tbsp	26	2	0
1oz quantity	130	9	1
1/2 cup, 1 3/4 oz	230	16	2
w. Romano (*Frigo*), grated, 1 oz	130	9	1

Note: Packaged grated and shredded Parmesan have more calories (per unit weight) than block Parmesan due to a lower moisture content.

	C	F	Cb
Pizza, shredded:			
Frigo, 1/4 cup, 1 oz	90	7	1
1 cup, 4 oz	360	28	4
Lowfat (*Frigo*), 1 oz	65	3	1
Port Du Salut, 1 oz	100	8	0.5
Port Wine (*Hickory Farms*), 1 oz	100	7	2.5
Pot (*Sargento*), 1 oz	25	0	1
Provolone: Regular, 1 oz	100	8	1
Reduced Fat, *Alpine Lace,* 1 oz	70	5	1
Pub (*Hickory Farms*), 1 oz	95	7	1
Quark: 40% fat, 1 oz	47	3	1
20% fat, 1 oz	32	1.5	1
Skim, 1 oz	22	0	1.5
Queso: Anego/Asadero/Blanco	105	9	1
Queso Chichuahua/De Papa	110	9	2
Queso De Taco, 1 oz	105	9	1
Ricotta Cheese:			
Whole Milk, 2 Tbsp, 1 oz	50	3.5	1
1/2 cup, 4 1/2 oz	225	16	4.5
Part Skim, 2 Tbsp, 1 oz	40	2.5	1
1/2 cup, 4 1/2 oz	180	12	4.5
Light/Low Fat, 2 Tbsp. 1 oz	30	1.5	2
1/2 cup, 4 1/2 oz	140	6	9
Fat Free (*Polly-O*), 1/2 c., 4 1/2 oz	100	0	4
Baked Ricotta, 2 oz portion	130	9	3
Romano: Block/Loaf, 1 oz	110	8	1
Grated (Pkg), 1 oz	120	9	1
1 Tbsp	26	2	0.5
Roquefort, 1 oz	105	9	0.5
Slim Jack (*Dorman's*), 1 oz	90	7	1
Sheep's Milk (*Hollow Rd Farm*)	45	3	1
Smoked: *Sargents* Smokestick	100	7	1
Hickory Farm, Smoky Lyte, 1 oz	80	6	1
Stilton, 1 oz	118	10	1
String (*Frigo/Kraft/Sargento*), 1 oz	80	5	1
String Lite (*Frigo*), 1 oz	60	2	1
Mootown Light (*Sargento*), 1 stick	50	2.5	0.5
Swiss: Regular, 1 oz	110	9	1
Reduced Fat: *Alpine Lace,* 1 oz	90	6	1
Dorman's/Kraft Light Naturals, 1oz	90	5	1
Weight Watchers, 3/4 oz slice	30	0	2
Taco, shredded, 1/4 cup			
(*Frigo/Kraft/Sargents*)	110	9	1
Tilsit (*Sargents*), 1 oz	100	7	0.5
Tybo (*Dorman's/Sargents*), 1 oz	100	7	0.5
Vermont (*Churny*), 1 oz	100	9	1
Wensleydale, 1 oz	108	9	0
Whey Cheese, 1 oz	125	8	9

Cheese Products   C   F   Cb

	C	F	Cb
Cheese Food:			
Average all flavors, 3/4 oz slice	70	5	1.5
1 oz slice	90	6	2
Alouette: Fr. Onion/Garl.,2 T., 0.8oz	70	7	1
Light Garlic, 2 Tbsp, 0.8 oz	50	4	1
Cracker Barrel, Cheddar, 1.1 oz	100	8	4
Delico: Alouette Cajun, 2 T, 0.8 oz	70	7	1
Garden Vegetable, 2 T, 0.8 oz	60	6	1
Handi-Snacks:			
Cheez 'n Breadsticks, 1 pkg	130	7	11
Cheez 'n Pretzels, 1 oz pkg	110	6	11
Cheez'n Crackers, 1.1 oz pkg	130	8	10
Mozzarella Stringchse Stick, each	80	6	0.5
Healthy Choice: Amer. Singles, 1 sl.	30	0	2
Heluva Good Cheese:			
American, 1 slice	45	5	2
Cheddar w. H/radish, 2 Tbsp, 1oz	90	7	3
Jalapeno: Aver., all brands, 1 oz	90	7	1
Kraft: American grated,1T., 0.2 oz	25	2	1
Singles, 1 slice, 3/4 oz	70	6	1
Free Singles, 1 slice, 0.7 oz	40	3	3
Pimento Spread, 2 Tbsp, 1.1 oz	80	6	3
Velveeta (Process Cheese Spread)			
Regular, 3/8" slice, 1 oz	100	6	3
Light, 3/8" slice, 1 oz	60	3	3
Lifeway: Farmers Cheese, 2 oz	75	5	2.5
Precious: String Chse Stuffsters, 1 oz	70	4.5	1
Roka Blue, 2 Tbsp, 1.1 oz	80	7	2
Rondele: Soft Spread., 2 T, 1 oz	100	9	1
Light, 2 Tbsp, 0.9 oz	60	4	2
SmartBalance: Crmy Cheddar, 1 sl.	40	2	2
SmartBeat: All flav., 1 sl., 0.6 oz	35	2	2
Spreadery: Vermont, 2 Tbsp, 1 oz	80	5	3
Neufchatel, all flavors, 2 T, 1 oz	80	7	1
Velveeta: Cheese, 1 slice, 1 oz	100	6	3
Light, 1 oz	60	3	3
Shredded, 1/4 cup, 1.3 oz	130	9	3
WisPride: Hickory Smoked Cup;			
Port Wine Ball/Cup, 2 T., 1.1 oz	100	7	4
Light, 2 T., 1.1 oz	80	3	5

Cheese Whiz (Sauce)

	C	F	Cb
Regular, 2 Tbsp, 33g	90	7	2
Light, 2 Tbsp, 33g	80	3	6
Squeezable, 2 Tbsp, 33g	100	8	4

Cheese Substitutes   C   F   Cb

Per 1 oz Unless Indicated

	C	F	Cb
Almond Rella (Nu Soya):			
Cheddar; Garlic & Herb, 1 oz	60	3	3
Borden: Taco-Mate, 1 oz	100	7	2
Delicia: American Colby	80	6	1
Dorman's Lo Chol: All types	100	7	1
Formagg:			
American Wh./Yellow, 1 sl. 0.7oz	60	4	0.5
Cheddar, 1 slice, 0.7 oz	60	4	0.5
Mozzarella (Old World), 1 oz	60	3	1
Parmesan Grated, 1 Tbsp, 1/4 oz	22	1.5	1.5
Provolone (Vintage), 1 oz	60	3	1
Swiss White, 1 slice, 0.7 oz	60	4	0.5
Frigo: Cheddar; Mozzarella, 1 oz	90	7	1
Georgio's: Imitation Cheddar;			
Mozzarella., shredded, 1/4 c., 1 oz	90	7	1
Golden Image: American 1 slice, 0.7 oz			
Mild Cheddar, 1 slice, 0.7 oz	70	5	1
Harvest Moon : Per 1/4 cup, 1.3 oz			
Shredded: American; Cheddar	120	9	3
Mozzarella	110	9	3
Nu Tofu: Mozzarella, 1 oz	70	4	2
Fat Free: Mozz./Ched./Jack, 1 oz	40	0	2
Sargento Classic Supreme:			
Cheddar, shredded, 1 oz	90	6	2
Mozzarella, shrd, 1/4 cup	80	6	0.5
Smart Beat, all varieties, 0.6 oz sl.	35	2	1
Soya Kaas: Regular, 1 oz	70	5	1
Fat Free, all varieties, 1 oz	40	2	1
Soyco: Almond/Oat/Rice Slices,			
1 slice, 0.7 oz	40	2	1
Veggy Singles, 1 slice, 0.7 oz	40	2	1
Grated Parmesan, 2 tsp, 5g	15	0.5	0
Tofu Rella: Per 1 oz			
Tofu Rella, average all varieties	180	2	39
Zero-Fat Rella, all varieties	45	0	3
Almond/Hemp/Rice Rella,			
average all varieties	70	3.5	3
Tofutti Better Than Cream Cheese	80	8	1
Weight Watchers: Fat Free Slices,			
All varieties, 3/4 oz slice	30	0	3
Grated Italian Topping, 1 Tbsp	20	0	2
White Wave, Soy A Melt:			
Cheddar/Mozz./Mont. Jack, 1 oz	80	5	1
Fat Free, 1 oz	40	0	3
Singles: Amer./Mozzrlla, 3/4 oz sl.	60	4	1
Yves Good Slice, 3/4 oz Slice	35	2	1

Cream Cheese

	C	F	Cb
Regular/Soft: 2 Tbsp, 1 oz	100	10	1
3 oz pkg	300	30	2
w. Chives/Herbs/Pimento, 1 oz	90	9	0.5
w. Fruit/Strawb./P'apple, 1 oz	90	8	5
Lox, 1 oz	90	9	0.5
Philadelphia Brand:			
Plain/Soft, 2 Tbsp, 1 oz	100	10	1
1/3 Less Fat, 1 oz	70	6	1
Light, 1 oz	70	5	2
Fat Free, 2 Tbsp, 1 oz	30	0	3
Flavor./Herbs/Fruit/Salmon, 1 oz	100	10	2
w. Smoked Salmon 1 oz	100	9	1
Light Blueberry, 2 Tbsp	70	4.5	5
Snack Bars: aver., all types, ea.	200	13	20
Whipped, 3 Tbsp, 1 oz	110	11	1
Alpine Lace: Fat Free, 2 T., 1 oz	30	0	1
Dominick's: Fat Free, 2 Tbsp, 1 oz	35	0	4
Light, 2 Tbsp, 1 oz	60	5	2
Weight Watchers, 2 Tbsp, 1 oz	40	2.5	1

Dips/Spreads

Per 2 Tbsp (1 oz) Unless Indicated

	C	F	Cb
Avocado/Guacomole	50	4	4
Baba Ghannouj (Eggplant/Sesame)	70	6	2
Birdseye: No Fat Veggie Dip, 1.1 oz	25	0	5
Breakstone: Sour Cream, all flav.	50	4	4
Chalco: Quéso Quesadilla; Cotija	120	10	0
Fresco, 2 Tbsp, 1 oz	70	8	0
Chef's Kitchen (Jewel): Dilly Dip	150	16	1
French Onion/Quarter; Spinach	70	6	2
Chi-Chi's: Con Quéso, 2 Tbsp	90	7	4
Hot/Medium/Mild/Acante, 2 T.	10	0	2
Dominick's: Port Wine & Cheddar	100	8	4
Eagle: Bean	35	2	2
French Onion Dip, aver. all brands	60	6	3
Frito Lay: Chili Cheese	45	3	3
French Onion	60	5	4
Bean/Jalapeno Bean	40	1	6
Jalapeno & Cheddar	50	3	3
Guacamole, 2 Tbsp, 1 oz	50	4	4
Guiltless Gourmet: Nacho Dip	25	0	5
Other varieties	30	0	5
Heluva Good Cheese:			
Cheese 'N Salsa	80	3	3
Clam/French Onion	50	5	2
Bacon/Homestyle/Ranch	60	5	2
Light Fr. Onion/Jalapeno Cheddar	40	2	3

Dips/Spreads (Cont)

Per 2 Tbsp (1 oz)

	C	F	Cb
Hummus: 2 Tbsp, 1 oz	50	1	5
1/2 cup, 4.5 oz	220	4.5	23
Hy-Top: Pimiento, 1 oz	90	8	3
Kaukauna: Nacho Cheese	90	7	4
Knudsen: Nacho Cheese	60	4	3
Sour Cream Bacon & Onion	60	5	2
Sour Cream French Onion	50	4	2
Kroger: The Big Dipper; all flavors	60	5	2
Kraft: Average all flavors	60	5	4
Premium: Bac. & On./Nacho Ch.	60	5	2
Other flavors	50	4	2
Philly flavors: Pineapple	100	9	1
Chive & Onion; Salmon	110	10	2
Cheesecake; Strawberry	110	9	5
Fat Free: Strawberry	45	0	6
Garden Veges	30	0	2
Lay's: Lowfat Sr. Cream, Onion	40	1	0
Louise's: (Fat Free) Honey Mustard	40	0	0
Sour Cream & Onion/Wh.Cheese	25	0	0
Marzetti: Blue Cheese	200	21	1
Light Ranch Veggie	60	7	5
Other flavors, average	140	14	2
Nalley's: All flavors, average	120	12	3
Naturally Fresh: All flavors, 1 oz	80	0	19
Old Dutch: Cheddar, Nacho	35	3	3
Old El Paso: Black Bean	25	0	5
Cheese'n Salsa: Mild; Medium	40	3	3
Lowfat, medium	30	1.5	3
Chunky Salsa varieties	15	0	3
Jalapeno Dip	30	1	4
Olys Bagel Spread: Berry	100	8	3
Honey Cinnamon; Raisin	100	8	6
Garden Veg; Garlic & Herb	90	9	1
Prices: Orig. Pimiento Cheese Spr.	80	7	2
Ruffles: French Onion; Ranch	70	6	4
Sealtest: French Onion	50	4	2
Snyder's: Mustard Pretzel	90	4	13
Supremo Chihuahua: Quéso Bianco	100	8	0
Quéso Fresco; Rancherito	80	6	0
TGI Fridays:Spinach,Chse, Artichoke	45	3.5	2
Tostitos Dip: Con Quéso	40	2	5
Medium/Mild/Hot	15	0	3
Tzatziki (Cucumber/Yoghurt Dip)	40	3	1
Wise: Jalapeno Bean	25	0	5
Taco	12	0	3

Salsa ~ See Page 80

Egg & Egg Dishes

Chicken Eggs

	C	F	Cb
Fresh Eggs			
Raw (weight with shell):			
Small, 40g	65	4	0
Medium, 44g	70	4	0
Large, 50g	75	4.5	0
Extra Large, 56g	80	5	0
Jumbo, 63g	90	5.5	0
Egg Yolk, 1 extra large	63	5	0
Egg White, 1 extra large	16	0	0
Dried Egg Powder			
Whole Egg, 1/4 cup, 1 oz	170	12	0
1 Tbsp	30	2	0
Egg White, 1/4 cup, 1 oz	105	0	0
Egg Yolk, 1/4 cup, 1 oz	195	18	0
1 Tbsp	27	2.5	0

Egg Substitutes

1/4 Cup (Equivalent to 1 Egg) ~ Zero Cholesterol.

	C	F	Cb
Better 'n Eggs (Papetti), 1/4 cup, 2 oz	30	0	0
Egg Beaters (Fleischmann's):			
Regular, 1/4 cup	30	0	1
Cheese Omelete, 1/2 cup	110	5	2
Vegetable Omelete, 1/2 cup	50	0	5
Egg Watchers (Tofutti), 2 oz	30	0	1
Eggstra, 1/2 envelope	50	2	0
Healthy Choice, 1/4 cup, 2 oz	25	0	0
Egg Substitute (Jewel), 1/4 cup	30	0	1
Scramblers (Morn Star), 1/4 cup	35	0	1
Second Nature: Regular, 1/4 cup	60	2	3
Fat Free, 1/4 cup, 60ml	30	0	1
Simply Eggs, 1/4 cup	35	1	0

Other Eggs

	C	F	Cb
Duck, 1 large, 2 1/2 oz	130	9.5	0
Goose, 1 large, 5 oz	280	19	0
Quail, 3 eggs, 1 oz	42	3	0
Turkey, 1 large, 3 oz	135	9.5	0
Turtle, 1 egg, 1 3/4 oz	75	5	0

Omega-3 Fat Enriched

	C	F	Cb
Eggs Plus (Pilgrim's Pride): 1 large	70	4.5	0

Note: Cholesterol content same as regular eggs, but Omega-3 fats inhibit blood cholesterol increase.
(Also see Cholesterol ~ Page 253)

Cooked Eggs

	C	F	Cb
Boiled Egg: Same as raw egg			
Fried Egg:			
With fat: 1 large egg	100	8	0.5
2 small eggs	175	13	1
No fat/nonstick pan, 1 large	80	5.5	0
Deviled Egg, 2 halves	145	13	0.5
Eggs Benedict (2) on toast or English muffin	860	56	25
Eggs Florentine (2) on toast or English muffin	890	59	25
Pickled Egg, 1 large	80	5.5	0
Poached Egg, 1 large	80	5.5	0
Scotch Egg, 1 egg	300	21	16
Scrambled Eggs: 1 large egg:			
w. 1 Tbsp milk + 1 tsp fat	120	9	1
w. 1 Tbsp skim milk/no fat	85	5.5	1
2 large eggs:			
w. 2 Tbsp milk + 2 tsp fat	260	20	2
w. 2 Tbsp skim milk/no fat	180	11	2

Omelets

	C	F	Cb
1 Egg: Plain (w. 1 tsp fat)	125	10	0.5
with 1/2 oz cheese	175	15	0.5
w. 1/2 oz cheese + 1/2 oz ham	200	16	0.5
2 Eggs: Plain (w. 2 tsp fat)	250	20	1
with 1 oz cheese	360	29	1
w. 1 oz cheese + 1 oz ham	410	32	1
3 Eggs: Plain (w. 1 Tbsp fat)	360	29	1.5
w. 2 oz cheese	580	47	2.5
w. 2 oz cheese + 2 oz ham	680	53	2.5
Extras: Tomato/Onion/Veges	20	0	4.5
Egg Substitute (*Eggbeaters*):			
2 eggs (1/2 cup) + 1 tsp fat	100	4	2
3 eggs (3/4 cup) + 2 tsp fat	160	8	3
Extras: 1 oz cheese	110	9	1
1 oz ham	50	3	1
Tom./Onion/Veges	20	0	4.5

Egg Nog

Per 1/2 Cup (4 fl.oz)

	C	F	Cb
Regular: *Borden*	160	9	16
Crowley	190	9	23
Hood (Goldeen)	180	8	22
Light: *Borden/Hood*	120	2	23
Fat Free: *Hood*	100	0	21

Breakfast Sides

	C	F	Cb
Toast: Plain, 1 thick slice	85	1	13
with 2 tsp butter/marg.	155	9	13
with 3 tsp/1Tbsp fat	190	13	13
English Muffin: Plain, 2 oz	130	1	26
with 3 tsp fat	230	12	26
Bacon, 2 strips	70	5	0
Ham: Lean, 2 oz	100	3	0
Hash Browns: 1/2 cup	125	6.5	14
1 cup serving	250	13	28
Sausages, 2 links (1 oz ea.)	180	16	1.5

Frozen Egg Dishes

	C	F	Cb
Downyflake: Scrambled Eggs			
w. Ham & Hash Browns, 1 pkg	360	26	17
w. Ham & Pecan Twirl	470	28	40
w. Hash Browns & Sausage	420	34	17
Pillsbury Toaster Scrambles, 1	170	11	14
Swanson Great Starts: Per Packet			
Scrambled Eggs: w. Burrito	200	8	25
w. Bacon & Home Fries	290	19	17
w. Home Fries	200	12	15
w. Sausage & Hash Browns	360	26	21
Low Fat	240	13	18
Low Fat/Chol Eggs: w. Pancakes	220	7	30
w. Canadian Bacon	240	6	33
Egg, Bacon, Cheese Muffin	290	15	25
Egg, Sausage & Cheese	460	28	37
French Toast Sticks w. Syrup	320	10	50
Pancakes w. Sausage	490	25	52
Sandwich Egg, Cheese	350	20	30
Sausage, Egg & Chse on Biscuit	460	28	37
Quaker Scrambled Eggs			
w. Cheese/Fried Potatoes	250	13	22
w. Sausage & Hash Browns	290	20	14
w. Sausage & Pancakes	270	14	21
Weight Watchers: Omelet	220	5	30

Frozen Egg Rolls

	C	F	Cb
Average All Brands (Chun King/La Choy)			
Chicken Egg Rolls: Mini, 5 rolls	165	6	24
Restaurant Style, 1 roll, 3 oz	170	5	25
Pork & Shrimp Egg Rolls:			
Mini, 5 rolls	175	5	23
Pork Restaurant Style, 1 roll	170	6	24
Shrimp Egg Rolls: Mini, 5 rolls	155	5	23
Restaurant Style, 1 roll	150	4	24

Fast Food/Restaurants

	C	F	Cb
Bojangles:			
Bacon/Egg/Chse S'wich	550	42	27
Burger King:			
Bisc. w. Sausage/Egg/Cheese	650	46	38
Croissan'wich Saus./Egg/Chse	500	36	26
Carl's Jr: Scrambled Eggs	180	14	1
Denny's: Eggs Benedict	695	46	34
Omelette: Ham 'n Cheddar	580	45	4
Veggie-Cheese	490	39	10
Sirloin Steak & Eggs	620	49	1
Hardee's: Bacon & Egg	570	33	45
Ham, Egg & Cheese	540	30	48
Ultimate Omelet	570	33	45
McDonald's: Egg McMuffin®	290	12	27
Bacon, Egg & Cheese Biscuit	480	31	31
Scrambled Eggs (2)	160	11	1
Perkins: Country Club Omelet	930	79	6
Roy Rogers: Ham & Egg Bisc.	470	26	44
Sausage & Egg Biscuit	560	35	44

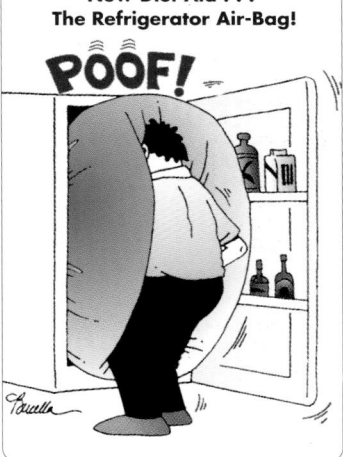

**New Diet Aid . . .
The Refrigerator Air-Bag!**

POOF!

This cartoon available as refrigerator magnet ~ See Page 287

Meat ✦ Beef

Note: Cooking reduces weight of meat by 20-45% due to water and fat losses. Average weight loss is 30%. Actual loss depends on cooking method and cooking time. Examples:

4 oz raw wt. = approx. 3 oz cooked wt.
4 oz cooked wt. = approx. 5.¹/₂ oz raw wt.

What 3 oz Cooked Meat Looks Like
- Half the size of this book (4¹/₄" x 3" x ³/₈" thick)
- Rectangular piece (4" x 2¹/₂" x ¹/₂" thick)
- Pack of cards (3¹/₂" x 2¹/₂" x ⁵/₈" thick)

Quick Guide · C · F · Cb

Steak

Sirloin (Choice Grade)
External fat trimmed to ¹/₄"
Broiled, Edible Portion (no bone)

Small Serving, 3 oz
(3 oz cooked, from 4-4¹/₂ oz raw)

	C	F	Cb
Lean + fat (¹/₄"), 3 oz	230	14	0
Lean + marbling, 3 oz	195	10	0
(External fat trimmed **before** cooking)			
Lean only, 3 oz	170	7	0
(No external fat or marbling)			

Medium/Regular Serving, 5 oz
(from approx. 7 oz raw)

	C	F	Cb
Lean + fat (¹/₄"), 5 oz	470	29	0
Lean + marbling, 5 oz	400	20	0
Lean only, 5 oz	350	14	0

Large Serving, 8 oz
(from 11-12 oz raw)

	C	F	Cb
Lean + fat, 8 oz	610	38	0
Lean + marbling, 8 oz	520	26	0
Lean only, 8 oz	454	18	0

Extra Large Serving, 12 oz
(from approx. 16-17 oz raw)

	C	F	Cb
Lean + fat (¹/₄"), 12 oz	915	57	0
Lean + marbling, 12 oz	780	39	0
Lean only, 12 oz	680	27	0

Pan Fried
Sirloin (choice), medium serving:

	C	F	Cb
Lean + fat (¹/₄"), 5 oz	450	32	0
Lean only, 5 oz	330	15	0

Other Steaks · C · F · Cb

Filet Mignon (Tenderloin):
1 medium steak, 6 oz raw wt.
Broiled, with ¹/₄" fat trim

	C	F	Cb
Lean + fat (¹/₄"), 4 oz	340	24	0
Lean only, 3¹/₂ oz	210	10	0

Broiled, (¹/₄" fat removed before cooking)

	C	F	Cb
Lean + marbling, 3¹/₄ oz	220	12	0
Lean only, 3 oz	180	8	0

New York/Club Steak:
Top Loin/Short Loin
1 steak, regular (9¹/₄ oz raw, ¹/₄" fat)

	C	F	Cb
Broiled: Lean + fat, 6¹/₄ oz	510	35	0
Lean + marbling, 5¹/₂ oz	330	16	0
Lean only, 5¹/₄ oz	310	14	0

Porterhouse Steak:
1 medium, 6 oz raw wt. (no bone)
Broiled:

	C	F	Cb
Lean + fat (¹/₄"), 4¹/₄ oz	370	27	0
Lean only, 3¹/₂ oz	220	11	0

T-Bone Steak:
1 medium, 8 oz raw wt.

	C	F	Cb
Broiled: Lean + fat	380	27	0
Lean only	220	10	0

Beef - Average All Cuts

Average All Retail Cuts · C · F · Cb
Edible weight (no bone)

Raw
(1 lb raw yields approx. 11-12 oz cooked)

	C	F	Cb
Lean + fat (¹/₄" trim), 1 oz	70	5.5	0
¹/₂ Pound, 8 oz	560	44	0
Lean only, 1 oz	40	2	0
¹/₂ Pound, 8 oz	320	16	0
Fat only, 1 oz	190	20	0

Cooked (No Added Fat)

	C	F	Cb
Lean + fat (¹/₄"), 1 oz	86	6	0
Small serving, 3 oz	260	18	0
Lean + marbling, (no ext. fat), 1 oz	78	5	0
Small serving, 3 oz	235	15	0
Lean only, 1 oz	60	3	0
Small serving, 3 oz	180	9	0
Fat only, 1 oz	193	20	0

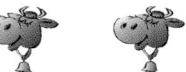

Beef - Individual Cuts

	C	F	Cb
Average All Grades			
Edible Weight (no bone)			
Brisket, whole, braised:			
Lean + fat ($1/4$"), 3 oz	330	27	0
Lean + marbling, 3 oz	250	17	0
Lean only, 3 oz	205	11	0
Chuck, blade, braised:			
Lean + fat ($1/4$"), 3 oz	290	22	0
Lean + marbling, 3 oz	285	20	0
Lean only, 3 oz	210	11	0
Flank: Raw, 4 oz	200	12	0
Braised, 3 oz	225	14	0
Broiled, 3 oz	190	11	0
Ribs, whole (ribs 6-12):			
Average all grades, roasted			
(1 lb raw yields $10^1/4$ oz roasted)			
Lean + fat ($1/4$")			
(3.6 oz w. bone, 3 oz no bone)	300	25	0
Lean only, 3 oz (no bone)	200	11	0
Round, bottom, braised:			
Lean + fat ($1/4$"), 3 oz	235	14	0
Lean only, 3 oz	180	7	0
Round, eye/tip, roasted:			
Lean + fat ($1/4$"), 3 oz	200	11	0
Lean, 3 oz	150	5	0
Round, top: *Per 3 oz*			
Braised, Lean + fat	210	10	0
Lean only	175	5	0
Broiled, Lean + fat	185	8	0
Lean only	155	4	0
Pan-fried, Lean + fat	235	13	0
Lean only	190	7	0

Ground Beef

	C	F	Cb
Raw: Reg. (73% lean), 4 oz	350	30	0
Lean (80% lean), 4 oz	300	24	0
Extra lean (85% lean), 4 oz	250	17	0
Healthy Choice (97% lean), 4 oz	130	4	0
Baked/Broiled: Reg., 3 oz	250	18	0
Lean, 3 oz	230	16	0
Extra lean, 3 oz	200	12	0
Pan-fried: Regular, 3 oz	260	19	0
Lean, 3 oz	230	16	0
Extra lean, 3 oz	200	12	0
Ground Beef Patties: Average			
Frozen, raw, 4 oz	320	26	0
Broiled, 3 oz	240	17	0

Quick Guide C F Cb

Roast Beef

	C	F	Cb
Round (Eye/Tip, average)			
Average All Cuts			
Small Serving, 3 oz			
(2 thin slices/1 thick slice)			
Lean + fat ($1/4$"), 3 oz	200	11	0
Lean only, 3 oz	150	5	0
Medium Serving, 5 oz, (3-4 thin slices)			
Lean + fat, 5 oz	330	18	0
Lean only, 5 oz	250	8	0
Large Serving, 8 oz, (3 thick slices)			
Lean + fat, 8 oz	530	29	0
Lean only, 8 oz	400	13	0

Roast Dinner Extras

	C	F	Cb
Gravy: Thin, 2 Tbsp	20	1	0.5
Thick, 2 Tbsp	50	2	0.5
1 Ladle/4 Tbsp	100	4	1
Veges: Beans, green, $1/2$ cup	20	0	5
Cauliflower w. cheese sauce, 4 oz	135	9	15
Corn, kernels, $1/4$ cup	35	0	9
Carrots, $1/4$ cup	20	0	3
Peas, $1/4$ cup	35	0	6
Pumpkin baked: w.fat, 4 oz	90	7	5
No added fat, 2 pces, 4 oz	25	0	5
Potato:			
Roasted w. fat, 1 small	155	8	30
Baked in Jacket, 1 large	220	0	50
with 1 Tbsp whipped butter	295	8	50
with Sour Cream, 2 Tbsp	270	6	51
Sweet Potato/Yam, 1 medium	80	0	20

"347 ~ 348 ~ 349..."

Meat • Lamb, Veal, Pork

Lamb | C | F | Cb

Choice Grade
Leg (Whole), roasted:

	C	F	Cb
Lean + fat, 3 oz	220	14	0
Lean only, 3 oz	160	7	0

Leg (Sirloin Half), roasted:

	C	F	Cb
Lean + fat, 3 oz	250	18	0
Lean only, 3 oz	175	8	0

Leg (Shank Half), roasted:

	C	F	Cb
Lean + fat, 3 oz	190	11	0
Lean only, 3 oz	155	6	0

Loin Chop, broiled:
1 chop (raw wt., $4^1/4$ oz):

	C	F	Cb
Lean + fat ($2^1/4$ oz edible)	200	15	0
Lean only (1.6 oz edible)	100	5	0

Rib Chop, broiled/roasted:
1 chop (raw wt., $3^1/2$ oz)

	C	F	Cb
Lean + fat ($2^1/2$ oz edible)	255	21	0
Lean only ($1^3/4$ oz edible)	120	7	0

Shoulder (Arm/Blade):

	C	F	Cb
Braised: Lean + fat, 3 oz	290	21	0
Lean only, 3 oz	240	14	0
Broiled: Lean + fat, 3 oz	240	16	0
Lean only, 3 oz	180	9	0
Roasted: Similar to Broiled			

Cubed Lamb (Leg/Shoulder):
For stew or kabob

	C	F	Cb
Raw, lean only, 8 oz	310	12	0
Braised, lean only, 3 oz	190	8	0
Broiled, lean only, 3 oz	160	6	0

New Zealand Lamb (Imported):
Similar calories and fat to domestic.

Veal

Edible Weights
Leg (Top Round):

	C	F	Cb
Braised: Lean + fat, 3 oz	180	6	0
Lean only, 3 oz	170	5	0
Pan-fried, breaded:			
Lean + fat, 3 oz	195	8	9
Lean only, 3 oz	175	6	9
Pan-fried, not breaded:			
Lean + fat, 3 oz	180	7	0
Lean only, 3 oz	155	4	0
Roasted: Lean + fat, 3 oz	135	4	0
Lean only, 3 oz	130	3	0

Veal (Cont) | C | F | Cb

Loin Chop: 1 chop, 7 oz raw wt.

	C	F	Cb
Braised: Lean + fat	230	14	0
Lean only	155	6	0
Roasted: Lean + fat	175	10	0
Lean only	125	5	0
Rib, roasted: Lean + fat, 3 oz	195	12	0
Lean only, 3 oz	150	7	0

Shoulder, Arm/Blade, roasted:

	C	F	Cb
Lean + fat, 3 oz	155	7	0
Lean only, 3 oz	145	6	0

Sirloin, roasted:

	C	F	Cb
Lean + fat, 3 oz	170	9	0
Lean only, 3 oz	145	6	0
Cubed for Stew, braised:			
Leg/Shoulder, lean only, 3 oz	160	4	0

(1 lb raw yields approx. $9^1/4$ oz cooked)

Pork

Figures based on NLMB data (1990)
Fresh Pork (Cooked Wt., no bone)
(4 oz raw wt. = approx. 3 oz cooked wt.)
Blade Steak, broiled:

	C	F	Cb
Lean + fat, 3 oz	220	15	0
Lean only, 3 oz	190	11	0

Country Style Ribs, broiled:

	C	F	Cb
Lean + fat, 3 oz	270	22	0
Lean only, 3 oz	205	13	0

Leg (Ham), roasted:

	C	F	Cb
Lean + fat, 3 oz	250	18	0
Lean only, 3 oz	180	9	0

(Ham, cured ~ See Cold Meats)
Loin Chops, broiled: Average
(From 1 chop: 5 oz raw wt. w.bone
or 4 oz raw wt., no bone)

	C	F	Cb
Lean + fat, 3 oz	200	11	0
Lean only, 3 oz	165	7	0

Rib Chops, broiled:

	C	F	Cb
Lean + fat, 3 oz	215	13	0
Lean only, 3 oz	180	7	0

Rib Roast, roasted:

	C	F	Cb
Lean + fat, 3 oz	210	13	0
Lean only, 3 oz	175	9	0

Loin Roast, roasted:

	C	F	Cb
Lean + fat, 3 oz	190	10	0
Lean only, 3 oz	160	7	0

Pork (Cont)	**C**	**F**	**Cb**
Sirloin Chop, broiled:			
Lean + fat, 3 oz	175	8	0
Lean only, 3 oz	155	6	0
Sirloin Roast, roasted:			
Lean + fat, 3 oz	215	14	0
Lean only, 3 oz	180	9	0
Tenderloin, roasted:			
Lean + fat, 3 oz	147	5	0
Lean only, 3 oz	140	4	0
Ground Pork			
Raw: Average, 1/4 lb, 4 oz	300	24	0
Broiled, 3 oz	245	18	0
Pan-fried, drained, 3 oz	250	19	0

Bacon	**C**	**F**	**Cb**
Raw: 1 med. slice (20 lb), 3/4 oz	125	13	0
1 thick slice (12 lb), 1 1/3 oz	210	22	0
(1 lb raw yields approx. 5 oz cooked)			
Broiled/Pan-Fried: 1 med. sl., 6 g	36	3	0
3 medium slices, 18g	110	9	0
2 thin slices, 1/2 oz	80	7	0
1 thick slice, 12g	70	6	0
Canadian-style: Cooked, 1 slice	43	4	0
As purchased, 1 slice, 1 oz	45	4	1
Bacon Bits, 1 Tbsp, 1/4 oz	20	1	0
Breakfast Strips: Broil., 1 sl., 12 g	50	4	0

Ham	**C**	**F**	**Cb**
Boneless Ham, cooked:			
Regular, (approx. 11% fat):			
Unheated (as purch.), 1 oz	52	3	0
Roasted, 3 oz	150	8	0
Extra Lean (5% fat):			
Unheated, 1 oz	37	2	0
Roasted, 3 oz	125	5	0
Whole Ham, cooked:			
Lean + fat (as purchased)			
Unheated, 1 oz	70	5	0
Roasted, 3 oz	345	26	0
Lean only, unheated, 1 oz	40	2	0
Roasted, 3 oz	135	5	0
Canned Ham: Similar to boneless ham			
Chopped, canned, 3 oz	260	21	0
Ham Patties, ckd, 1 pty, 2 1/4 oz	205	18	1
Ham Steak, extra lean, 2 oz	70	2	0
Luncheon Slices~ See Cold Meats: Page 50			

Game Meats	**C**	**F**	**Cb**
Bison Steak, lean, 6 oz (raw)	210	4	0
Boar (wild), roasted, 3 oz	140	4	0
Caribou, roasted, 3 oz	140	4	0
Deer/Venison, roasted 3 oz	135	3	0
Rabbit: Roasted, 3 oz	130	6	0
Stewed, 1 cup, diced, 5 oz	300	14	0

Variety & Organ Meats	**C**	**F**	**Cb**
Brains: Braised, 3 oz	130	9	0
Pan-fried, 3 oz	200	14	0
Chitterlings, pork, simmered, 3oz	260	25	0
Ears, pork, simmered, 1 ear	180	12	0
Feet, pork: Simmered, 3 oz	165	11	0
Cured, pickled, 3 oz	170	14	0
Hormel, 2 oz	80	6	0
Head Cheese (Pork Snouts/Ears/Vinegar/Spices):			
1 oz slice	50	4	0
Heart: Average, braised, 3 oz	140	5	0
Jowl, pork, raw, 4 oz	750	80	0
Kidneys, simmered, 3 oz	130	4	0
Liver: Raw, 4 oz	160	5	3
Braised, 3 oz	140	4	3
Pan-fried, 3 oz	200	9	3
Pancreas, braised, 3 oz	200	13	0
Pork Cracklins, 0.5 oz	80	6	0
Pork Hocks, 1 piece, 6 oz	340	23	0
Scrapple, pork, 1 oz	60	4	4
Spleen, braised, 3 oz	130	4	0
Stomach, pork, raw, 4 oz	180	11	0
Sweetbreads: Beef, ckd, 3 oz	270	20	0
Lamb, cooked, 3 oz	150	5	0
Tail, pork, simmered, 3 oz	340	31	0
Tongue, braised, 3 oz: Veal	170	9	0
Beef/Lamb/Pork, average	240	17	0
Tripe, beef, raw, 4 oz	110	5	0
Lean + fat	310	25	0

> *In eating, one third of the stomach should be filled with food, one third with drink, and the rest left empty.*
>
> ~ Gitten, the Talmud

Sausages, Franks

Fresh Sausages

	C	F	Cb
Pork/Beef: *Average All Types*			
Small: Raw, 4" link, 1 oz	120	12	1.5
Broiled/Pan-fried	50	4	1.5
Medium: Raw, 2 oz	235	23	2.5
Broiled/Pan-fried	100	8	2.5
Large: Raw, 3 oz	360	36	3.5
Broiled/Pan-fried	150	12	3.5
Italian: Raw, 3.2 oz	315	28	1.5
Cooked, 4 oz	215	17	1.5

Note: Fat is lost in broiling/pan frying.
(Cooked wt. = approx. 60-70% raw wt.)

Franks & Weiners

	C	F	Cb
Beef: *Average All Brands*			
Regular/Smoked: *Per Frank*			
4 oz link	280	22	5
2.6 oz link	240	19	2
2 oz link (8/16 oz pkg)	180	17	2
1.6 oz link (10/16 oz pkg)	140	13	1
1.5 oz link (8/12 oz pkg)	135	12	1
1.2 oz link (10/12 oz pkg)	110	10	1
1 oz link (16/16 oz pkg)	90	8	0.5
Small/Cocktail (50/lb), each	30	3	0.5
Light/Fat Reduced: *Best's Kosher,*	50	1	5
Oscar Mayer, 2 oz link	110	8	2
Hebrew National (97% FF), each	45	1.5	2
Healthy Choice (Jumbo Frank)	70	1.5	4
Fat-Free: *Ball Park* (1),1.76 oz	50	0	6
Pork: *Country Style,* 2 oz panfried	240	22	1
Chorizo, 5 sausages, 2.5 oz	280	26	3
El Popular, 2 oz cooked	210	17	3
Jimmy Dean, cooked, 2 oz	240	21	0
Oscar Mayer (2), 1.7 oz, ckd	170	15	1
Light, 2 oz link	110	8	2
Turkey Franks: *Ball Park,* 1.75 oz	40	0	6
Empire Kosher, 2 oz	90	6	1
Foster Farms, 2 oz	130	11	0
Louis Rich: Reg., (10/16 oz pkg), 2 oz	110	8	2
(8/12 oz pkg), 1½ oz	80	6	2
Mr Turkey, smoked, 2 oz	90	5	3
Shelton's: 1 frank, 1.2 oz	80	6	1
Chicken Franks (*Shelton's*), 1.2 oz	95	8	1
Empire Kosher, 2 oz	100	7	1
Foster Farms, 2 oz	140	12	0
Scott Petersen, 1.2 oz	80	6	1
Zacky Farms, 2 oz	150	13	0

Smoked Sausages

	C	F	Cb
Ball Park: Knockwurst(1) 4 oz	360	33	4
Beef Corn Dog(1) 2.6 oz	220	12	21
Butterball (w. Turkey), 2 oz	60	0	6
Eckrich, 2 oz	180	16	4
Healthy Choice, 2 oz	70	1.5	6
Lemington Foods: 2 oz link	180	15	3
Skinless, 3 oz link	250	21	5
Bacon & Cheddar, 3 oz pce	250	20	7
Scott Petersen: Skinless, 3 oz link	280	24	5

Vegetarian Sausages

See Vegetarian Section ~ Pages 70 - 72

Breakfast Sausages/Biscuits

	C	F	Cb
Healthy Choice			
Breakfast Sausage, 2 patties, 1.6 oz	50	1.5	3
Jimmy Dean			
Sausage Biscuit 2	390	25	29
Mini Burgers, 2	270	14	23
Saus. Egg & Cheese, Biscuit, 1	390	27	28
Minyard: Pork Sausage Biscuit, 1	200	12	16
Owens Border Breakfast			
2 Sausages, Egg, Cheese, Tacos	330	11	42
2 Hot Sausages, Biscuits	370	23	26
Knob Sausages, 2 oz, ckd	210	18	0
Swift Premium			
Morning Makers: *Per 3.5 oz*			
Egg & Cheese, 1 pce	240	8	30
Ham, Egg & Cheese	250	10	31
Sausage, Egg & Cheese	250	8	32

WILL-POWER TONIC ~ RECIPE ~

- 1 Cup of Desire
- 1 Quart of Determination
- 1 Tbsp of Common Sense
- 1 Tbsp of Stick-to-itiveness
- 1 Tbsp of Foresight
- 1 Cup of Energy

Bagel, Corn & Hot Dogs

	C	F	Cb
Hot Dogs, Ready-To-Go			
Includes Ketchup/Relish; No Mayo			
Small (1 oz frank/ 1 oz roll)	200	8	24
Regular (1½ oz frank/ 2 oz roll)	310	13	39
Large (2 oz frank/ 2 oz roll)	360	18	40
Super/Giant (3 oz frank/3 oz roll)	540	26	59
Corn Dogs			
Beef/Pork Frank: Average, 2.6 oz	250	17	21
Mini, each	65	4.5	5
Turkey: *Gobblers! (Shelton's)*	220	11	27
Bagel Dogs			
Best's Kosher: 1 dog, 1 oz	320	11	43
Mini, 1 piece, 0.8 oz	60	2	8
Vienna Beef: 1 piece, 1 oz	85	3.5	7
Weinerschnitzel (Franchise Outlets)			
Carbohydrate figures ~ author estimates only.			
Chili Dog, 1 serve	295	16	38
w. Lowfat Frank	230	5	38
Chili Cheese Dog	350	21	40
w. Lowfat Frank	280	9	40
Corn Dog	290	23	25
Deluxe Dog	275	14	38
w. Lowfat Frank	220	3.5	38
Kraut Dog	265	14	37
Mustard Dog	260	14	37
Relish Dog	280	14	37
Western Dog	380	23	40

Also See Fast-Foods Section

Toppings/Extras

	C	F	Cb
American Chse, 1 slice, 1 oz	110	9	1
Catsup, 1 Tbsp	16	0	4
Chili (w. Beans), ¼ cup	70	3.5	9
Mustard, 1 Tbsp	20	0	1
Pickle Relish, 1 Tbsp	20	0	5
Sauerkraut, ½ cup	20	0	5

Deli & Luncheon Meats

	C	F	Cb
Beef Jerky:			
Bridgeford Beef Jerky, 1 oz	50	1	3
Beef Stick (5.5 oz stick), 1 oz	140	12	1
Beef Steak, 1 oz	50	1	0
Beef & Cheese (Giant Size), ½ pkg, 1.5 oz	170	14	1
Pepperoni Sticks, 2, 1 oz	140	12	1
Pepperoni (1" diam.), 1 oz	130	12	1
Teriyaki, 1.25 oz pkg	80	1	8
Original; Hot 'n Spicy	70	1	5
Berliner (pork/beef), 1 oz	65	4	0.5
Beerwurst (Beef):			
Small (2.75"diam), ¹⁄₁₆" slice	20	2	0
Large (4"diam), ⅛" slice	75	7	0.5
Beerwurst (Pork):			
Small (2.75"diam), ¹⁄₁₆" slice	15	1	0
Large (4"diam), ⅛" slice	55	4	0.5
Bologna, Beef & Pork:			
Regular: 1 thin slice, 1 oz	90	8	1
1 thick slice, 1.6 oz	145	13	1
Light *(Oscar Mayer),* 1 sl., 1 oz	60	4	2
Red. Fat *(Hebrew Nat.),* 1 oz	65	6	0
Fat Free *(Osc. M.),* 2 sl., 1.6 oz	40	0	1
Healthy Choice, 1 oz	35	1	3
Weight Watchers, 2 sl., ¾ oz	35	2	0
Turkey, average, 1 oz	60	5	0.5
Chicken *(Tyson),* 1 slice	45	4	0.5
Ring *(Boar's Head),* 2 oz	160	13	0.5
Blood Sausage, 1 oz	100	9	0.5
Bratwurst:			
Average, 1 oz	90	8	0.5
Boar's Head, cook., 1 wurst, 4 oz	300	25	0
Bob Evan's, Beer, 2.6 oz link	270	21	1
Braunschweiger (Pork/Liver/Sausage),			
Oscar Mayer, 1 oz slice	100	9	1
Chicken, *Average All Brands*			
1 thick or 2 thin slices, 1 oz	30	1	1
Chicken Roll, 1 slice, 1 oz	90	4	1.5
Corned Beef:			
Average, full fat, 1 oz	70	5	1.5
*Healthy Choice, Hillshire Farm,*1oz	30	1	0.5
Hebrew National, 4 slices, 2 oz	90	4.5	0
Loaf, jellied, 1 oz	45	2	0
Hash, canned, average, 1 oz	50	3	2
Dutch Brand Loaf, average, 1 oz	70	5	1.5

Continued Next Page

	C	F	Cb
Ham, Luncheon:			
Baked/Boiled, sliced, 1 oz	30	1	0.5
Chopped: *Eckrich* (97% FF), 1 oz	25	1	1
Armour, canned, 1 oz	35	1.5	0.5
97% Fat Free, 1 oz	25	1	1.5
Healthy Choice Deli Traditions:			
Baked, 2 sl., 2 oz	60	1.5	1
Larger Slice, 1 slice, 1 oz	30	1	1
Hormel (Black Label), 1 oz	70	6	0
Oscar Mayer, 1 oz slice	60	3	1
Honey/Brown Sugar, aver., 1 oz	30	1	0.5
Healthy Choice Deli Traditions:			
2 slices, 2 oz	60	1.5	2
Prosciutto, average, 1 oz	70	5	1
Ham & Cheese Loaf, aver., 1 oz	70	5	0.5
Head Cheese (Osc. Mayer), 1 oz sl.	50	4	0
Honey Loaf (Osc. Mayer), 1 oz sl.	35	1	2
Italian Sausage, 2.6 oz	270	21	1
Kielbasa (Polish Sausage), 1 oz	85	7	0.5
Scott Petersen, 3.4 oz link	320	27	4
Beef, 2.8 oz link	290	25	4
Boar's Head, 1 oz	60	5	0
Kippered Beefsteak:			
(Hickory Farms), 3 slices, 0.75 oz	50	1	1
Knackwurst, 1 oz	90	8	0.5
Liverwurst, 1 oz	95	8	0.5
Liver Pate, fresh, average, 1 oz	110	10	3.5
Luncheon Loaf (Foods Co), 1 oz	80	7	2
Mortadella, 1 oz	90	7	0.5
Olive Loaf, average, 1 oz	70	5	3
Oscar Mayer, 1 oz slice	70	6	2
Pastrami (Beef), average, 1 oz	40	2	0.5
Healthy Deli, 1 oz	34	1	0.5
Hillshire (DeliSelect), 6 sl., 2 oz	60	1	1
Turkey Pastrami, 1 oz	30	1	1
Peppered Beef, 1 oz slice	40	2	1
Pepperoni: 5 slices, 1 oz	135	12	0
Pickle Loaf, average, 1 oz	80	6	1
Pickle & Pimiento Loaf			
(Oscar Mayer), 1 oz	80	6	3
Polish Sausage: See Kielbasa			
Proscuitti, average, 1 oz	70	5	1
Hormel, 1 oz	90	7	1
Roast Beef, lean, 1 oz	40	1	0.5
Healthy Choice, all types 2oz	60	1	1
Salami: Beef, average, 1 oz	80	7	1
Beer: average, 1 oz	70	6	0.5
Cotto: *Oscar Mayer,* 1 slice, 1 oz	70	5	1

	C	F	Cb
Salami (cont)			
Dry: Hard, aver. 3 slices, 1 oz	110	10	0.5
Oscar Mayer, 2 slices, 1.6 oz	120	10	1
Genoa: average, 1 oz	110	10	1
Stick (Best's Kosher), 2, 1.75 oz	180	15	2
Italian: (Bridgeford), 1 oz	120	11	0
Turkey: average, 1 oz	55	4	1
Spam: Original, 2 Tbsp, 1 oz	70	6	0
Summer Sausage: *Bridgeford,* 1 oz	100	9	0
Oscar Mayer, 1 slice, 0.8 oz	70	7	0
Treet (Armour), canned, 1 oz	100	9	1.5
Turkey: average, 1 oz slice	30	1	0.5
³/₄ oz slice	22	0.5	1
Turkey Breast:			
Butterball Fat Free, 2 sl, 2 oz	50	0	2
Deli Thin Smoked, 1 sl., 1 oz	25	0	2
Hillshire Deli Select, 6 sl., 2 oz	50	0.5	2
Louis Rich Carvery Board,			
3 slices, (52g), 1.8 oz	50	0.5	1
Free, 2 slices, 2 oz	50	0	2
Healthy Choice, 2 sl., 2 oz	60	2	2
Hearty Deli Rst'd, 2 sl., 2 oz	50	0.5	1
Honey Roasted, 2 sl., 2 oz	70	2	2
Oven Roasted, 2sl, 2oz	45	0	1
Honey Rst & Smoked, 2oz	60	0	2
Salsa Turkey Breast, 2oz	60	1	2
Turkey Ham, 1 slice, 1 oz	35	1.5	0.5
Turkey Pastrami, 1 oz	35	1.5	0.5
Turkey Roll, 1 oz	40	2	0.5
Turkey Loaf, 1 oz	30	1	0.5
Vegetarian Deli:			
Worthington, Yves ~ Page 70			

Meat Spreads

Average All Brands Per ¼ cup (2 oz)	C	F	Cb
Chicken	120	8	2
Ham, deviled	160	14	0
Liverwurst	170	14	3
Roast Beef	140	11	0
Sandwich Spread	140	10	8
Turkey	110	7	2

Paté

	C	**F**	**Cb**
Canned: *Average All Brands*			
Chicken Liver, 1 Tbsp, 1/2 oz	30	2	1
2 Tbsp, 1 oz	60	4	2
Foie Gras, goose liver, 1 oz	130	12	2
Wells, liverpate, 2 1/8 oz	190	16	3
Fresh (Refrigerated):			
Average all types, 1 oz	110	10	2
Marcel Henri, 2 oz serving	220	20	2
Pate de Campagne, 1 oz	105	9	1
Chicken Liver w. Port Wine, 1 oz	100	9	1
Duck Truffle w. Port Wine, 1 oz	120	12	1
Coeur de France:			
Smoked Salmon Pate, 1 oz	45	3.5	1
Spinach Pate w. Roquefort, 1 oz	50	4	1
Garden Fresh Vegetable Pate:			
Mushroom, Artichoke & Spinach in Puff Pastry, 2 oz	110	7	8

Lunch Packs

	C	**F**	**Cb**
Lunchables *(Oscar Mayer)* Per Package:			
Beef Tacos/Butterfinger/Drink	490	15	69
Bologna/Chse/Crackers/Cookies	470	31	31
Bologna/Chse/Crack./M&M's/Drink	530	27	60
Chsy Chip Nachos/Choc Fudge/Drink	540	26	70
Cinnamon & Fruit Roll/Drink	510	12	98
Cinnamon Rolls	370	11	65
Deluxe Turkey/Chicken	390	22	26
Grilled Burgers/Choc Balls/Cola	460	14	67
Ham & Swiss/Crackers/Drink	350	9	51
Hot Dogs/Choc Balls/Drink	450	19	64
Lean Ham/Chedd./Crackers/Cookie	420	21	39
Lean Ham/Chse/Crack./Snickers/Drk	440	18	54
Lean Ham/Swiss Chse/Crackers	340	18	21
Lean Turkey/Cheese/Cracker/ Reese's Peanut Butter/Drink	430	18	51
Lean Turkey Brst./Chedd. Crackers	340	19	22
Lean Turkey/Chse/Crack./Skittles/Drink	410	14	61
Waffles & Sausage/ Fruity Pebbles Bar/Drink	510	13	94
Nachos: Cheese & Salsa	380	21	39
Cheesy Crisp	380	23	35
w. Capri Sun/Nestle Crunch	570	29	70
Tacos: Beef Taco & Cheese	310	11	34
w. Capri Sun/Butterfinger	470	13	67
Mega Lunchables: *Per Package*			
2 Pepp. Pizza/Reese's P.B.Cup/Cola	760	28	105
2 Extra Cheesy Pizza/M&Ms/Drink	700	25	104
Soft Pizzastix + Twix	650	16	111
Ultimate + Shock Tarts/Cola	780	32	113
Sandwiches:			
Ham, Turkey, Cheddar	470	22	47
Oven Rst. Turkey & Chse Sub	410	17	45
Smoked Ham & Cheddar Sub	380	14	44
Smoked Turkey & Chedd. Bagel	380	4	63
Pizza:			
Deep Dish w. Reese Cup	760	28	105
Sauce & Mozzarella Cheese	300	13	38
Pepperoni Flavored Sausage, 3	310	14	30
Pizza/Nestlé Crunch/Drink	450	15	62
Munch-A-Bunch *(Jewel)*: Per 4 oz Package			
Bologna/Chse/Crackers/Cookies	430	29	27
Other varieities, average	350	19	29
Smuckers: **Snackers**, 3.96 oz pkg	610	24	88
StarKist: Tuna Salad & Crackers	190	6	25
Chunk White Tuna w.Mayo	230	9	17

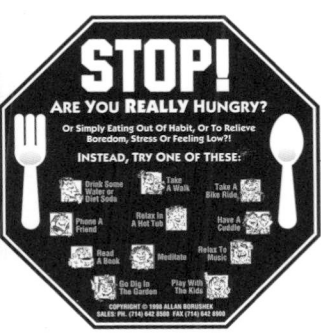

Chicken

Quick Guide

Chicken

From 3lb ready-to-cook chicken

Breast/Wing Quarter

	C	F	Cb
Roasted: With skin	300	15	0
Without skin	190	5	0
Fried, batter dipped	480	26	18

Leg Quarter: Thigh & Drumstick

	C	F	Cb
Roasted: With skin	265	15	0
Without skin	180	8	0
Fried, batter dipped	430	26	16

KFC ~ See Fast-Foods Section.

Average - All Meats

Average of Light & Dark Meats
Per 4 oz Serving (no bone)

	C	F	Cb
Roasted: With skin	270	15	0
Without skin	215	8	0
Stewed: With skin	250	14	0
Without skin	200	8	0
Fried: Batter-dipped	330	20	11
Flour coated	305	17	3.5

Chicken Parts

Broilers or Fryers: Edible Weights (no bone)

Breast: *Per 1/2 Breast*

	C	F	Cb
Raw: With skin, 5 oz	245	13	0
Without skin, 4 1/4 oz	130	2	0
Roasted: With skin, 3 1/2 oz	195	8	0
Without skin, 3 oz	140	3	0
Stewed: With skin, 4 oz	210	8	0
Without skin, 3 1/4 oz	140	3	0
Fried: Batter-dipped, 5 oz	370	19	12
Flour coated, w. skin, 3 1/2 oz	220	9	7

Drumstick: *Per Drumstick*

	C	F	Cb
Roasted: With skin, 2 oz	125	6	0
Without skin, 1 1/2 oz	75	2	0
Fried: Batter-dipped, 2 1/2 oz	195	11	7
Flour coated, 1 3/4 oz	120	7	1
Stewed: With skin, 2 oz	115	6	0
Without skin, 1 1/2 oz	80	3	0

Thigh Portion: Edible Wt. (no bone)

	C	F	Cb
Raw: With skin, 3.3 oz			
(4 1/4 oz with bone)	200	14	0
Without skin, 2.4 oz	80	3	0
Roasted: With skin, 2 1/4 oz	155	10	0
Without skin, 2 oz	110	6	0

Thigh Portion (Cont)

	C	F	Cb
Stewed: With skin, 2 1/2 oz	160	10	0
Without skin, 2 oz	105	5	0
Fried: Batter-dipped, 3 oz	240	14	8
Flour coated, 2 1/4 oz	165	9	2

Wing: *Per Wing*
Raw Weight 3.2 oz (with bone)

	C	F	Cb
Raw: With skin	110	8	0
Without skin	35	1	0
Roasted: With skin	105	7	0
Without skin	45	2	0
Fried: Batter-dipped	160	11	5
Flour coated	105	7	1
Stewed: With skin, 4 oz	100	7	0
Neck: Simmered, with skin	95	7	0
Without skin	30	2	0

Skin Only: *Skin from 1/2 Chicken*

	C	F	Cb
Raw skin, 2 3/4 oz	275	26	0
Roasted skin, 2 oz	255	22	0
Stewed skin, 2 1/2 oz	260	24	0
Fried, Flour coated, 2 oz	280	24	5
Fried, Batter-dipped, 6 3/4 oz	750	55	45

Roasters
Average of Light & Dark Meat:

	C	F	Cb
Roasted: With skin, 4 oz	250	15	0
Without skin, 4 oz	190	8	0
Light Meat: Without skin, rst.	175	5	0
Dark Meat: Without skin, rst.	206	10	0

Stewing Chicken
Stewed: Per 4 oz Serving
Average of Light & Dark Meat:

	C	F	Cb
With skin	325	21	0
Without skin	270	14	0
Light Meat: Without skin	240	9	0
Dark Meat: Without skin	295	17	0

Capon Chicken

	C	F	Cb
Roasted: With skin, 4 oz	260	13	0
1/2 Chicken, with skin	1460	74	0

Chicken Offal & Stuffing

	C	F	Cb
Giblets, simmered, 1 cup	230	7	1.5
Fried, flour-coated, 1 cup	400	20	6
Gizzard, simmered, 1 cup	220	5	1.5
Heart, simmered, 1 cup	270	12	0.5
Liver: Raw, 4 oz	140	5	3.5
Simmered, 1 cup	220	8	1
Liver Pate Fresh, 1 Tbsp, 1/2 oz	60	2	1
Stuffing: Average, 1/2 cup	200	2	22

Chicken Products

Tyson	C	F	Cb
Chicken Chunks: Regular, (6)	280	20	19
Breast, (6)	220	19	11
Southern Fried, (6)	260	19	11
Breast Patties: Regular, each	190	12	11
Chick 'n Quick/Chedd., 74g ea.	220	14	12
Crispy Baked, each	80	0	9
Thick 'n Crispy, each	200	19	10
Southern Fried, each	180	12	8
Nuggets: Breaded White Meat, (6)	250	18	12
Wings: Flavored, average, (3)	170	10	1
BBQ Style, (3)	200	13	2
Stir Fry Kit: Chicken, 2³/4 c. froz.	430	4.5	73
Wraps: Southwest Black. 1¹/2	560	12	82
Mandarin Sesame, 1¹/2 wraps	560	12	82
M/wave S/wiches: Breast, 119g	320	15	33
Stove Top: *Per Serving*			
Chicken Stuffing Mix: 1 oz	110	1	20
¹/2 cup prep.	170	9	20

Duck, Goose, Quail

	C	F	Cb
Duck: roasted, with skin, 3 oz	285	24	0
Without skin, 3 oz	170	10	0
¹/2 whole duck, with skin	1300	108	0
Goose: roast, with skin, 3 oz	260	19	0
Without skin, 3 oz	200	11	0
Pheasant: ¹/2 bird, raw	720	37	0
Quail: 1 whole, raw	210	13	0

Turkey

Fryer-Roasters

Roasted: *Per 3 oz Serving*			
Light Meat: With skin	140	4	0
Without skin	120	1	0
Dark Meat: With skin	155	6	0
Without skin	140	4	0
1/4 of Whole Turkey: (Approx. 3¹/4 lbs raw wt. w/out neck and giblets; 2 lb 6 oz cooked wt.)			
Roasted: With skin	1400	46	0
Without skin	1030	18	0
Ground Turkey, Raw: (4oz raw wt. = 3oz ckd wt.)			
Regular (85% lean), 4 oz	180	10	0
Lean (90% lean), 4 oz	160	8	0
Breast, no skin, 4 oz	115	1	0

Turkey Parts

Roasted, Edible Weights (no bone)	C	F	Cb
Breast (¹/4): (from 17¹/4 oz raw wt. w/bone)			
With skin, 12 oz (no bone)	525	11	0
Without skin, 10³/4 oz	415	2	0
Back (¹/2): With skin, 4¹/2 oz	265	13	0
Without skin, 3¹/2 oz	165	5	0
Leg (Thigh & Drumstick): (from 1 lb raw wt. w/bone)			
With skin, 8¹/2 oz (no bone)	420	13	0
Without skin, 7³/4 oz	355	8	0
Wing: (from 7¹/4 oz raw wt. w/bone)			
With skin, 3 oz (no bone)	185	9	0
Without skin, 2 oz	100	2	0
Neck: Simmered, 1 neck (9 oz w. bone)	275	11	0
Giblets, simm., 1 cup, 5 oz	240	7	3

Young Hens (Roasted)

	C	F	Cb
Light Meat: With skin, 3 oz	175	8	0
Without skin, 3 oz	135	3	0
Dark Meat: With skin, 3 oz	200	11	0
Without skin, 3 oz	165	7	0
Young Toms — Similar to Young Hens			

Turkey Products

	C	F	Cb
Banquet ~ Frozen Meals, Page 57			
Circle L: Boneless Turk Bacon,3 oz	120	9	1
Louis Rich			
Fat Free Breast of Turkey			
Rotiss'd/Smoked/Rstd, 2 oz	60	0	1
Turkey Ham & Chunks, cooked:			
Breast & White Turkey, 2 oz	60	1	2
Turkey Ham/Pastrami, 2 oz	70	3	1
Turkey Salami, 2 oz	100	8	0
Luncheon Slices ~ See Cold Meats, Page 50			
Franks: Medium, 1¹/2 oz	80	6	2
Large, 2 oz	110	8	3
Smoked Sausage/Kielbasa, 1 oz	45	2	2
Turkey Nuggets, cooked, each	65	4	4
Turkey Patties, cooked, each	220	13	13
Turkey Sticks, cooked, each	75	5	4
Swanson ~ Frozen Meals, Page 61			
Turkey Store			
Gobble Stix: Honey, each	25	0	1
Lean Burger Patties, 1 patty	180	8	5
Lean Italian Sausage, 1 link	190	8	2

Quick Guide

Fresh Fish   Ⓒ Ⓕ Ⓒⓑ

Low Oil (Less than 2.5% fat)
White/pale colored flesh. Examples:
Cod, Flounder, Haddock, Halibut, Monkfish
Perch, Pike, Pollock, Snapper, Sole, Whiting.

Per 4 oz Edible Portion

	C	F	Cb
Raw, 4 oz (no bones)	90	1	0
Steamed, Broiled, Baked	130	1	0
Fried: Lightly Floured	210	8	3.5
Breaded	260	12	8
In Batter	320	16	27

Medium Oil (2.5-5% fat)
Pale colored flesh. Examples:
Bluefin Tuna, Catfish, Kingfish, Salmon (Pink),
Swordfish, Rainbow Trout, Yellowtail.

	C	F	Cb
Raw, 4 oz (no bones)	140	5	0
Baked, Broiled, 4 oz	175	6	0
Fried, 4 oz	230	11	8

High Oil (Over 5% fat)
Darker colored flesh. Examples:
Albacore Tuna, Bluefish, Herring, Mackerel,
Orange Roughy, Salmon (Atl./Chinook/Sockeye),
Sardines, Trout, Whitefish.

	C	F	Cb
Raw, 4 oz (no bones)	230	16	0

Cooking Yields (Fin Fish):
4 oz Raw wt. = 3 1/2 oz Cooked wt.
4 oz Cooked wt. = 5 oz Raw wt.

Calorie & Fat Variations
The amount of fat/oil in fish varies with the
species, season and locality. Within the same fish,
fat/oil content is generally higher towards the
head.

Fish & Shellfish   Ⓒ Ⓕ Ⓒ

Edible Weights: (no bones/shell)

	C	F	C
Abalone: Raw, 4 oz	120	1	7
Anchovy: Paste, 1 Tbsp, 1/4 oz	15	1	0.5
Cnd. in oil, drnd., 5 only, 3/4 oz	40	2	0
Pickled, 1 oz	50	3	0
Barracuda (Pacific), raw, 4 oz	130	3	0
Bass: Black, raw, 4 oz	105	1	0
Striped, raw, 1 fillet, 5 1/2 oz	150	4	0
Blue Fish, raw, 1 fillet, 5 1/4 oz	185	6	0
Butterfish, raw, 4 oz	165	9	0
Calamari, breaded/fried, 1 serve	360	21	10
Carp, raw, 4 oz	145	6	0
Catfish: Raw, 4 oz	130	5	0
Fried, bread., 1 fillet, 3 oz	200	12	7
Caviar: black/red, 1 Tbsp, 16g	40	3	0.5
Clams: Raw, 3 oz (4 lge/9 sm)	65	1	2
Fried, breaded, 3 oz	170	10	9
Canned, 3 oz	125	2	4
Minced, 1/4 cup, 2 oz	25	0	0.5
Cod, Atl./Pacific: Raw, 4 oz	95	1	0
Baked/Broil., 1 fill., 6 1/4 oz	135	2	0
Canned, 3 oz	90	1	0
Minced, 1/4 cup, 2 oz	25	0	0
Crab: Alaska King, raw, 4 oz	95	1	0
1 leg, cooked, 4 3/4 oz	130	2	0
Blue, raw, 1 crab (1/3 lb whole crab, 3/4 oz flesh)	18	<1	0
Canned, 1/2 cup, 2 1/2 oz	65	<1	0
Dungeness, 1 crab, 5 3/4 oz edible (from 1 1/2 lb whole crab)	140	2	2
Imitation Crab Legs/Stix, 3oz	80	1	8.5
Crayfish, raw, 4 oz (edible)	100	1	0
Croaker, raw, 4 oz	120	3	0
Cuttlefish, raw, 4 oz	90	1	1
Dolphinfish, raw, 4 oz	95	1	0
Eel: Raw, 4 oz	210	13	0
Smoked, 2 oz	190	16	0
Flounder/Sole, raw, 4 oz	120	<1	0
Gefilte Fish: See Kosher Foods ~ Page 163			
Grouper, raw, 4 oz	105	1	0
Haddock: Raw, 4 oz	100	<1	0
Broiled, 1 fillet, 5 1/4 oz	170	1	0
Smoked, 2 oz	22	<1	0
Halibut, raw, 4 oz	125	3	0
Herring: Atlantic, raw, 4 oz	180	10	0
Pickled, 2 pieces, 1 oz	60	4	2

Herring (Cont): Pickled	C	F	Cb
In Sour Cream, 1 oz	50	5	1
Party Snacks, 1/4 cup, dr., 2 oz	120	5	0
Rollmops, 11/2 oz	110	8	6
Canned: Plain w. liq., 4 oz	235	15	0
in Tomato Sauce, 4 oz	200	12	1
Smoked, kippered, 4 oz	245	14	0
Jellyfish: Raw, 4 oz	30	<1	0
Salted, 4 oz	40	<1	0
Kingfish, raw, 4 oz	120	3.5	0
Ling, raw, 4 oz	100	<1	0
Lobster, Northern: Raw, 4 oz	105	1	0.5
1 Lobster, 61/4 oz			
(from 11/2 lb whole lobster)	135	1.5	0.5
Cooked, plain, 5 oz	140	1	2
Lobster Newberg, 3/4 cup	360	20	9
Lobster Thermidor, 1 serv.	370	22	15
Lobster Salads, 1/2 cup	220	13	5
Lox, Regular/Nova, 4 oz	65	2	0
Mackerel: Atlantic, raw, 4 oz	235	16	0
Jack, can., 1/2 cup, 31/3 oz	150	6	0
King, raw, 4 oz	120	2	0
Pacific/Jack, raw, 4 oz	180	9	0
Spanish, raw, 4 oz	160	7	0
Mahi-Mahi, raw, 4 oz	140	5	0
Monkfish, raw, 4 oz	75	1	0
Mullet, striped, raw	135	4	0
Mussels: Raw, 4 oz (edible)	100	2	4
1 cup, 51/4 oz (edible)	130	3	5
Cooked, moist heat, 3 oz	150	4	6
Ocean Perch, raw, 4 oz	90	1.5	0
Octopus, common, raw, 4 oz	95	1	2
Orange Roughy, raw, 4 oz	145	9	0
Cals may be much lower. Over 90% of total fat is waxester which may not be metabolized)			
Oysters: Common, raw, 3 oz	70	1	3.5
Eastern raw:			
6 medium, 3 oz	60	2	3
1 cup, 83/4 oz	170	6	8.5
Fried/bread., 6 medium, 3 oz	170	11	10
Pacific, raw, 1 med., 13/4 oz	40	1	2
Oysters Rockfeller, 3 oysters	220	13	12
Perch, average, raw, 4 oz	105	2	0
Pollock, raw, 4 oz	100	1	0
Pompano, Florida, raw, 4 oz	190	10	0
Porgy/Scup, raw, 4 oz	130	4	0
Rockfish, Pacific, raw, 4 oz	110	2	0
Roe, raw, 1 oz	40	2	0.5

Salmon:	C	F	Cb
Raw: Chinook, 4 oz	205	7	0
Atlantic; Coho/Silver, 4 oz	160	7	0
Chum; Pink, 4 oz	135	4	0
Red/Sockeye, 4 oz	190	10	0
Smoked Salmon: Average, 2 oz	65	1	0
Pacific Supreme, 2 oz	100	4	0
Canned Salmon: *Average All Brands*			
Pink: 1 oz	40	2	0
1/4 cup, 63g (2.2 oz)	90	5	0
33/4 oz can, whole	155	8.5	0
71/2 oz can, whole	300	17	0
Skinless/boneless, 1/4 c., 2 oz	70	2	0
Red Sockeye: 1 oz	50	3	0
1/4 cup, 63g (2.2 oz)	110	7	0
33/4 oz can, whole	190	12	0
Atlantic, 1/2 cup, 31/2 oz	230	14	0
Chinook/King, 1/2 cup	210	14	0
Chum, 1/2 cup, 31/2 oz	140	5	0
Coho/Silver, 1/2 cup	155	5	0
Atlantic Steaks: Small, 8 oz	320	14	0
Medium, 12 oz	480	21	0
Large, 16 oz	640	28	0
Salmon Cake, take-out, 3 oz	240	15	6
Sardines: Canned: *Average All Brands*			
In Oil, undrained, 1 oz	85	7	0
Drained of oil, 1 oz	60	3	0
33/4 oz can, drained, (31/4 oz)	190	11	0
1 lrg/2 med. 3"/5 small, 0.8 oz	50	3	0
In Tom./ Mustard Sce, 1 oz	45	3	0
33/4 oz can (8 sardines)	170	11	0
Scallop: Raw, 6 lg./14 sm., 3 oz	75	<1	2.5
Breaded/fried, 6 lge, 3 oz	200	10	9
Shark: Raw, 4 oz	150	6	0
Batter-dipped, fried, 4 oz	260	16	7
Shrimps: Raw, in shell, 1/2 lb	140	2	1.5
Raw, shelled, 3 oz (12 lge)	90	1.5	0.5
Bread./fried, 3 oz (11 lge)	210	11	10
Canned, 2 oz	60	1	0.5
Smelt, Rainbow, raw, 4 oz	115	3	0
Snapper, raw, 4 oz	115	1	0
Sole, Lemon, raw, 4 oz	90	1	0
Squid, raw, 4 oz	105	1	3.5
Surimi, Imt. Crablegs/Shrimp, 4 oz	110	1	7.5
Swordfish, raw, 4 oz	140	5	0
Trout, Rainbow, raw, 4 oz	135	4	0
Smoked, 2 oz	110	6	0

Fish - Fresh/Canned/Frozen

Fish (Cont)

	C	F	Cb
Tuna:			
Raw, Bluefin, 4 oz	165	6	0
Skipjack, Yellowfin	120	1	0
Canned: *Average All Brands*			
In Water, drained:			
Chunk/Solid, 2 oz can	60	0.5	0
3 oz can	90	1	0
6 oz can	150	1.5	0
In Oil, drained:			
Chunk Light, 2 oz	110	5.5	0
6 oz can, drained	275	14	0
Solid White, 2 oz	90	2.5	0
6 oz can, drained	225	6.5	0
Tuna Salad: Deli Style, 1/2 c., 4oz	300	24	15
Whitefish, raw, 4 oz	155	7	0
Whiting, raw, 4 oz	100	1.5	0

Frozen Fish Products

	C	F	Cb
Fisher Boy			
Quik Stix: 6 sticks, 3 oz	200	11	16
Quik Bake Crunchy Fish Portions:			
2 portions, 3.2 oz	200	10	19
Fish Rings, 7 rings, 3.2 oz	230	12	20
Salmon Fillet, 1 pce, 3.8 oz	100	2.5	1
Gorton's			
Fish Sticks: Breaded, 6, 3 oz	210	12	17
Crunchy Fish Fillets: Breaded *(Per Fillet)*			
Lemon Pepper	135	9	9
Garlic & Herb; Hot & Spicy	125	7	10
Grilled: It. Herb; Lemon Butter	130	6	2
Cajun Blackened; Lemon Butter	120	6	1
Battered: Parmesan	130	7.5	10
Plain, 1 fillet	120	6.5	10
Garlic & Herb, 1 fillet	125	6.5	11
Lemon Pepper, 1 fillet	135	9	9
Homestyle Baked:			
Au Gratin, 1 fillet, 4.6 oz	230	12	14
Primavera, 1 fillet, 4.6 oz	120	5	4
Fish Portions: 1 portion, 2 1/2 oz	170	11	12
Popcorn Shrimp, 20 shrimp, 2 oz	240	13	22
Tenders: 3 1/2 piece, 4 oz	250	14	20
Kroger Fish Portions: *Per 2 Pieces, 4 oz*			
Batter Dipt, 2 pces, 4 oz	260	14	22
Crispy Breaded, 2 pces, 4 oz	270	18	18
Louis Kemp: Crab Delights,			
Surimi, 1/2 cup, 2.5 oz	80	0	10

Frozen Fish Products (Cont)

	C	F	Cb
Mrs Paul's			
Battered: Fish Sticks, 6	240	11	13
Fish Portions, 2	280	17	22
Batter Dipped: Fish Sticks, 2	330	17	28
Crispy Crunchy: Fish Sticks, 5	200	14	20
Fish Fillets, 2	250	13	11
Breaded Fish Portions, 2	240	12	20
Crunchy Batter: Fish Fillets, 2	280	13	23
Flounder Fillets, 2	260	14	24
Haddock Fillets, 2	250	12	25
Healthy Treasures:			
Fish Sticks, breaded, 4 sticks	140	6	14
Fish Cakes, 2 cakes, 4 oz	190	7	24
Light Seafood Entrees: Fish Dijon	200	5	17
Fish Florentine	220	8	10
Fish Mornay	230	10	12
Sea-Pak			
Crunchy Clam Strips, 1 pkt, 5 oz	410	2.5	41
Oven Crunchy Butterfly Shrimp,			
4 shrimp, 3 oz	200	9	20
Popcorn Fish, 7 pces, 3 oz	240	11	23
Popcorn Shrimp, 15 pces, 3 oz	210	12	18
Van De Kamp's			
Fish Sticks: Breaded, 6 stix, 4 oz	290	17	23
Battered Fillets: 2.6 oz Fillet	180	11	12
Crisp & Healthy: Breaded,			
1 fillet, 1.8 oz	85	1.5	12
Grilled: Italian Herb, 1, 4 oz	130	6	2
Breaded Butterfly Shrimp, 7, 4 oz	300	14	32
Lemon Pepper, 1, 3.6 oz	130	6	0
Salmon, Creamy Dill, 1	90	2.5	1
Tuna, Barbecue, 1, 1.8 oz	100	0.5	5
Tuna, Sesame Teriyaki, 1	110	1.5	4

"You're eating too much fish!"

Frozen Entrees & Meals

Advantage\10 ~ See Page 70

Amy's • Boca Burger

See Page 70

Banquet

Meals: Per Meal

	C	F	Cb
Beef Enchilada	380	12	54
Boneless Pork Rib	400	19	39
Chicken Fingers & BBQ Sce, 9 oz	340	16	36
Chicken Fried Beef Steak	400	20	39
Chicken Nugget	410	21	42
Chicken Parmigiana	290	15	27
Fettuccine & Meatballs, Wine Sce	280	7	42
Fish Stick Meal, 6.6 oz	300	13	33
Fried Rice w. Chicken & Egg Rolls	330	9	51
Meat Loaf	280	16	23
Mexican Style Enchilada Combo	360	11	55
Our Original Fried Chicken	470	27	35
Pepperoni Pizza Meal	480	23	56
Pork Cutlet	410	24	39
Roasted Honey Turkey	270	12	29
Salisbury Steak Meal, 9.5 oz	340	19	28
Turkey Mostly White Meat	290	10	34
White Meat Fried Chicken	470	28	40
Yankee Pot Roast, 9.4 oz	230	10	20

The Hearty One: Per Meal

	C	F	Cb
Beef Enchilada, 15.65 oz	520	16	73
Boneless Pork Rib Dinner, 15.25 oz	720	38	62
Chicken Fried Beef Steak, 16 oz	820	50	63
Fried Chicken Dinner, 14.7 oz	910	55	70
Salisbury Steak Dinner, 16.5 oz	780	54	47
Turkey Dinner, 17 oz	630	10	57

Family Pack: Per Serving

	C	F	Cb
Big Wings: Firehouse, (2) 3 oz	200	14	1
Smokehse BBQ, 2 pces, 2.75 oz	200	14	4
Hot 'n' Spicy Wings (4) 2.75 oz	220	15	6

Pot Pies, each: Beef

	C	F	Cb
Beef	330	15	38
Chicken	350	18	36
Turkey	370	20	38

Budget Gourmet

Dinner: Per Meal

	C	F	Cb
Angel Hair Pasta w. Tom. Meat Sce, 8 oz	230	5	38
Beef Cheddar Melt w. Pot. Wedges, 9 oz	350	21	24

Budget Gourmet (Cont)

Dinner (Cont):

	C	F	Cb
Italian Style Meatballs & Vege.	280	12	28
Low Fat Pasta in Wine & Mushr.	270	7	39
Mandarin Chicken	240	6	38
Potatoes Mozzarella in Sce	300	16	33

Light Entrees: Beef Stroganoff

	C	F	Cb
Beef Stroganoff	290	7	30
Orange Glazed Chicken	300	2	51

Regular Entrees

	C	F	Cb
Chicken & Egg Noodles	370	21	31
Chicken w. Fettuccine	340	14	40
Pepper Steak w. Rice	290	8	37
Roast Beef Supreme	300	13	35
Swedish Meatballs	550	34	42
Three Cheese Lasagna	390	16	36

Value Classics

	C	F	Cb
Chinese Style Veg. & White Chick.	250	6	40
Fettucini Alfredo w. Four Cheeses	480	22	40
Fettucini Primavera w. Chicken	260	7	36
Homestyle Macaroni & Cheese	280	9	38
Lasagna Mozzarella	360	11	40
Lasagne w. Meat Sauce	300	9	40
Macaroni & Chse w. Cheddar	310	7	45
Rigatoni in Cream Sce & Chicken	230	5	37
Spaghetti Marinara	290	6	43
Spicy Szechuan Vege & Chicken	290	9	41
Stir Fry Rice & Vegetables	410	18	44

Hearty (14 oz):

	C	F	Cb
Chicken a la King	520	21	56
Fettucini Alfredo w. 4 Chs/Chick.	520	25	50
Golden Fried Chicken Supreme	390	19	42
Oriental Rice w. Veg. & Chicken	645	33	67
Penne Pasta w. Chicken	450	11	63
Tex-Mex Rice & Beans	470	14	69

Celentano

	C	F	Cb
Ravioli: Cheese	260	6	40
Low Fat Cheese, 4.2 oz	280	3.5	46
Mini Round Cheese, 12	260	5	41
Meat Ravioli	270	5	44
Eggplant: Parmigiana, 10 oz pkg	350	28	17
Rollettes, 1, 7.2 oz	230	18	11
Great Choice Rollettes, 10 oz pkg	290	20	17
Lasagne: Lasagne 1/2 tray, 7 oz	270	12	29
Great Choice: Low Fat, 10 oz tray	290	6	40
Lasagne Primavera, 10 oz tray	260	4.5	39
Manicotti, 2 pcs, 10 oz pkg	340	16	34

Frozen Entrees & Meals (Cont)

See Page 56

Celentano (Cont) C F Cb

	C	F	Cb
Stuffed Shells: w. sauce, 3 shells, 10 oz pkg	320	15	31
w/out sauce, 4 shells, 6.25 oz, 1/2 pkg	320	12	36
Great Choice:			
Low Fat, 3 shells, 10 oz pkg	250	6	32
Broc. Stuffed Shells, 10 oz pkg	230	4.5	32
Tortellini:			
Cheese, 1 cup, 5 oz	420	8	68
Meat, 1 cup, 5 oz	340	4	55
Specialty Pastas:			
Baked Ziti, 9 oz pkg	250	13	24
Cavatelli, 1 cup, 5 oz	400	1.5	77
Gnocchi, 1 cup, 5 oz	210	0.5	38

Croissant Pockets

	C	F	Cb
Chicken Broccoli & Cheese	320	13	41
Egg, Sausage & Cheese	340	16	38
Ham & Cheddar	330	14	40
Pepperoni Pizza	360	17	40
Philly Steak & Cheese	350	16	40
Supreme Pizza	350	17	41
Turkey & Ham w. Swiss	320	13	39

Empire Kosher

Express Meal

	C	F	Cb
Chicken Fajita, 1	130	2.5	15
Chicken w. Pasta, 1 cup	140	2	17
Chicken Stir-Fry, 1 cup	160	2.5	20
Pierogies:			
Potato Cheese, 5.3 oz	250	4	44
Potato Onion, 5.3 oz	245	4	47
Pies: Chicken Pie, 8 oz	440	21	41
Turkey Pie, 8 oz	470	23	45
Blintzes: Cheese, 2	200	6	29
Blueberry, 2	190	4	36
Potato Pancakes: mini, 12, 3 oz	150	7	19

Fisher Boy • Gorton's

See Page 56

GardenBurger

See Page 70

Green Giant C F Cb

Create A Meal: Prepared

	C	F	Cb
Beef & Broccoli Stir Fry, 1 1/3 cup	290	13	15
Beefy Noodle, 1 1/4 cup	350	14	31
Cheesy Pasta & Veg, 1 1/4 cup	420	21	29
Chicken Alfredo, 1 1/4 cup	400	13	36
Garlic & Ginger Stir Fry, 1 1/2 cup	270	7	25
Garlic Herb Chicken, 1 1/4 cup	380	15	30
Homestyle Stew, 1 cup	340	16	24
Lo Mein Stir Fry, 1 1/4 cup	320	7	33
Mushroom Wine Chicken, 1 1/4 c.	390	13	31
Oven Roasted: Garlic Herb, 1 3/4 c.	350	9	35
BBQ Chicken, 1 1/3 cup	350	9	37
Chicken & Stuffing, 1 1/3 cup	370	11	36
Lemon Pepper Chick., 2 2/3 cup	310	8	30
Parmesan Herb Chicken, 1 3/4 cup	340	11	29
Skillet Lasagna, 1 1/4 cup	340	13	31
Sweet & Sour Stir Fry, 1 1/4 cup	340	7	43
Szechuan Stir Fry, 1 1/4 cup	310	14	20
Teriyaki Stir Fry, 1 1/4 cup	230	6	18

Healthy Choice

Entrees: Beef Macaroni	C	F	Cb
Beef Macaroni	220	4	34
Cheddar Broccoli Potatoes	280	7	41
Cheese Ravioli	260	5	44
Cheesy Rice & Chicken	230	4	34
Chicken & Broccoli Bread Stuff	310	7	50
Chicken Enchiladas	310	7	46
Chicken Olé	270	4	42
Fettuccini Alfredo	240	5	37
Ham & Cheese Bread Stuff	320	5	48
Homestyle Chicken & Pasta, 9 oz	270	6	32
Italian Style Meatball	330	5	52
Lasagna Bake	280	6	43
Macaroni & Cheese	250	6	36
Manicotti w. 3 Cheeses	300	9	40
Philly Beef Steak	310	5	50
Tuna Casserole, 9 oz	240	7	30
Duos: Grilled Chick. Brst & Pasta	240	6	26
Breaded Chicken & Macaroni Chse	270	6	34
Salisbury Steak & Mashed Pot.	210	6	23
Turkey Breast w. Mash. Potatoes	200	5	19
Bowl Creations: *Per Bowl*			
Beef & Broccoli	300	8	41
Cheese Tortellini	320	7	50
Chicken Broccoli Alfredo	280	6	34
Chicken Teriyaki w. Rice	300	5	45

Healthy Choice (Cont)

Bowl Creations (Cont):

	C	F	Cb
Country Chkn Bake w. Hash Brown	260	7	28
Homestyle Chili w. Beans, Rice	380	6	59
Orange Beef	340	9	46
Roasted Red Pepper Chicken	340	7	50
Shrimp & Vegetables	290	5	44
Turkey Divan	270	7	30

Dinners:

	C	F	Cb
Beef Pot Roast	330	9	41
Beef Stroganoff	330	9	40
Chicken Enchilada	270	6	42
Chicken Teriyaki w. Rice	270	6	37
Country Breaded Chicken	350	9	51
Country Herb Chicken	280	6	40
Herb Baked/Lemon Pepper Fish	340	7	54
Mesquite Beef w. BBQ Sauce	320	9	38
Mesquite Chicken BBQ	290	5	45
Roasted Chicken Breast	230	6	23
Sesame Chicken Breast	360	7	54
Stuffed Pasta Shells	370	6	60
Traditional Breast of Turkey	320	5	49
Traditional Meatloaf	330	7	52

Medleys:

	C	F	Cb
Beef Teriyaki	330	7	48
Chicken Carbonara	310	5	39
Chicken Piccata	270	5	40
Country Glazed Chicken	250	5	31
Mandarin Chicken	280	3.5	43
Oriental Style Chicken	240	5	28
Rigatoni w. Broccoli & Chicken	280	7	34
Spiral Pasta & Beef Tips	300	7	40

Hot Pockets

Per Pocket

	C	F	Cb
Bacon, Egg & Cheese, 2 pc	340	18	34
Barbecue Sauce w. Beef	340	12	47
Beef & Cheddar	290	14	28
Beef Fajita	330	14	37
Cheeseburger	320	10	46
Chicken & Cheddar w. Broccoli	300	12	38
Chicken Melt	350	16	39
Four Cheese Pizza, 1 pce	360	15	45
Ham & Cheese	310	12	40
Jalapeno Steak & Cheese, 1 pce	330	15	37
Meatballs w. Mozzarella	310	11	39
Pepperoni & Sausage Pizza	340	16	39

Hot Pockets (Cont)

Per Pocket

	C	F	Cb
Pepperoni Pizza	340	14	43
Philly Steak & Cheese, 1 pce	320	13	38
Sausage, Egg & Cheese, 2 pce	360	20	32
Sausage Pizza	370	18	40
Turkey & Ham w. Cheese	310	11	41
Toaster Breaks: *Per Piece, 2.1 oz*			
Pizza: Double Cheese	170	8	21
Pepperoni	180	9	22
Sausage & Pepperoni	170	8	21
Juniors: Average all types, 1 pce	150	6	19

Kid Cuisine

	C	F	Cb
Cheese Pizza	430	11	71
Circus Show Corn Dog, 8.8 oz	490	20	30
Cosmic Chicken Nuggets	440	16	50
Fantastic Fish Sticks, 7 oz	370	14	48
Game Time Taco Roll-Up, 7.35 oz	420	18	55
Hamburger Pizza	390	12	60
High Flying Fried Chicken	440	19	48
Magical Macaroni & Cheese	410	13	63
Parachuting Pork Ribettes, 7.55 oz	380	15	43

La Choy See Egg Rolls ~ Page 43

Lean Cuisine

Everyday Favorites

	C	F	Cb
Angel Hair Pasta	240	4	43
Baked Chicken Florentine	220	4.5	32
Cheese Cannelloni	250	6	30
Cheese Lasagne	240	4.5	37
Cheese Ravioli	260	7	38
Chicken Chow Mein w. Rice	240	3.5	37
Chicken Enchilada Suiza w. Rice	280	5	48
Chicken Fettucini	270	6	33
Chicken Lasagna	280	7	34
Classic Cheese Lasagne	290	7	34
Deluxe Cheddar Potato	260	7	37
Fettucini Alfredo	280	7	40
Grilled Chicken w. Penne Pasta	250	5	29
Hunan Beef & Broccoli	240	3.5	40
Lasagna w. Meat Sauce	300	8	38
Macaroni & Cheese	290	7	42
Macaroni & Beef	260	5	38
Mandarin Chicken	240	4	36

Lean Cuisine (Cont)

Everyday Favorites (Cont)

	C	F	Cb
Oriental Style Dumplings	290	6	49
Penne Pasta w. Tomato	260	3.5	47
Rst Chick. w. Lem. Pepper Fettuccine	250	7	32
Santa Fe Style Rice & Beans	300	5	54
Spaghetti w. Meat Balls	270	6	37
Spaghetti w. Meat Sauce	300	5	51
Stuffed Cabbage w. Whipped Pot.	210	8	25
Swedish Meatballs w. Pasta	290	7	35
Teriyaki Stir-Fry	290	4	45
Three Bean Chili	280	8	43
Vegetable Egg Roll, 9 oz	300	5	57
Vegetable Lasagna	260	7	33

Hearty Portions

	C	F	Cb
Cheese & Spinach Manicotti	350	8	50
Chicken & BBQ Sauce	370	6	60
Chicken Fettuccine w. Broccoli	400	9	49
Jumbo Rigatoni w. Meatballs	440	9	64
Roast Chicken	330	5	43
Roast Turkey Breast Dinner	320	6	43
Salisbury Steak Dinner	300	6	40

Cafe Classics: Baked Chicken

	C	F	Cb
Baked Chicken	240	4.5	33
Baked Fish	290	6	40
Beef Peppercorn, 8.75 oz	260	7	32
Beef Portabello, 9 oz	220	7	24
Beef Pot Roast	190	6	19
Cheese Lasagna w. Chicken	270	8	34
Chicken a l'Orange	230	1.5	33
Chicken Breast in Wine Sauce	220	5	23
Chicken Carbonara	260	8	29
Chicken in Peanut Sce	260	6	32
Chicken Mediterranean	260	4	38
Chicken Parmesan	300	6	41
Chicken Piccata	300	9	41
Chicken w. Basil Cream Sce	290	7	37
Fiesta Grilled Chicken	260	4.5	25
Glazed Chicken w. Veg. Rice	230	5	25
Glazed Turkey Tenderloins	260	4.5	41
Grilled Chick. w. Pasta, 9 3/8 oz	250	5	29
Herb Roasted Chicken	200	3.5	24
Honey Roasted Pork, 9.5 oz	240	5	31
MeatLoaf w. Whipped Potatoes	260	7	28
Oriental Beef, Vege & Rice	210	3.5	30
Salisbury Steak	290	9	26
Shrimp & Angel Hair Pasta, 10 oz	280	5	44

Skillet Sensations: Per 1/2 Pkt

	C	F	Cb
Beef Teriyaki & Rice	290	4	50

Lean Cuisine (Cont)

Skillet Sensations (Cont)

	C	F	C
Chicken Oriental	280	4	43
Chicken Primavera	300	4	51
Garlic Chicken	340	4.5	56
Herb Chicken & Rst. Potatoes	250	4	38
3 Cheese Chicken	350	9	43

Lean Pockets

	C	F	C
Chicken Parm./Broccoli Supreme	300	7	44
Meatballs & Mozzarella	300	7	44
Philly Steak & Cheese	290	7	43
Turkey/Broccoli	230	7	30
Other flavors	290	7	42

Marie Callender's

Meals & Dinners

	C	F	C
Beef Pot Roast & Noodles, 1/2 pkt	290	9	33
Beef Tips & Mush. Sce, 13.6 oz	430	19	39
Cheese Ravioli in Marinara Sauce w. Spirals & Garlic bread, 1 c. + 1 oz brd	370	14	51
Cheesy Rice Chick. Broccoli, 12 oz	390	13	44
Chicken Cordon Bleu, 1 dinner	590	25	58
Chicken Parmigiana, 1 dinner	620	28	63
Chili/Cornbread, 1 c. + 1 1/2 oz br.	350	13	45
Chunky Chicken & Noodle, 1 meal	520	30	42
Country Fried Chick. & Gvy,1 din.	610	27	61
Country Fried Pork Chop, 1 dinner	550	27	50
Escalloped Noodles/Chicken, 1 c.	270	16	38
Fettucine Alfredo & Garlic Brd, 1 cup + 1 oz bread	460	27	71
Fettucine w. Broccoli & Chick., 1 c.	410	24	37
Grilled Chick. Brst w. Mash. Pot.	340	18	20
Ham Steak w. Macar. & Chse, 1 din.	450	9	61
Lasagna w. Meat Sauce, 1 cup	370	18	34
Meatloaf & Gvy w. Mashed Pot.	540	30	42
Roast Chicken & Vegies, 1/2 pkt	260	6	36
Salisbury Steak & Gravy, 1 dinner	550	25	51
Spagh. & Meat Sce,1 c. + 1 oz brd	260	10	37
Sweet & Sour Chicken, 1 dinner	530	9	56
Turkey w. Gravy/dress., 1 dinner	530	17	51

Pot Pies:

	C	F	C
Chicken; Yankee, 10 oz	680	44	51
Turkey, 10 oz	710	46	56
Chicken & Broccoli, 10 oz	780	48	49
Chicken Au Gratin, 10 oz	720	48	53

Michelina's | C | F | Cb

Per Serving

	C	F	Cb
Black Bean Chili w. Rice, 8 oz	300	4	58
Chicken a la King	280	8	39
Chili-Mac, 8 oz	280	9	36
Fettucine & Meatballs in Marsala	250	7	34
Fettucine Alfredo	380	15	45
Four Cheese Lasagna, 8 oz	290	7	42
Gr., Egg Noodles & Swedish M'ball	360	13	45
Lasagna Pollo	280	9	33
Lasagna Primavera	270	10	34
Lasagna w. Meat Sce, 9 oz	290	7	40
Linguini w. Clams & Sauce	310	4.5	55
Macaroni Cheese	360	14	40
Meatloaf, Gravy, Mash. Potato	290	16	22
Noodles Stroganoff w. Beef, 8 oz	350	15	39
Noodles w. Chicken, 8 oz	300	10	40
Penne Pasta w. Mushroom Sce	280	8	41
Penne Pollo	290	8	39
Pepper Steak & Rice	260	4.5	46
Rigatoni Pomodoro	220	2.5	40
Risotto Parmigiana	460	21	50
Salisbury Steak Mashed Potato	300	13	33
Shells & Cheese	360	12	45
Spagh. & Meatballs Pomodoro Sce	300	8	43
Spaghetti Marinara, 8 oz	250	2.5	47
Spaghetti w. Tomato Basil Sce	250	3	46
Stuffed Cheese Rigatoni	260	8	36
Yu Sing: Chicken Fried Rice	360	8	58
Chicken Lo Mein	220	3.5	34
Garlic Chicken	250	2.5	42
Sweet & Sour Chicken	340	4	67
Teriyaki Beef	240	2	51

Natural Touch

See Page 71 ~ Vegetarian

Old El Paso

	C	F	Cb
Burrito: Bean & Cheese	300	9	44
Beef & Bean	320	10	47
Pizza, all types	250	9	30
Chimichanga, all types	350	18	38

Ore-Ida

Lil' Calzones: Per 3 Pieces, 2.8 oz

	C	F	Cb
Saus., Pepperoni & Chse, 2.8 oz	200	6	22

Ore-Ida (Cont) | C | F | Cb

Blasts: Per 6 Pieces, 3 oz

	C	F	Cb
3 Cheese, 6 pce, 3 oz	200	4.5	25
Cheese, Sausage & Pepperoni	200	5	25
Pepperoni & Cheese	220	7	25

Deep Dish Minis: Per 2 Pieces

Pepperoni & Cheese, 3.5 oz	280	12	26
Chse, Saus & Pepperoni, 3.6 oz	240	10	27

Bagel Bites: Per 4 Pieces, 3 oz

Cheese & Pepperoni, 4 pc, 3 oz	210	7	25
Chse, Saus. & Pepperoni, 4 pc, 3 oz	200	6	27

Ortega

	C	F	Cb
Beef Taco Filling, 1/3 cup, 2 oz	100	6	4
Nacho Beef Bake, 1/4 pkt, 9 oz	400	20	36
Spanish Rice & Beans, 10 oz pkt	400	17	44
Beef Enchilada, 9.3 oz pkt	360	13	49
Cheese Enchilada, 9¾ oz pkt	410	15	55
Chicken Enchilada, 9½ oz pkt	400	16	51
Skillet Fajitas: Steak, 1/2 c., 2 oz	35	1	3
Chicken, 3/4 cup, 2½ oz	45	1	4
Nachos Ckn Supreme, 1/2 pkt, 11 oz	380	11	49

Rosina

	C	F	Cb
Meatballs: (1 oz balls) 3 oz	250	19	5
Italian Saus. Bites, 4 bites, 2 oz	180	15	1
Light Meatballs (3/4 oz balls) 4	150	7	5
Swedish Meatballs, 6 balls, 3 oz	260	19	5
Turkey Meatballs, 3 balls, 3 oz	170	9	7

Stouffer's

Entrees:

	C	F	Cb
Beef, Rst Pot. & Peppers	300	6	44
Broccoli & Beef	320	5	51
Cheddar Cheese & Chicken Bake	450	21	41
Cheddar Pasta w. Beef & Tom.	450	19	45
Cheese Ravioli	380	13	51
Cheesy Spaghetti Bake	460	21	47
Chicken & Dumplings	280	8	33
Chicken a la King	350	13	41
Chicken Pie, 10 oz	540	33	38
Chili w. Beans	270	10	30
Classic/Cheese Manicotti	360	16	34
Creamed Chicken	260	19	8
Creamed Chipped Beef	160	11	6
Escalloped Chick. & Noodles, 10 oz	430	27	30

Stouffer's (Cont)

	C	F	Cb
Entrees: Fettucini Alfredo	520	28	50
Fish Fillets w. Mac. Cheese, 9 oz	430	21	37
Five Cheese Lasagna	360	13	40
Grilled Chicken & Vegetables	400	9	54
Lasagna Bake	370	12	47
Lasagna w. Meat Sauce, $10^1/2$ oz	370	14	40
Macaroni & Beef	420	20	40
Macaroni & Chse, w. Broccoli	350	16	36
Macaroni Cheese, 1 cup	380	17	40
Meat Lasagna, 1 cup	270	10	28
Penne Pasta & Chicken Bake	340	14	37
Roasted Garlic Chicken	320	11	39
Salisbury Steak, 16 oz	570	24	47
Salisbury Steak & Macaroni Chse	410	19	34
Spaghetti w. Meat Sauce	350	12	46
Spaghetti w. Meatballs	440	15	56
Stuffed Pepper, 10 oz	200	5	27
Swedish Meatballs	480	24	43
Tuna Noodle Casserole	320	10	37
Turkey Tetrazzini	360	17	33
Veal Parmagiana	630	26	68
Veg. & Chicken Pasta Bake	380	11	46
Vegetarian Lasagne	410	18	42
Yankee Pot Roast	320	9	41
Side Dishes: Corn Souffle	170	7	21
Creamed Spinach	160	12	8
Escalloped Apples	180	3	38
Potatoes au Gratin	130	6	15
Scalloped Potatoes	140	5	18
Spinach Souffle	150	10	10
Welsh Rarebit	120	9	5
Slowfire Classics: Beef Stew, 11 oz	290	12	24
Cheesy Pizzatini, 12 oz	410	18	47
Chicken Minestrone Stew, 12 oz	260	6	30
Chunky Beef & Bean Chili, 11 oz	330	13	28
Homestyle Chicken & Noodles, 12 oz	380	14	39
Hearty Portions:			
Beef Pot Rst, 16 oz	370	11	44
Chicken Fettuccini, $16^3/4$ oz	640	24	67
Country Fried Beef Steak, 16 oz	560	25	61
Fried Chicken Breast, $15^1/8$ oz	520	16	66
Meatloaf w. Potatoes, 17 oz	480	23	46
Pork w. Roast Potatoes, $15^3/8$ oz	570	15	75
Roast Turkey Breast	490	20	52
Family Style Favorites: Per Serving			
Chick. & Broc. Pasta Bake, 1/5 pkt	340	17	28
Grandma's Chick. & Veg. Rice Bake	360	15	36

Stouffer's (Cont)

	C	F	Cb
Skillet Sensations: Per 1/2 Pkg			
Chicken & Dumplings	280	8	33
Chicken Alfredo	490	16	63
Homestyle Beef	360	11	34
Homestyle Chicken	390	13	47
Teriyaki Chicken	340	3	59
Homestyle: Beef Pot Roast	250	8	30
Baked Chicken in Gravy/Potato	260	11	18
Breaded Pork Cutlet	420	23	27
Chick. Breast w. Mushr. Gravy	360	15	32
Fried Chicken & Mashed Potato	400	17	38
Meatloaf & Whipped Potato	360	21	28
Salisbury Steak in Gravy/Onions	350	16	27
Veal Parmigiana	410	16	48

Swanson

	C	F	Cb
4 Compartment Meals			
Boneless Pork Rib, 10.5 oz	470	19	58
Boneless White Meat Fr. Chicken	430	16	49
Chicken Nuggets	590	25	71
Classic Fried Chicken, $11^1/2$ oz	600	31	58
Country Fried Beef Steak w. Gravy	460	22	47
Fish 'N Chips	490	20	59
Herb Roasted Chicken	310	7	44
Mexican Style Comb., 13.25 oz	470	18	59
Salisbury Steak	340	15	35
Stuffed Baked Turkey	450	15	59
Turkey Brst. w. Stuffing & Gravy	330	6	50
Veal Parmigiana, $11^1/4$ oz	390	18	40
Yankee Pot Roast	250	4.5	39
Pot Pies: Pot-Topped Beef, 12 oz	450	22	47
Potato-Topped Chicken, 12 oz	440	21	51
Deep Dish Chicken, 1/2 pkt, 8.5 oz	430	20	48
Hungry Man Dinners: Mexican	690	27	78
Boneless Pork Rib	770	38	78
Boneless Rst. Chick. Herb Gravy	500	12	65
Boneless White Meat Fried Chick.	430	16	49
Classic Fried Chicken, $16^1/2$ oz	790	40	75
Country Fried Beef Steak	660	33	66
Fisherman's Platter, 13 oz	640	25	80
Fried Chicken Dinner, 11 oz	430	16	48
Salisbury Steak	610	33	46
Sirloin Beef Tips	440	15	53
Stuffing Baked Turkey	450	15	59
Traditional Pot Roast	360	6	48
Turkey, mostly white meat	510	15	64

TGI Friday's

	C	F	Cb
uffalo Wings, 3 pc, 3 oz	100	7	1
otato Skins, 3 pc, 2.8 oz	170	9	16

Uncle Ben's

asta Bowl: Per 12 oz

	C	F	Cb
Chicken Fettuccini Alfredo	350	7	47
Parmesan Shrimp Penne	380	7	58
Tomato Sausage Rotini	420	8	67
Bowl, Mini (8 oz): Beef Taco Olé	350	15	42
Cheeseburger! Cheeseburger!	360	17	38
Cheesy Mac & Cheese	390	16	49
Chicken & Veggie	240	3.5	37
Crazy Cartwheels & Meatballs	330	11	47
Pepperoni Pizza	330	15	34
Noodle Bowls: Honey Ging. Chkn	430	5	69
Orange Glazed Beef	440	8	70
Spicy Peanut Chicken	420	8.5	58
Spicy Thai Style Chicken	400	8	60
Rice Bowls: Chicken Fried Rice	410	7	65
Cajun Style Chicken & Sausage	350	7	61
Turkey, Wild Rice & Cranberries	360	4	61
Mexican Bowl: Beef Fajita, 12 oz	300	4.5	45
Fiesta Chicken, 12 oz	350	6	55
Southwest Style Chkn, 12 oz	330	5	54

Weight Watchers

Smart Ones: Per Meal

	C	F	Cb
ngel Hair Pasta	180	2	32
roccoli & Chse Baked Pot., 10 oz	250	6	39
hick. Chow Mein; Fiesta Chicken	205	2	34
hicken Enchiladas Suiza, 9 oz	270	9	33
hicken Oriental	230	4.5	34
r. Rigatoni w. Broccoli & Chicken	240	3.5	39
ettuccini Alfredo w. Broc., 9.25 oz	270	6	39
esta Chicken, 8.5 oz	210	2	35
rilled Salisbury Steak	260	10	24
oney Mustard Chicken, 8.5 oz	210	3.5	38
asagna Bolognese	240	2.5	43
asagna Florentine, 10.5 oz	290	8	36
emon Herb Chicken Piccata	210	2	31
lac. & Chse; Ravioli Florentine	220	2	43
asta & Spinach Romano	260	8	35
enne Pasta w. Sundr. Tom., 10 oz	300	8	43
avioli Florentine, 8.5 oz	220	2	43
oast Turkey Medallions, 9 oz	200	7	33
anta Fe Style Rice & Beans, 10 oz	300	8	49

Weight Watchers (Cont)

Smart Ones (Cont): Per Meal

	C	F	Cb
Spaghetti & Meat Sce/Bolognese	280	5	43
Spaghetti Marinara, 9 oz	280	7	46
Spicy Penne & Ricotta	280	6	45
Spicy Penne Mediterranean	260	6	40
Spicy Szechuan Veg. & Chicken	220	2	39
Swedish Meatballs, 9 oz	290	7	34
Tuna Noodle Gratin	270	6	40
Ziti Mozzarella, 9 oz	290	7	47
Main Street Bistro Selections: Per Meal			
Basil Chicken, 9 oz	280	7	35
Bean & Beef Salsa Verde Bowl	290	8	37
Beef & Vege Rice Bowl	260	5	38
Chicken & Veges Carribean	230	3	37
Chicken Carbonara, 9.5 oz	300	6	36
Chicken Fettuccine	300	8	39
Fajita Chicken Supreme, 9.25 oz	280	7	33
Fire-Grilled Chick. & Vegies, 10 oz	280	5	40
Golden Baked Garlic Chick., 10 oz	280	6	40
Oven Rst Veg. Primavera, 10 oz	300	8	46
Oven Roasted Chicken	300	7	38
Slow Roast Turkey Breast, 10 oz	220	7	20
Southwestern Style Chicken Bowl	230	2.5	35
Yukon Gold Pot. & Corn Chowder	260	8	38
Pizza: 5.5 oz each	390	12	50

Wolfgang Puck's

Per Meal

	C	F	Cb
Breaded Chick. Parmagiana, 12 oz	540	21	58
Chick. & Spinach Pasta Wrap	460	11	68
Chicken Bolognese & Spaghetti	480	22	48
Chicken Pappardelle	460	18	47
Eggplant Parmesan	370	28	14
4 Cheese Lasagna; Meat Lasagna	490	22	51
4 Cheese Macaroni	610	33	51
Italian Sausage Pasta Wrap	700	29	67
Meat Lasagne, 12 oz	490	22	51
Meatloaf in Wine Sauce	560	32	36
Mushroom & Spinach Ravioli	260	18	54
Mushroom Lasagna/Tortellini	440	17	53
Penne Pasta w. Beef & Vege	410	18	38
Radiatore Pasta Primavera	310	10	41
Spicy Chicken Lasagna	470	21	45

Worthington ~ See Page 72

Frozen Pizza

Amy's: Per 1/3 Pizza	C	F	Cb
Cheese; Spinach; Pesto	300	12	38
Roasted Vegetable, 4 oz	270	8	43
Soy Cheese; Veggie Combo, aver.	280	10	37
Mushroom & Olive	250	9	33

Celeste

Large Pizza: Per 1/4 Pizza	C	F	Cb
Cheese	320	16	32
Deluxe; Pepperoni	350	20	34
Suprema, 1/5 pizza	290	16	27
Large Premium Pizza: Per 1/4 Pizza			
Cheese	350	18	33
Deluxe; Pepperoni	390	22	34
Sausage/Pepperoni	380	22	33
Pizza For One: Per Pizza			
Cheese; Vegetable	420	21	45
4-Cheese Orig.; Pepperoni	475	27	41
Deluxe; 4-Cheese Zesty	470	25	45
Sausage	530	27	52
Suprema	500	27	49
Rising Crust: Per 1/6 Pizza			
4-Cheese	320	11	39
Pepperoni	380	16	43
Suprema; Three Meat	385	17	40

Connie's Pizza (Chicago Deep Dish)

	C	F	Cb
Cheese, 1/4 pizza, 4.5 oz	300	12	34
Sausage, 1/4 pizza, 4.6 oz	300	11	39
Spinach Mushroom, 1/4 pizza, 5 oz	310	12	30

Di Giorno

Rising Crust Pizza	C	F	Cb
Large: Per 1/6 Pizza			
Four Cheese	320	11	39
Pepperoni; Three Meat	390	17	41
Supreme	400	17	41
Small (Individual) Size:			
Pepperoni, 12.75 oz	300	13	33
Supreme, 14.3 oz	300	14	34
Vegetable, 13.8 oz	900	39	90

Dominick's

Per 1/6 Pizza	C	F	Cb
Four-Cheese, 5 oz	290	9	38
Italian Sausage/Supreme, 5 oz	320	13	38

Healthy Choice: French Bread Pizza

	C	F	Cb
Cheese; Pepperoni, 6 oz	340	5	50
Supreme, 6.35 oz	330	5	51
Vegetable, 6 oz	280	4	44

Freschetta Per Slice	C	F	C
8" Pizzas: 4 Cheese, 1/4 pizza	390	14	4?
Pepperoni, 1/2 pizza	420	17	48
Garlic Chicken, 1/3 pizza	260	9	3?
Supreme, 1/3 pizza	290	12	33
12" Pizzas: 4 Cheese, 1/5 pizza	380	15	4?
Vegetable Primavera, 1/5 pizza	350	13	45
4 Meat, 1/5 pizza	340	14	3?
Pepperoni; Saus. & Pepperoni, 1/6	350	15	3?
Special Deluxe; Supreme, 1/6	350	15	4?
Sauce Stuffed Crust: 4 Chse, 1/5	310	10	4?
Sausage & Pepperoni, 1/5	340	13	4?
Supreme, 1/5 pizza	350	13	4?

Home Run Inn: Per 1/4 Pizza

	C	F	C
Cheese, 4.5 oz	390	30	3?
Sausage, 5 oz	400	22	3?
Sausage & Mushroom, 5.5 oz	390	23	2?

Jack's Pizza

Original 12": Per 1/4 Pizza	C	F	C
Canadian Style Bacon	280	10	3?
Cheese, 1/3 pizza	360	13	4?
Hamburger; Saus.; Spicy Italian, 1/4	300	14	2?
Pepperoni	330	15	3?
Original 9": Per 1/2 Pizza			
Pepperoni; Sausage, average	380	18	3?
Great Combinations (12"): Per 1/4 Pizza			
Bacon Cheeseburger; Dble Cheese	380	19	3?
Pepperoni; Sausage, average	400	19	4?
Sausage & Mushroom	310	15	2?
Other types, average	350	18	3?
Great Combinations (9"): Per 1/2 Pizza			
Double Cheese	430	21	3?
Pepperoni & Sausage	380	18	3?
Naturally Rising (12"): Per 1/6 Pizza			
Canadian Style Bacon; Cheese	290	10	3?
Other types, average	340	16	3?
Naturally Rising (9")			
Cheese, 1/3 pizza	300	10	3?
Comb. w/Saus. & Pepperoni, 1/4	300	14	2?
Pepperoni; Sausage, 1/3 pizza	360	16	3?
The Works, 1/4 pizza	280	12	2?
Pizza Bursts: All types, 6 pieces	250	13	2?

Jeno's Crisp 'n Tasty: Per Pizza

	C	F	C
Canadian Style Bacon; Cheese	450	19	1?
Combination; Sausage; Supreme	520	28	1?
Hamburger; Three Meat	500	25	1?
Pepperoni	510	27	1?

64

	C	F	Cb
Lean Cuisine			
French Brd Pizza: Deluxe, 6 1/8 oz	330	9	44
Pepperoni, 5 1/2 oz	300	7	44
Cheese, 6 oz	340	8	46
Marie Callender's: *French Bread Pizza*			
Hearty Pepperoni	570	28	50
Smothered 4 Cheese	530	24	50
Super Supreme	510	23	50
Pepperidge Farm			
Croissant & Pastry Pizza:			
Cheese	390	20	39
Deluxe	450	27	40
Pepperoni	420	23	39
Pillsbury			
Microwave: Cheese, 1/2 pizza	240	10	28
Pepperoni, Combination, 1/2 pizza	310	15	29
Sausage, 1/2 pizza	280	13	29
French Bread Pizza: Cheese (1)	370	15	41
Sausage & Pepperoni, 1 pizza	430	19	46
Sausage, 1 pizza	410	16	48
Power Dogz Pizza For Kids			
Gonzo's Cheeseburger Max, each	460	20	48
T's Poppin' Pepperoni, each	500	24	46
Shaggy's Cheezy Cheese, each	420	14	46
Red Baron: 4 Cheese, 1/4 pizza	430	21	45
Pepperoni, 1/4 pizza, 154g	450	23	41
Special Deluxe, 1/5 pizza	340	17	34
Supreme, 1/5 pizza	350	18	38
Deep Dish Singles: Pepperoni	540	31	47
Supreme, 1/5 pizza	490	27	46
Stouffer's: *French Bread Pizzas, 1/2 Pkg*			
Bacon Cheddar/Deluxe Pizza	430	21	45
Cheese; Vegetable Deluxe	370	16	47
Cheeseburger; Pepperoni	430	20	45
Extra Cheese	400	16	50
Pepperoni & Mushr./Sausage	440	21	50
Sausage & Pepperoni/White Pizza	460	23	45
Three Meat	460	21	48
Tombstone: *Original 12" Pizza*			
Canadian; Extra Cheese, 1/4	350	14	36
Pepperoni, 1/4 pizza	400	21	35
Other varieties, average, 1/5	320	15	29
12" Special Order: Per 1/5 Pizza			
Four Cheese	400	19	37
Other varieties, average	360	18	32

	C	F	Cb
Tombstone (Cont)			
Original 9" Pizza (Cont):			
Deluxe; Hamburger; Saus., 1/3	280	13	27
Extra Cheese, 1/2 pizza	380	16	40
Pepperoni varieties, aver., 1/3	310	16	27
Double Top:			
Two Cheese, 1/5 pizza	380	19	29
Other varieties, average, 1/6	330	18	25
Oven Rising: Per 1/6 Pizza			
All types, average	330	15	34
Thin Crust: 3 Cheese; Italian, 1/4	370	22	26
4 Meat Combo, 1/4 pizza	380	23	26
Pepperoni, 1/4	400	25	25
Supreme; Supreme Taco, 1/4	370	23	27
For One: average all types	550	32	42
For One (1/2 Less Fat): Cheese	360	10	43
Vegetable, 1 pizza	360	9	48
Totino's			
Party Pizza: Per 1/2 Pizza			
Cheese; Can Bacon; Vegetable	320	14	34
Combination; Zesty Italiano	390	21	35
Hamburger	380	20	34
Sausage & Mushr.; Three Meat	380	19	34
Sausage; Bacon; Pepperoni	380	21	34
Supreme	380	20	35
Pizza Family Size			
Cheese, 1/3 pizza	360	16	39
Combination, 1/4 pizza	310	17	29
Pepperoni, 1/3 pizza	410	22	38
Sausage, 1/4 pizza	300	16	29
Pizza Rolls: Per 6 Rolls			
Combination	230	12	23
Pepperoni	240	12	24
Sausage	230	11	24
Supreme; Cheese	210	10	25
Three Meat	220	10	24
M'wave Pizza For One: Cheese	240	11	26
Pepperoni; Sausage	290	16	26
Supreme	300	17	26
Wolfgang Puck's			
Per 1/2 Pizza: Mushroom & Spinach	270	8	36
Pepperoni & Mushroom	390	15	43
Spicy Chicken	360	16	36
Supreme	400	17	37
4 Cheese	360	15	40
Per 1/4 Pizza: BBQ Chicken	370	13	41
Pepperoni	360	15	34

Canned & Packaged Meals

Banquet	C	F	Cb
Homestyle Bake: *Prepared, Per Serving*			
Creamy Turkey & Stuffing	260	12	29
Cheesy Ham & Hashbrowns	240	11	31
Country Chkn, Potato, Biscuit	380	13	55
Italian Pasta w. M'balls, Garlic Br.	370	16	46

B & M			
Baked Beans: *Per 1/2 Cup (4 1/2 oz)*			
Bacon & Onion w. Brown Sugar	190	2	36
Baked Beans w. Pork	180	2	33
Barbeque; Vegetarian	170	1	33
w. Natural Honey; Red Kidney	170	2	30
Yellow Eye Baked Beans	180	3	30

Betty Crocker			
Chicken Helper: *Per 1 Cup Prepared*			
Chicken & Herb Rice	260	7	26
Homestyle Chkn & Biscuit	440	11	53
Southwestern Chicken	240	5	29
Average other flavors	300	9	28
Hamburger Helper: *Per Cup, Prepared*			
Bacon Cheeseburger; 3-Cheese	380	17	35
Beef Pasta; Beef Stew, average	260	10	25
Cheddar & Broccoli	350	15	33
Cheddar Cheese Melt	310	12	31
Cheeseburger Macaroni	360	15	31
Cheesy Hashbrowns; Chili; Pizza	290	10	31
Double Cheese Pizza	330	13	35
4-Cheese Lasagna; Stroganoff	330	14	31
Lasagna; Ravioli; Sthwestern Beef	290	10	32
Philly Cheesesteak	330	17	25
Potato Buds: Plain, 1/3 cup mix	80	0	18
As prepared, 1/2 cup	160	8	19
Suddenly Salad: *Per 3/4 Cup, Prepared*			
Classic	250	8	38
Ranch & Bacon	330	20	30
Roasted Garlic & Parmesan	260	11	33
Tuna Helper : *Prepared as Directed, Per Cup*			
Cheesy Pasta	310	14	32
Creamy Pasta	300	13	31
Tuna Melt; Creamy Broccoli	310	12	34

Campbell's: *Per 1/2 Cup, 4 1/2 oz*			
Barbecue; Old Fashioned Beans	170	2.5	29
Brown Sugar & Bacon Beans	170	3	29
Chili Beans	130	3	21
New England Beans	180	3	32
Pork & Beans in Tomato Sauce	130	2	24

Campbell's (Cont)	C	F	Cb
Supper Bakes: *1/6 Box, Prepared*			
Lemon Chick. w. Herb Rice	340	7	43
Herb Chick. w. Rice	330	7	40
Garlic Chicken w. Pasta	370	7	44
Savory Pork Chops	380	18	31

Chef Boyardee			
Microwave Cup Meals: *Per Bowl*			
Beef Ravioli	190	3.5	28
Lasagna; Pasta w. Chick. & Veg.	220	6	34
Pasta w. Meatballs	230	8	30
Rice w. Beef & Veges.	250	7	38
Spaghetti & Meatballs	210	7	28
Pull Ring 7 oz Can: Beef Ravioli	170	4	27
Spaghetti w. Meatballs	210	8	27
Homestyle 15 oz Can: *Per Cup, 9 oz*			
Cannelloni; Rigatoni	250	10	31
Chicken Alfredo w. Pasta	250	12	24
Ravioli Primavera	230	6	40
Pull Ring 16 oz Can: *Per Cup*			
Beef/Cheese Ravioli	220	5	38
99% Fat Free Beef Ravioli	210	1	41
Spaghetti w. Meatballs	270	10	32
Lasagna Dinner Kit: *Per Serving*	290	7	44
Cheese Pizza Kit: *Per Serving*	300	5	51
Chef Jr: Micro Ravioli, 8 3/4 oz	210	5	33
Flying Saucers & Aliens, 9 oz	240	1.5	40
Other varieties, 1 cup, 9 oz	200	0.5	43

Dennison's Chili: *Per 1 Cup Serving (15 oz Can)*			
Chili Con Carne With Beans:			
Original; Hot, 1 cup	350	15	36
Chunky; Hot & Chunky	320	12	32
Beef Chili w. Beans (99% Fat Free)	220	2	27
Mild Green w. Beans	370	17	32
Vegetarian w. Beans (99% FF)	180	1	35
No Bean Chili Con Carne	330	18	21

Dinty Moore (Hormel Foods)			
1 1/2 lb Can: Beef Stew, 1 cup	230	14	16
7 1/2 oz Can: Beef Stew	190	10	15
Noodles & Chicken	200	9	21
American Classics: *Per 10 oz Microwave Bowl*			
Beef Pot Roast	200	3	24
Chicken & Noodles	270	8	28
Chkn Brst/Rst Beef & Gravy w. Pot.	240	5	24
Hearty Lasagna	340	16	24
Salisbury Steak w. Potato	300	13	24
Turkey & Dressing w. Gravy	290	8	32

Dr. McDougall's: Per Cup	C	F	Cb
Pasta w. Beans, Mediterranean	180	1	29
Pinto Beans & Rice, Sthwestern	190	2	38
Ramen Noodles; Chicken; Beef	140	1	39
Rice & Pasta Pilaf	210	1	36
Eden: Per 1/2 Cup, 4 1/2 oz			
Baked Beans w. Sorghum, Mustard	150	0	27
Black Soy Beans	90	1.5	9
Chili Beans w. Jalapeno & Peppers	130	0	21
Ginger Blacks w. Ginger, Lemon	120	0	21
Lentils w. Onion, Bay Leaf	90	0	13
Fantastic			
Cup Meals: Per Packet			
Bombay Curry Rice & Beans	250	1.5	53
Cajun Rice & Beans	230	3	46
Cha-cha Chili	220	1	37
Chili Ole, average	260	2.5	48
Ready, Set, Pasta!, average	230	3.5	41
Spanish Rice & Beans	210	1.5	49
Tex Mex Rice & Pinto Beans	240	2.5	48
Vegetarian Chili	160	1	27
Noodles: Average	140	1	27
Couscous: Black Bean Salsa	240	1.5	46
Creole Vegetable	220	1.5	41
Nacho Cheddar	120	2	21
Sweet Corn	180	1	36
Franco-American: Per Cup			
Life w. Louise Pasta	190	2	36
Spaghetti in. Tom Sce w. Cheese	210	2	41
Spaghettios: in Tomato & Cheese	190	2	36
w. Sliced Franks/Meatballs	260	11	32
Beef Ravioli	230	3.5	42
Green Giant: Per Cup, 4.5 oz			
Pork & Beans w. Tomato Sce	240	2	46
Spicy Chilli Beans	220	2	40
Hungry Jack Potatoes			
Casseroles: 1/2 cup, average	150	5	24
Idaho Mashed: 1/2 cup, aver.	155	5	21
Inst. Potato Flakes: 1/3 cup	80	0	18
Pot. Pancake Mix, 2 T., Made Up	90	1.5	16
Hormel: Per Cup			
Kid's Kitchen: Beans 'N Wieners	310	13	37
Beefy Macaroni	190	6	23
Cheesy Macaroni 'N Beef	260	7	33
Cheezy Mac 'N Cheese	260	11	30
Mini Beef Ravioli	240	7	34

Hormel: Per Cup	C	F	Cb
Kid's Kitchen (Cont):			
Noodle Rings & Chicken	150	5	16
Spaghetti Rings w. Meatballs	230	7	35
Microwave Cup: Beef Stew	190	10	15
Chicken & Noodles	200	9	16
Low Calorie	110	2.5	16
Chili w. Beans	220	6	27
Chili no Beans	190	8	15
Lasagna w. Meat Sauce	210	6	29
Scalloped Potatoes & Ham	240	14	20
Spaghetti w. Meat Sce	220	7	31
Chili, 15 oz Can: Per Cup			
With Beans: Reg./Hot/Chunky	270	7	34
Homestyle Chili	330	19	24
Turkey (99% Fat Free)	200	3	26
Vegetarian (99% Fat Free)	200	1	38
No Beans, 1 cup	210	9	17
Hy Top: Per Serving			
Deluxe Shells & Ched. Chse Dinner	410	16	51
Refried Beans, 1/2 Cup	150	2.5	24
Cans: Per 1 Cup			
Spagh. Rings & Tom. Meatballs	410	16	51
Spagh. Rings in Tomato Sce	190	0.5	40
Spaghetti w. Tom. Sce & Chse	180	0	39
1 1/2lb Can: Beef Stew, 247g	190	7	18
15oz Can: Corned Beef Hash	430	28	28
Chili w. Beans, 270g	510	32	34
Kraft Pasta Dinners: Per Cup, Prepared			
Deluxe: Four Cheese	320	10	44
Sharp Cheddar	270	4	38
Macaroni & Cheese:	320	10	44
Light	290	4.5	48
Light (Only 1 T. fat + skim milk)	290	6	47
Child's/Cartoon Pack	410	19	47
Easy Mac, 1 pouch	250	7	38
Velveeta: All varieties	360	13	46
Oven Classic Chicken Bake: 1/6 Pkt, Prepared			
Au Gratin; Traditional Roast	340	11	33
Herb & Garlic	320	8	34
Homestyle BBQ	360	8	43
Honey Mustard	380	10	43
Lemon	370	7	48
Roasted Garlic	310	10	28
Lipton Packet Meals: Per Cup, Prepared			
Rice & Sauce: Spanish	270	7.5	47
Cheddar Broccoli; Chicken	280	9	46

If no fat used in prep'n, deduct 55 Cals and 6g Fat

Canned & Packaged Meals (Cont)

Lipton Packet Meals (Cont)

	C	F	Cb
Per Cup, Prepared			
Noodles & Sauce: Butter/& Herb	310	14	42
Chicken Flavor; Chick. Broccoli	300	11	42
If no fat used in prep'n, deduct 55 Cals and 6g Fat			
Pasta & Sauce: Creamy Garlic	350	13	47
Crmy Mushr./Tom.; Zesty Ched.	320	11	43
Mild Ched. Chse; Rst Garlic Chick.	290	10	40
Roasted Garlic Olive Oil w. Tom.	270	8.5	42
Other varieties, average	290	9	40
If no fat used in prep'n, deduct 55 Cals and 6g Fat			
Recipe Secrets: Golden Onion	50	1	9
Onion	20	0	4
Onion & Mushroom; Savory Herb	30	0.5	6
Vegetable	30	0	9
Sizzle & Stir: *1/6 Pkt, Prepared*			
3 Cheese Alfredo Chkn & Penne	410	15	29
Savory Herbed Chicken & Pasta	340	9	28
Spanish Garlic; Teriyaki Stir Fry	360	9.5	34

Lunch Basket: *Per Serving*

	C	F	Cb
Microwave: Dumplings 'n Chicken	140	5	21
Hearty Beef Stew	170	9	17
Lasagna w. Meat Sauce	160	3	19
Pasta 'n Chick. w. Veg	150	5	22

Manischewitz: Taco Dinner

	C	F	Cb
Manischewitz: Taco Dinner	290	12	38
Vegetarian Chili, *3/4 cup*	145	1.5	31

Maruchan: *Per Pkt*

	C	F	Cb
Instant Noodles: all flavors, aver.	280	12	37
Instant Wonton, all flavors	200	12	19
Oriental Noodle, all flavors	290	12	38
Ramen flavors, *1/2 pkt*, 1 1/2 oz	180	7	26
Wonton flavors, *1/3 pkt*	90	5	9

Near East: *Prepared as Directed, Per Cup*

	C	F	Cb
Couscous: Original Plain	230	2	46
Chicken & Herbs	270	6	51
Toasted Pine Nut	230	6	40
Creamy Parmesan	280	7	48
Roasted Garlic; Broccoli	220	4	41
Roasted Pecan & Garlic	240	9	37
Rice Pilaf	190	0.5	42

Nile Spice: *Per Cup*

	C	F	Cb
Couscous: Lentil Curry	200	1.5	36
Minestrone	180	1.5	34
Parmesan	200	3	34

Nissan

	C	F	Cb
Cup Noodles, all types, average	300	14	38

Old El Paso: *Per Serving*

	C	F	Cb
One Skillet Mexican (Prepared):			
Rice Burrito, (1)	190	4	35
Salsa; Taco, average, (2)	460	16	56
Refried Beans: Reg., Black, *1/2 c.*	100	0.5	19
w. Green Chilies	100	0.5	19
w. Cheese, *1/2 cup*	130	3.5	18
w. Sausage, *1/2 cup*	200	13	14
Fat Free varieties, *1/2 cup*	100	0	18
Mexe/Pinto Beans, *1/2 cup*	110	0.5	19
Black/Garbanzo Beans, *1/2 cup*	100	1	17
Dinner Sets (Prep'd): Soft Taco	390	19	33
Burrito (1)	270	12	27
Hard & Soft Taco (2)	360	17	32
Shells, Taco Sce, Seasoning (2)	310	18	19
Fajita (2)	330	10	35
Taco Dinner (2)	300	17	19
Side Dishes: *Per Serving*			
Canned: Chili with Beans, 1 cup	240	11	19
Spanish Rice, 1 cup	140	1	30
Tamales in Chili Gravy (1)	320	19	19
Boxed: Chsy Mexican Rice *1/3 pkt*	250	2	55
Spanish Rice, *1/3 pkt*	280	4.5	55

Pasta-Roni: *Per Cup, Prepared*

	C	F	Cb
Angel Hair Pasta Primavera	330	16	39
Broccoli	340	15	41
Broccoli Au Gratin	280	10	41
Butter & Garlic	260	8	40
Chicken; Shells & White Cheddar	310	13	41
Chicken & Broccoli; Parmesano	370	16	49
Chicken & Garlic (Lowfat)	210	3	39
Creamy Garlic	420	25	41
Fettucini Alfredo: Reduced Fat	310	8	50
Garlic & Olive Oil w. Vermicelli	360	16	48
Homestyle Chicken	230	6	39
White Cheddar & Broccoli	400	19	41

	C	F	Cb
Pritikin: Vegetarian Chili, 1 cup	160	1	27
Progresso: Beef Rav., 1 c., 9 oz	260	5	45
Cheese Ravioli, 1 cup, 9 oz	220	2	43
Italian Style Zucchini, *1/2 c.*, 4.2 oz	50	2	

Ramen Noodles: *Per Serving*

	C	F	Cb
Beef/Chicken Flavor, 3 oz	190	8	27
Baked Noodle: *1/2 Block*, 1 1/2 oz	140	1	30
Noodles: Fat Fried Shrimp, 1 1/2 oz	170	6	26
Other Flavors, 1 1/2 oz	160	6	26
Fried Cup: Beef, 1 packet, 2.2 oz	290	11	4
Lowfat: Average, 2 oz	215	1.5	4

Meals (Cont) • Soy & Tofu Products

Rice-A-Roni: *Per Cup, Prepared*	C	F	Cb
Beef; Herb & Butter	310	9	52
Broccoli Au Gratin	370	17	47
1/3 Less Salt	320	11	50
Chicken	310	9	52
1/3 Less Salt	280	5	53
Lowfat	210	3	41
Chicken & Broccoli	230	6	41
Chicken & Garlic; Chkn Teriyaki	260	9	41
Chicken & Mushroom	360	14	52
Fried Rice	320	11	51
Long Grain & Wild Rice	240	6	43
Red Beans & Rice	290	7	51
Rice Pilaf; Risotto	310	9	51
Savory Chicken Vegetable	210	3	41
Spanish Rice	270	8	46
White Cheddar & Herbs	340	13	48
(Reduced Fat Recipe: If only 1 Tbsp fat is used			
instead of 2 Tbsp, deduct 35 calories and 4g fat.)			

Stagg Chili: *15 oz Can: Per 1 Cup*			
Chili w. Beans: Classic/Dynamite	330	17	28
Country Brand/Laredo	320	16	29
Rancho House Chicken	290	9	32
No Beans: Steakhouse/Double	330	21	16
99% Fat Free: 4-Bean Chili	200	1	37
Turkey Ranchers/Silvarado Beef	240	3	31

Sweet Sue: Chkn & Dumpling, 1 c.	240	7	31
Canned Whole Chicken:			
w/out giblets, 2 oz	80	5	0

Taco Bell: *Per 1/2 Cup*			
Home Originals: Refried Beans	140	2.5	22
Fat Free Beans w. Green Chilles	120	0	23

Trader Joe's			
Quiche: Broccoli & Cheddar, 6 oz	490	33	33
Mexicaine, 6 oz	510	36	29
Spinach & Mushroom, 6 oz	470	30	32

Tuna Helper ~ *See Betty Crocker, Page 66*

Wolf			
Chili w. Beans: 227g Can	300	16	27
15 oz Can, 1 cup, 254g	330	18	30
Chili No Beans: 227g Can	390	27	18
15 oz Can, 1 cup, 248g	420	30	20
Chunky Beef w. Beans:			
15 oz Can, 1 cup, 254g	300	15	28
No Beans, 1 cup, 246g	330	22	18

Soybean Products

	C	F	Cb
Cheeses (Soy): See Page 40			
Miso, 1/2 cup, 5 oz	280	8	39
Cold Mountain: Red, 1 T., 0.5 oz	25	1	3
Mellow White, 1 Tbsp, 0.5 oz	35	0.5	6
Natto, 1/2 cup, 3 oz	190	10	13
Tempeh, 1 piece, 3 oz	170	6	14
Fried, 3 oz	250	14	14
SoyBoy, White Wave ~ See Page 70			
Soybean Protein (TVP), 1 oz	90	0	7
Soy Drinks ~ See Page 23			

Tofu

	C	F	Cb
Azumaya Tofu:			
Soft (Silken), 3 oz	45	2	4
Firm, 3 oz	60	2.5	3
Extra Firm, 3 oz	75	3.5	10
Age (Tofu Puff), 1/2 oz	40	1.5	2
Nama-Age (Fried Tofu), 3 oz	130	5	8
Calco: Tasty Tofu, 3 oz	50	3	2
Hinoichu Tofu:			
Soft, 3 oz, 1" slice	45	2.5	5
Reg. (Japanese), 3 oz, 1" slice	60	3	6
Firm (Chinese), 3 oz, 1" slice	60	3	6
Extra Firm, 3 oz	90	5	10
Mori-Nu Tofu (Silken):			
Soft, 4 oz	60	3	3
Firm, 4 oz	70	3	3
Extra Firm, 4 oz	70	3	2
Nasoya Tofu: Soft, 3 oz	60	3	2
Silken, 3 oz	50	2	2
Firm, 3 oz	80	4	2
Extra Firm, 3 oz	90	5	1
Chinese 5 Spice Tofu, 3 oz	80	4	2
Pulmuone Tofu: Soft, 3 oz	45	2	5.5
Silken, 3 oz	45	2	5.5
Firm, 3 oz	55	2.5	6
SoyBoy:			
Firm Organic, 3 oz	100	5	2
X-Firm Organic, 3 oz	120	6	2
X-Firm LowFu, 3 oz	90	2	6
TofuLin, 2 oz	100	5	4
Baked, Seasoned, Smoked, 2 oz	100	5	3
Carribean Tofu, 2 oz	100	5	3
Tree of Life: Firm Raw, 3 oz	100	5	2
Reduced Fat, 3 oz	90	4	4
Tofu Stir Fried, 4 oz	120	8	3

Vegetarian Meals & Products

Advantage\10	C	F	Cb
Vegetable Burgers:			
Southwestern-style, 1 patty, 3 oz	140	1	24
Mushroom, 1 patty, 3 oz	130	1.5	22
Pizzas: Per 5 oz Slice			
Vegetarian Sausage & Mushroom	250	2.5	40
Vegetarian Pepperoni	250	2.5	40
Roasted Vegetable Pizza w/o Chse	210	2.5	39
Entrees: Per 10 oz Container			
Caribbean Sweet 'n Sour	280	3	50
Mediterranean Pasta	230	2	44
Pasta Santa Fe	230	1.5	44
Vegetable Szechwan	250	2.5	39

Amy's Kitchen (Frozen): Per Serving	C	F	Cb
Pot Pies: Broccoli, 7^1/2 oz	430	22	46
Country Vege, 7^1/2 oz	370	16	47
Mexican Tamale, 8oz	220	3	41
Non-Dairy Vegetable, 7^1/2 oz	320	9	50
Shepherd's Pie, 8 oz	160	4	27
Vegetable (Non Dairy), 7^1/2 oz	420	19	54
Entrees: Chse Enchilada, 4.75 oz	210	12	13
Blk Bean Vege. Enchilada, 4.75 oz	130	4	20
Cheese Lasagna, 10.25 oz	310	11	37
Lasagna (Family Pack), 7 oz serving	200	8	27
Macaroni & Cheese, 9 oz	390	16	50
Macaroni & Soy Cheeze, 9 oz	360	14	42
Pasta Primavera, 9^1/2 oz	320	12	39
Ravioli w. Sauce, 8 oz	340	12	44
Vege./Tofu Lasagne w. Chse, 9^1/2 oz	300	10	41
Burgers: Californian, 2^1/2 oz	100	3	17
Chicago Veggie, 2^1/2 oz pattie	100	4	9
Texas Veggie, 2^1/2 oz pattie	130	2.5	15
Burritos: Bean & Rice, 6 oz	270	6	48
Bean & Cheese, 6 oz	280	8	43
Black Bean Vegetable, 6 oz	320	8	54
Breakfast Burrito, 6 oz	230	5	38
Asian Meals: Thai Stir Fry, 9.5 oz	270	11	36
Asian Noodle Stir Fry, 10 oz	240	4.5	41
Skillet Meals: Per 1 Cup			
Country Cheddar	250	11	27
Pasta & Vegetables Alfredo	220	8	27
Teriyaki Stir Fry	320	2.5	64
Whole Meals: Cannelloni, 9 oz	260	11	35
Black Bean Enchilada, 10 oz	250	8	41
Country Dinner, 11 oz	380	12	60
Cheese Enchilada, 9 oz	330	14	38
Chili & Cornbread, 10.5 oz	320	6	59
Veggie Loaf, 10 oz	260	5	47

Amy's Kitchen (Cont)	C	F	Cb
Pocket Sandwich:			
Broccoli & Cheese	270	10	37
Cheese Pizza, 4^1/2 oz	290	9	38
Mediterranean Vegetable, 4^1/2 oz	220	7	33
Roasted Vegetable, 4^1/2 oz	220	8	35
Spinach Feta, 4^1/2 oz	200	7	27
Tamale, 4^1/2 oz	250	7	39
Vegetable Pie, 5 oz	230	6	37
Veggie Pizza, 4^1/2 oz	240	5	35
Pizza: Per ^{1}/3 Pizza			
Cheese; Spinach; Pesto	300	12	38
Roasted Vegetable, 4 oz	270	8	43
Soy Cheese; Veggie Combo, aver.	280	10	38
Mushroom & Olive	250	9	33

Boca Burger	C	F	Cb
Burgers: All American, 2.5 oz	110	3.5	6
Original	90	1	6
Grilled Vegetable	80	1	6
Roasted Onion; Salsa	90	1	8
Roasted Garlic	100	2	7
Sausages: Italian (1), 2.5 oz	120	6	6
Smoked; Bratwurst, average	130	6	7
Breakfast: Patties, (1), 1.4 oz	80	4	5
Bkfst Links, (2), 1.5 oz	100	4	4
Crumbles: Orig. Burger, ^{1}/2 c., 2 oz	80	0.5	7
Chik'n: Patties, (1), 2.5 oz	150	6	12
Chik'n Nuggets: (4), 3 oz	190	7	16

Gardenburger: Per 2^1/2 oz Patty	C	F	Cb
The Original	120	3	18
Flame Grilled: Hamburger Style	120	4	7
Chik'n Grill	100	2.5	5
Gourmet Style: Santa Fe	130	2.5	20
Fire Rsted Vege; Savory Mushr.	120	2.5	18
Veggie Medley	90	0	18
Hamburger Style: Classic	90	1	8
Sautéed Onion	90	0	8

Health Valley: Fat-Free Beans & Chili,	C	F	Cb
Chili Burrito/Enchilada, 1^1/2 cup	80	0	15
Chili in a Cup, all types, ^{3}/4 cup	120	1	21
Chili, Fajito flavored, ^{1}/2 cup	80	0	15
Honey Baked Beans, ^{1}/2 cup	110	0	25
Mild/Spicy Vegetarian Chili:			
all flavors, ^{1}/2 cup	80	0	15
Ken & Robert's: Veggie Burger	130	1	26
Veggie Pockets, average, 4.5 oz	250	8	39

Litelife (Frozen)	C	F	Cb
Smart Deli Slices, 3 slices, 1 1/2 oz	50	0	2
Smart Dogs, 1 link, 1 1/2 oz	45	0	1
Tofu Pups, 1 link, 1 1/2 oz	60	2.5	2
Wonderdogs, 1 1/2 oz	55	1	1

Loma Linda

Canned & Dry Foods:

	C	F	Cb
Big Franks, 1 link, 1.8 oz	110	7	2
Lowfat, 1 link, 1.8 oz	80	3	3
Chicken Supreme Mix, 1/3 cup mix	90	1	6
Chik Nuggets, 5 pieces, 3 oz	240	16	13
Fried Chik'n/Gravy, 2 pcs, 3 oz	160	10	4
Gravy Quik, 1 Tbsp mix (1/4 pkt)	20	0	4
Linketts, (1), 1 1/4 oz	70	4.5	1
Little Links, 2 links, 1.6 oz	90	6	2
Nuteena, 3/8" slice, 2 oz	160	13	6
Ocean Platter, 1/3 c. dry mix, 1 oz	90	1	8
Patty Mix, 1/3 cup dry mix, 1 oz	90	1	6
RediBurger, 5/8" slice, 3 oz	120	2.5	7
Sandwich Spread, 1/4 cup, 2 oz	80	4.5	7
Savory Din. Loaf, 1/3 cup, dry mix	90	1.5	7
Soyagen, 1/4 c. (1 oz) dry (make 1 c.)	130	6	12
Swiss Stake, 1 piece, 3 1/4 oz	120	6	8
Tender Bits, 6 pieces, 3 oz	110	4.5	7
Tender Rounds, 6 pieces, 2 3/4 oz	120	5	5
Vege Burger, 1/4 cup, 2 oz	70	1.5	2
Vita Burger Chunks, 1/4 cup, 3/4 oz	70	1	6
Vita Burger Granules, 3 T., 3/4 oz	70	1	6

Morningstar Farms

	C	F	Cb
Better'n Burger, 1 pattie, 3 oz	80	0	8
Better'n Eggs, 1/4 cup, 2 oz	20	0	0
Breakfast Links, 2 links, 1 1/2 oz	60	2	3
Breakfast Patties, frozen (1), 1 1/4 oz	80	3	3
Refrigerator Pack (1), 1 oz	60	2.5	3
Breakfast Strips, 2 strips	60	4.5	2
Buffalo Wings, 5 nuggets, 3 oz	200	9	16
Burger-Style Recipe Crumbles, 2/3 c.	80	2.5	4
Chik Nuggets, 4 nuggets	160	4	17
Chik Patties, 1 pattie	150	6	15
Corn Dog (Meat Free), 1 link	150	4	22
Mini, 4 pieces, 2.7 oz	170	4.5	21
Garden Vege Patties (1), 2 1/2 oz	100	2.5	9
Restaurant, 1 pattie, 3 1/2 oz	150	3.5	13
Grillers, 1 pattie, 2 1/4 oz	140	6	5
Ground Meatless, 1/2 cup, 2 oz	60	0	4
Hard Rock Café Veggie Burger, 1	170	8	18

Morningstar Farms (Cont)	C	F	Cb
Harvest Burgers (1), 3.2 oz	140	4.5	8
Quarter Prime Patties (1), 2 3/4 oz	140	2	6
Oven Rstd Veggie Burger, froz., (1)	120	3	9
Saus. Recipe Crumbles, 2/3 c., 2 oz	90	3	5
Scramblers, 1/4 cup, 2 oz	35	0	2
Spicy Black Bean Burger, 1 pattie	110	1	16
Veggie Dog, 1 link, 2 oz	80	0.5	6
Breakfast Sandwiches:			
Muffin/Scramblers/Pattie/Cheese	280	3	35
Muffin/Scramblers/Pattie	240	2.5	32
Stuffed S'wich, all types, average	290	8	42
Dry Products			
Garden Veggie Burger Kit, 1/4 pkg	80	0	6
Sth.West.Veggie Burger, 1/4 pkg	90	0	9

Midland Harvest

Fat Free & Lowfat Dry Mix:

	C	F	Cb
Taco Filling & Dip, 2.7 oz	50	0	7
Chili Fixin's, 8 oz	160	1	24
Sloppy Joe Fixin's, 3.6 oz	70	0	11
Burger Loaf Dry Mix: Per 3.2 oz	120	4	8
Frozen Patties: Sausage, 2 oz	80	4	5
Other varieties, 3.2 oz	120	4	8

Natural Touch

Frozen Products

	C	F	Cb
Dinner Entree, 1 pattie, 3 oz	220	15	2
Garden Vege Pattie, 1 pattie	170	8	18
Hard Rock Cafe Burg., 1 pattie, 3 oz	220	15	2
Lentil Rice Loaf, 1" slice, 3 oz	170	9	14
Nine Bean Loaf, 1" slice, 3 oz	160	8	13
Okara Pattie, 1 pattie, 2 1/4 oz	110	5	4
Spicy Black Bean Burger, 1 pattie	110	1	15
Vegan Burger, 1 pattie, 2 3/4 oz	70	0	6

Canned & Dry Products

	C	F	Cb
Kaffree Roma, 1 rounded tsp, 2g	10	0	2
Loaf Mix, 4 Tbsp dry mix (1/4 pkt)	100	0.5	10
Roasted Soy Butter, 2 Tbsp, 1.1 oz	170	11	10
Stroganoff Mix, 4 Tbsp, (1/4 pkt)	90	3.5	10
Toaster Squares: Date Walnut (1)	200	3	32
Blueberry (1)	180	2	30
Tuno, 1/3 cup, drained, 2 oz	60	2	2
Vegetarian Chili, 1 cup, 8 oz	170	1	21

New Menu (Vitasoy)	C	F	Cb
VegiBurgers, 3 oz	110	1	12
VegiDogs, 1 link, 1.5 oz	45	0	1
Tofumate (Season. Mixes): 1/4 pkt	25	0	4

SoyBoy			
Breakfast Links, 1 link, 1 oz	65	2.5	6
5-Grain Tempeh	135	6	9
Leaner Weiners, 1 weiner, 1.5 oz	55	0	2
Not Dogs, 1 link, 1.5 oz	95	3	10
Ravioli Rosa/Verde, 1 cup, 3.5 oz	180	3	29
Soysage, 2 oz	120	5	12
Soy Tempeh, 3 oz	150	6	9
Tofu Ravioli, 1 cup, 3.5 oz	180	3	31

White Wave			
Seitan: Chicken w. Broth, 5 oz	130	0	12
Traditional, 4 oz	140	0	4
Tempeh: Five Grain, 1/3 pkg	140	4	15
Original, 1/3 block, 2.7 oz	140	4	12
Sea Veggie, 1/3 block, 2.7 oz	120	3	11
Wild/Soy Rice, 1/3 block, 2.7 oz	140	5	13
Tofu: Baked: All flavors, 2 oz	120	6	3
Organic: Soft/Firm, 1/5 pkg, 3.2 oz	90	6	1
Fat-Reduced, 1/5 pkg, 3.2 oz	90	4	4
Extra Firm, 1/4 pkg, 3 oz	80	5	1
Soy Milks & Yogurts ~ See Pages 23, 26			

Worthington			
Frozen Products			
ChikStiks, 1 piece, 1 1/2 oz	110	7	3
Crispy Chic Patties, 1 pattie	170	9	15
Fillets, 2 pieces, 3 oz	180	10	8
FriPats, 1 pattie	130	6	4
Golden Croquettes, 4 pieces	210	10	14
Leanies, 1 link	100	7	2
Prosage Links, 2 links	60	2.5	2
Prosage Patties, 1 pattie, 38g	80	3	2
Stakelets, 1 piece, 2 1/2 oz	140	8	6
Stripples, 2 strips, 1/2 oz	60	4.5	2
Canned & Dry Products			
Chic-Ketts, 2 slices (3/8"), 2 oz	120	7	2
Chicken, 2 slices, 2 oz	80	4.5	1
Chili, 1 cup, 8 oz	290	15	21
Low Fat Chili, 1 cup, 8 oz	170	1	21
Choplets, 2 slices, 3 1/4 oz	90	2	3
Corned Beef, 4 slices, 2 oz	140	9	5
Country Stew, 1 cup, 8 1/2 oz	210	9	20
Diced Chik, 1/4 cup, 2oz	40	0	1
Dinner Roast, 3/4" slice, 3 oz	180	12	5

Worthington (Cont)	C	F	Cb
Canned & Dry Products (Cont)			
FriChik, 2 pieces, 3 oz	120	8	1
Low Fat FriChik, 2 pcs, 3 oz	80	3	1
Multigrain Cutlets, 2 sl., 3 1/4 oz	100	2	5
Numete, 3/8" slices, 2 oz	130	10	5
Prime Stakes, 1 piece, 3 1/4 oz	120	7	4
Prosage Roll, 5/8" slice, 2 oz	140	10	2
Protose, 3/8" Slice, 2 oz	130	7	5
Salami, 3 slices, 2 oz	130	8	2
Saucettes, 1 link, 1.3 oz	90	6	1
Savory Slices, 3 slices, 3 oz	150	9	6
Sliced Chik, 3 slices, 3 oz	70	0.5	1
Smoked Beef, 6 slices, 2 oz	120	6	6
Smoked Turkey, 3 slices, 2 oz	140	10	3
Super Links, 1 link, 1.7 oz	110	8	2
Tuno, 1/2 cup (drained), 2 oz	80	6	2
Turkee Slices, 3 slices, 3 1/4 oz	190	14	3
Vegetable Skallops, 1/2 cup, 3 oz	90	1.5	4
Vegetarian Burger, 1/4 c., 2 oz	60	2	2
Vegetarian Cutlets, 1 slice, 2.2 oz	70	1	3
Veja Links, 1 link, 1 oz	50	3	1
Low Fat Veja Links, 1 link	40	1.5	1
Wham, 2 slices, 1 1/2 oz	80	5	1

Yves Veggie Cuisine			
Breakfast: Brkfast Links, 2, 1.8 oz	60	0	3
Breakfast Patties, 1, 2 oz	70	2	4
Canadian Veg. Bacon, 3 sl, 2 oz	80	0	2
Burgers: Veggie Burger, 1, 3 oz	120	2	9
Garden Vegetable Patties, 1, 3 oz	90	0	11
Blk Bean & Mushroom, 1, 3 oz	100	0	13
Veggie Chick 'N Burger, 1, 3 oz	120	3	6
Dogs: Good Dog, 1, 52g	70	1.5	2
Veggie Dog, 1, 46g	60	0	1
Jumbo Veggie Dog, 76g	100	1.5	7
Tofu Dog, 1, 38g	45	0.5	2
Veggie Grand Round: 1/2 cup, 3 oz	90	0	8
Veggie Entrees: *Per 300g Tray*			
Country Stew	170	0	24
Chili; Macaroni; Penne, average	230	2	38
Lasagne	300	3	51

Homemade & Restaurant

Restaurant & Take-Out	C	F	Cb
Per 8 fl.oz			
Bean Medley	200	3	34
Beef Consomme	30	0	2
Borscht (w. Cream)	130	8	14
Bouillabaisse	400	15	10
Chicken & Corn	290	14	20
Chicken & Wild Rice	80	4	9
Chicken Consomme	50	0	2
Chicken Curry	180	8	18
Chicken Jambalaya	160	7	8
Chicken Noodle	80	2	12
w. Chicken	160	4	12
Chicken Soup	80	2	6
Chili with Beans	250	12	25
Clam Chowder	240	15	17
Corn & Crab	120	3	18
Corn Chowder	150	8	16
Cream of Broccoli	200	12	20
Cream of Potato	220	12	20
Cream of Mushroom	290	21	20
Creamy Pumpkin	210	10	26
Fish Chowder	220	15	6
French Onion	420	15	25
Gazpacho	60	0	13
Lentil Soup	250	9	28
Lobster Bisque	320	15	10
Matzo Ball (w.1 large ball)	180	7	24
Minestrone	140	2	14
Mulligatawny	300	15	4
Pea & Ham	240	10	25
Potato & Bacon	170	7	19
Shark Fin Soup	220	6	4
Spicy Shrimp Soup, 1 bowl	160	7	10
Split Pea Soup	150	6	18
Vegetable (Fat Free)	75	0	18
Vegetable Beef	80	2	10
Vichyssoise	200	9	15
Watercress	90	4	13

● Ethnic & Restaurant Section: Pages 161-165
● Fast Foods/Restaurant Section: Pages 167-250
(Arby's, Au Bon Pain, Boston Market, Dunkin' Donuts, Denny's, Schlotzsky's, Sizzler, Souplantation, Sweet Tomatoes)

Homemade Soups: Calculate calories, fat and carbohydrates from ingredients.

Bouillon Cubes & Powders

	C	F	Cb
Bouillon Cubes: Aver. all types			
Regular, 1 cube	8	0	1
Low Sodium (LiteLine)	12	0	1
Powders: Average, 1 tsp	8	0	1
Herb-Ox: Instant Broth & Seasoning,			
Beef, 1 envelope	10	0	2
Chicken, vegetarian	10	0	2
Herbs, Spices: 1 tsp	5	0	1
Soup Oyster Crackers			
40 small/20 large, $^1/_2$ oz	60	2	8

Amy's

	C	F	Cb
Per 1 Cup ($^1/_2$ Can)			
Black Bean Vegetable	110	1	22
Cream of Mushroom, $^3/_4$ cup	120	9	10
Cream of Tomato, 1 cup	100	2	17
Lentil	130	4	19
Minestrone	90	1.5	17
No Chicken Noodle	90	3	12
Split Pea	100	0	19

Barnum & Bagel

	C	F	Cb
Frozen Soup: Per 1 Cup Serving			
Chicken Noodle	100	1.5	17
Chicken Matzo Ball	100	5	11
Minestrone	140	2	24
Mushroom Barley; Vegetable	130	1	26
Sweet & Sour Cabbage	160	1	36

Bean Cuisine

	C	F	Cb
Made as Directed: Per 1 Cup Serving			
Florentine/Country Bean; Barcelona	210	1.5	29
Basque Beans; Italian Market Bean	195	1.5	30
13 Bean Bouillabaisse	240	0	18

Betty Crocker

	C	F	Cb
Bowl Appetit!: Per 2.7 oz Serving			
Cheddar Broccoli Rice	300	8	52
Herb Chicken Veg. Rice	260	4	50
Macaroni & Cheese	370	12	54
Pasta Alfredo	360	11	51
Southwestern Rice	260	3	52
3-Cheese Rotini	370	12	52
Tomato Parmesan Penne	350	8	57

Soups (Cont)

Campbell's

Red & White Label   **C** **F** **Cb**
Per 1 Cup Prepared (from 1/2 Cup Condensed)

	C	F	Cb
Bean & Bacon	180	5	25
Beef Broth	15	0	1
Beef w. Vegetable & Barley	80	2	11
Broccoli Cheese	110	7	9
Californian Veg.; Chicken Gumbo	60	1	10
Cheddar Cheese	130	8	11
Chicken Broth	30	2	1
Chicken Noodle/w. Stars	70	2	9
Chicken Vegetable	80	2	12
Clam Chowder Manhattan	60	0.5	12
Clam Chowder New England	100	2.5	15
Cream of Asparagus; Celery	110	7	9
Cream of Broccoli; Shrimp	100	6	9
Cream of Chicken & Broccoli	120	8	11
Cream of Chicken Dijon	130	8	12
Cream of Mushroom	110	7	9
Double Noodle in Chicken Broth	100	2.5	15
French Onion	70	2.5	10
Golden Mushroom	80	3	10
Minestrone	100	2	16
Split Pea w. Ham; Green Pea	180	3.5	28
Tomato	80	0	18
Tomato Bisque	130	3	24
Tomato Noodle	120	1	25
Tomato Rice (Old Fashioned)	120	2	23
Vegetable	90	1	16
Vegetable & Beef; Turkey Noodle	80	2	10
Won Ton	45	1	5

Healthy Request (Blue Label): *Per 10 3/4 oz Can*

	C	F	Cb
Average all varieties	80	2	10

16 oz Can: *Per 1/2 Can Serving*

	C	F	Cb
Hearty Chicken & Rice	110	2.5	16
Hearty Chicken Noodle	100	3	14
New England Clam Chowder	120	3	17
Split Pea & Ham	170	1.5	29

Simply Home: *Per 1 Cup Serving*

	C	F	Cb
Chicken & Pasta; Chicken Noodle	90	1	14
Chicken w. Rice	100	1	19
Country Vegetable	110	0.5	23
Minestrone	140	1	27

Soup To Go: *Per 10 3/4 oz Ctn*

	C	F	Cb
Chicken Rice	140	1.5	25
Garden Vegetable	130	1	25
Hearty Chicken Noodle	100	1.5	16
Vege. Beef w. Pasta	130	1.5	22

Campbell's (Cont)

Chunky (Red Can):   **C** **F** **Cb**
19 oz Can: Per 1/2 Can Serving

	C	F	Cb
Baked Potato w. Cheddar, Bacon	180	8	23
Baked Potato w. Steak, Cheese	200	9	21
Beef w. White & Wild Rice	140	1.5	23
Cheese Tortellini	110	2	18
Chicken & Dumplings	190	10	16
Chicken Broccoli Cheese	200	12	18
Chicken Chowder Mushroom	210	12	18
Chicken Corn Chowder	250	15	18
Classic Chicken Noodle	130	3	16
Grilled Chicken Veg. & Pasta	110	2	17
Grilled Sirloin Steak & Vegies	120	2	20
Hearty Chicken & Vegetable	90	2	12
New England Clam Chowder	300	18	26
Potato Ham Chowder	220	14	16
Savory Chicken & Rice	140	3	18
Sirloin Burger	180	7	20
Tomato Cheese Ravioli & Veges	150	3	26
Vegetable	160	4	15
Vegetable Beef	150	5	17

10 1/2 oz Can: All flavors, 1 cup   120   3   20

Select: *Per 1 Cup (approx. 1/2 Can)*

	C	F	Cb
Chicken & Pasta w. Garlic	110	2	17
Chicken Rice/Vegetables	100	1.5	18
Creamy Potato w. Garlic	180	9	21
Fiesta Vegetable	120	0.5	24
Grilled Chicken w. Tomato & Veg.	100	1.5	17
Honey Rst Chkn w. Golden Potato	110	1	17
Minestrone	120	2.5	21
New England Clam Chowder	190	13	14
Fat Free	110	3	17
Roast Chicken w. Rotini & Penne	110	2	17
Tomato Garden	100	0.5	22
Vegetable	110	1	20

Soup & Recipe Mixes (Dry): *Per 1 Tbsp*

	C	F	Cb
Chicken Noodle/w. Broth	30	0.5	5
Onion	20	0	5

College Inn

	C	F	Cb
Beef/No Fat Broth, 1 cup	20	0	0
Chicken Broth/Lower Sodium, 1 c.	25	1.5	1

Cup-A-Ramen

	C	F	Cb
Beef; Cajun Chicken, 1 cup	310	16	36
Chicken ; Shrimp, 1 cup	320	17	36

Dominick's | C | F | Cb
Canned:			
Tomato, condensed, 1/2 cup	80	0.5	18
Chicken Broth: Regular, 1 cup	15	0.5	0
Reduced Salt, 1 cup	15	0	0

Dr McDougall's
Cup Mix:			
Minestrone & Pasta, 1 cup	180	1	31
Ramen Noodles, 1 container, 43g	150	0.5	29
Split Pea w. Barley, 1 cup	200	2	36
Tamale Pie w. Baked Chips, 1 cup	200	1.5	39
Tortilla Soup w. Baked Chips, 1 c.	190	1.5	37

Fantastic Cup Soups
Per 1 Cup			
Country Lentil	230	1	41
Creamy Soups: Average	150	2.5	27
5 Bean	230	1	43
Jumpin' Black Bean	210	1	39
Minestrone	150	1	29
Split Pea	190	1	35
Vegetable Barley	150	0.5	29

Goodman's
Soup Mixes (Prep.): Per 1 Cup			
Alphabet Vegetable	45	0	9
Noodle Soup: Regular	45	0.5	9
Salt Free	50	0.5	9
w. Vegetables	45	0	9
Onion Soup	30	1	5

Hain
Canned: Per 1 Cup			
Homestyle Naturals:			
Chicken Broth	25	2	3
Chicken Noodle	150	3	24
Chunky Tomato	80	0.5	18
Minestrone	110	2	20
Healthy Naturals:			
Black Bean	90	0	18
Mushroom Barley	130	1.5	26
Vegetable Broth	30	0	8
Vegetarian Lentil	120	1	20
Vegetarian Split Pea	170	1	30
Wild Rice	80	1.5	15

Healthy Choice | C | F | Cb
Per 1 Cup			
Baked Potato, 1 cup	140	2	25
Bean and Ham	160	1.5	29
Chicken & Roast Garlic	130	2	21
Chicken Corn Chowder	150	2.5	29
Chicken Pasta	110	2.5	19
Chicken w. Rice	100	2	16
Chunky Beef & Potato	110	1	21
Classic Italian Beef & Pasta	100	1.5	17
Country Vegetable	100	0.5	22
Creamy Potato & Ham	140	2.5	25
Creamy Tomato	100	1.5	21
Fiesta Chicken	90	1	16
Garden Vegetable	120	0.5	27
Hearty Chicken	130	2	21
Hearty Chili Beef	190	2	34
Lentil	150	1	29
Mediterranean Bean w. Pasta	120	1.5	22
Minestrone	120	1	24
New England Clam Chowder	120	1	22
Old Fashioned Chick. Noodle	150	0.5	27
Split Pea & Ham	170	2	28
Turkey w. White & Wild Rice	100	1.5	17
Vegetable Beef	120	1	20
Vegetable Clam	80	0.5	17
Zesty Gumbo	100	2	15

Health Valley
Bean Vegetable, 1 cup	140	0	32
Beef Broth, 1 cup	20	0	0
Chicken Broth, 1 cup	45	1.5	0
Garden/Tomato Vegetable, 1 cup	80	0	17
Real Minestrone; Italian Plus, 1 c.	80	0	20
Split Pea & Carrots, 1 cup	110	0	17
Country Corn & Vegetable, 1 cup	70	0	17
Carotene varieties, average, 1 cup	70	0	17
Lentil & Carrots, 1 cup	90	0	25
Pasta Soups:			
Pasta Fagioli, 1 cup	120	0	25
Other varieties, 1 cup	110	0	23
Organic:			
Black Bean; Split Pea	110	0	25
Mushroom Barley; Potato Leek	60	0	15
Lentil; Tomato; Minestrone, 1 c.	90	0	20
Vegetable, 1 cup	80	0	18
Dry Soups: 1/3 cup, average	120	0	24

### Hormel	C	F	Cb
Microwave Cup Hearty Soup: *1 cup, 7 1/2 oz*			
Chicken w. Vegetable & Rice	110	2	17
Beef Vegetable	90	1	15
Beef & Ham	190	4	29
Chicken Noodle	110	2.5	13
Chicken w. Vegetable & Rice	110	2	17
Beef Vegetable	90	1	15
Beef & Ham	190	4	29
Chicken Noodle	110	2.5	13

### Hy-Top Soups			
Condensed (10 1/2 oz Can): *Per 1/2 Cup*			
Chicken w. Rice	70	1.5	11
Chicken Noodle	60	2	8
Cream of Chicken	100	5	10
Cream of Mushroom	110	7	10
Tomato	70	0	16
Vegetable	80	2	12

### Knorr's Soup			
Taste Breaks: *Per 1.6 oz Cup*			
Black Bean	190	1	36
Chicken Noodle/Vegetable	120	2	21
Corn Chowder	140	3	26
Hearty Lentil	200	1	38
Navy Bean	130	0.5	25
Potato Leek	130	2.5	22
Split Pea	150	0.5	29
Vegetarian Vegetable	160	1	32
Noodle Cups: *Per 2.1 oz Cup*			
Fettuccine Alfredo	230	4	41
Fettuccine w. Creamy Basil Sce	220	4	40
3-Cheese Macaroni	230	3.5	41

### Lipton			
Cup-a-Soup: *Per Envelope*			
Broccoli & Cheese	70	3	9
Cream of Chicken	70	2	12
Creamy Chicken Vegetable	80	4.5	10
Chicken Noodle	50	1	8
Recipe Secrets Mixes: *Per Serving*			
Golden Onion	50	1	9
Onion Mushroom	30	0.5	5
Savory Herb w. Garlic; Vegetable	30	0	7
Noodle	60	2	9

### Manischewitz	C	F	Cb
Condensed:			
Per 1/3 Cup (Unprepared)			
Chicken	15	0.5	2
w. 3 Matzo Balls	80	4	9
Four Bean	70	1	13
Lentil	140	2	24
Minestrone	90	1.5	16
Per 8 fl.oz Serving (Prepared)			
Borscht w. Beets	90	0	21
Borscht Low Calorie	25	0	6
Instant Cup (Mrs Manischewitz): *Per Cup*			
Black Bean	200	1	37
Chicken Noodle	140	2	26
Chicken Rice	130	1	28
Hearty Lentil	140	1	26
Minestrone	210	1.5	39
Potato Leek	100	1	39

### Near East			
Per Serving			
Black Bean; Split Pea	195	1.5	34
Chicken; Sweet Corn	120	2.5	20
Chili & Corn	160	3	25
Country Mushroom	140	2.5	26
Italian Tomato	140	4	21
Lentil; Mediterranean Pasta	180	2	34
Minestrone; Parmesan Pasta	160	3	32
Potato Leek; Tomato & Rice	130	3	21
Primavera Pasta	190	2.5	36
Red Beans & Rice	190	2.5	36

### Nile Spice			
Per Cup			
Chicken Flavored Vegetable	110	1.5	21
Lentil	180	1.5	31
Minestrone	140	1	30
Potato Leek	110	3	19
Red Beans & Rice	170	1	36
Split Pea	200	1	35
Tomato & Rice	140	2.5	27

### Pacific Foods			
Ready To Eat: *Per Cup (8 fl.oz)*			
All Natural Chicken Broth	15	0	2
Organic Vegetable Broth	0	0	0

Progresso

Per 1 Cup Serving

	C	F	Cb
Basil Rotini Tomato	120	1.5	22
Bean & Ham	160	2	25
Beef Barley	130	4	13
Beef Minestrone/Noodle	140	3	16
Cheese & Herb Tortellini Tomato	140	3	23
Chickarina	130	5	12
Chicken & Wild Rice	100	1.5	15
Chicken Barley	110	1.5	16
Chicken Broth	20	1.5	1
Chicken Minestrone	110	1.5	15
Chicken Noodle	90	2	9
Chicken Rice w. Vegetable	90	2	13
Chicken Vegetable	90	1.5	13
Creamy Cheddar Chicken	210	9	23
Creamy Tomato & Garlic	150	6	23
Escarole in Chicken Broth	25	1	3
French Onion	50	1.5	9
Green Split Pea	170	3	25
Hearty Black Bean	170	1.5	30
Hearty Chicken & Rotini	90	1.5	12
Hearty Penne in Chicken Broth	80	1	14
Herb & Rotini Vegetable	100	1	19
Home Style Chicken w. Veges	90	1.5	11
Italian Herb Shells Minestrone	120	1.5	22
Lentil	140	2	22
Macaroni & Bean	160	4	23
Manhattan Clam Chowder	110	2	11
Minestrone	120	2	21
Minestrone Parmesan	100	2.5	16
New England Clam Chowder	190	10	21
Oregano Penne Italian Style Vege.	90	2	15
Peppercorn Penne Vegetable	110	2	19
Potato Broccoli	165	6.5	21
Potato w. Ham & Cheese	170	7	21
Roasted Chicken Garden Herb	70	1.5	9
Roasted Chicken Italiano	80	1.5	10
Roasted Chicken Rotini	80	1.5	11
Roasted Garlic Pasta Lentil	120	1.5	20
Roasted Potato & Garlic	180	9	23
Southwestern Style Corn Chowder	200	7	29
Spicy Chicken & Penne	110	1.5	14
Split Pea w. Ham	150	4	20
Steak & Baked Potato	130	2.5	18
Steak & Mushrooms/Vegetables	100	2	13
Tomato; Tomato Basil	100	2	19
Tomato Vegetable Italiano	90	2	15

Progresso (Cont)

	C	F	Cb
Tortellini in Chicken Broth	70	2	10
Turkey Noodle	90	1.5	11
Turkey Rice w. Vegetable	110	1	18
Vegetable	90	1	17
Vegetarian Vegetable	100	0.5	20
Zesty Herb Tomato	130	3.5	21

99% Fat Free: Per 1 Cup Serving

	C	F	Cb
Beef Barley	130	2	20
Beef Vegetable	160	2	24
Chicken Noodle	90	1.5	13
Chicken Rice w. Veges	110	2	16
Creamy Chicken Broccoli	90	2	13
Lentil; Minestrone	130	1.5	20
New England Clam Chowder	110	1.5	18
Roast Chicken, all types	90	1.5	12
Split Pea	170	1.5	29
Tomato Garden Vegetable	100	1.5	19
Vegetable	70	1	13
White Cheddar Potato	100	1.5	20

Pritikin

Per Cup

	C	F	Cb
Black Bean w. Rice	200	1	37
Chicken Flavored Vegetable	160	1	27
Minestrone	130	0.5	25
Potato Broccoli	110	0	22

Ralph's

	C	F	Cb
Chicken Broth, 1 cup	30	1	3
Fat Free/Reduced Salt, 1 cup	20	0	2

Ramen Noodles   ~ See Page 68

Rokeach

15 oz Can (Ready to Serve): Per Serving

	C	F	Cb
Barley & Mushroom	110	1	23
Chicken Consomme	50	4	0
Cream of Mushroom	120	7	13
Minestrone	170	1	32
Potato	100	1	20
Seven Bean	130	1	24
Split Pea & Egg Barley	190	1.5	35
Vegetable	110	1.5	22

Shari's

	C	F	Cb
Cream of Tomato, 1 cup	80	0	17
Great Plains Split Pea, 1 cup	150	0	26
Indian Black Bean & Rice, 1 cup	150	1	30
Italian White Bean, 1 cup	170	1	32
Spicy French Green Lentil, 1 cup	130	0	22
Spicy Mexican Bean, 1 cup	210	1	38
Tomato w. Red Bell Pepper, 1 cup	100	0	19
Vegetarian French Onion, 1 cup	60	0	9

Shelton's

Canned: Per Cup

	C	F	Cb
Black Bean & Chicken	170	4	22
Turkey Meatball; Chicken Noodle	90	3	11
Chicken Tortilla	110	1.5	16
Chicken Broth	35	2.5	0

Streit's

Instant Soups: Per Serving

	C	F	Cb
Chicken Flavor; Mushr. & Barley	70	0.5	11
Garden Vegetable	70	0.5	13
Mild Chili; Split Pea	60	0	14
Tomato Minestrone; Veg. Chicken	80	0.5	18

Swanson

Canned: Per Cup

	C	F	Cb
Beef Broth	20	1	1
Chicken Broth	30	2	1
100% Fat Free	15	0	1
Vegetable Broth	20	1	3

Tabatchnick

Frozen: Per Serving (1 bag, 7 1/2 oz)

	C	F	Cb
Barley Mushroom	70	0	13
Cream of Broccoli/ Spinach	90	4	11
Old Fashioned Potato	70	0	16
Pea	180	2	31
Vegetable	110	1	20
Yankee Bean	160	2	27

Uncle Ben's

Hearty Soup Mix: Per Serving (1/3 pkg)

	C	F	Cb
Black/Red Bean & Rice	150	2	28
Southwest Vegetable	90	1	19
White Bean & Pasta	100	1.5	18

Weight Watchers

	C	F	Cb
Chicken Noodle, 10 1/2 oz	150	2	25
Chicken & Rice, 10 1/2 oz	110	1.5	17
Minestrone, 10 1/2 oz	130	2	23
Vegetable, 10 1/2 oz	130	1	27
Instant Beef/Chicken Broth, 1 pkg	10	0	2

Westbrae

Canned: Per Cup Unless Indicated

	C	F	Cb
Alabama Black Bean Gumbo	80	0	23
Calif. Unchicken Broth, 3/4 cup	15	0.5	2
Chattanooga Corn Chowder	110	1	23
French Country Onion, 3/4 cup	60	0	12
Great Plains Savory Bean	70	0	20
Irish Isle Potato Leek	110	1	23
Monte Carlo Cr. Mushroom, 3/4 c.	70	3	10
Natural Wellington Unbeef	60	0	13
Rocky Mount. Crmy. Unchick., 3/4 c.	70	3	10
Santa Fe Vegetable	120	0	23
Savanna Unchicken Rice	60	0.5	11
Spicy Southwest Vegetable	90	0	23
Tuscany Tomato	60	0	9
Versailles Garden Vegetable	70	0	15

Wolfgang Puck

Canned: Per 1 Cup

	C	F	Cb
Chicken & Egg Noodles	150	5	16
Chicken & Vegetables	140	5	17
Chicken w. Pasta & Mushrooms	130	4.5	15
Chicken w. Sweetcorn	200	10	20
Creamy Chicken	210	12	15
Hearty Potato & Cheddar	260	18	16
Hearty Vegetable Beef	140	6	13
New England Clam Chowder	240	13	18
Old World Minestrone	180	7	24
Rst Chicken w. Wild Rice	150	5	13
Spicy 7 Bean w. Italian Sausage	230	11	22
Thick Country Vegetable	170	7	23

Enjoy nutritious soup as part of a meal or as a snack.

Soup is an excellent filler - especially to beat the 4.30pm snack syndrome. Choose low fat varieties.

Herbs & Spices • Condiments

## Herbs & Spices	C	F	Cb
Per 1 Teaspoon: Average all types	5	0	1
Allspice, ground	5	0	1
Chili Powder	8	0	1
Cinnamon, ground	6	0	2
Curry Powder	6	0	1
Garlic Powder	9	0	2
Nutmeg, ground	12	0	1
Onion Powder	7	0	2
Parsley, dried	4	0	1
Pepper, black/red/white, aver.	6	0	1
Saffron	2	0	0
Tumeric, ground	8	0	1
Seeds: Fenugreek	12	0	2
Mustard, Poppyseed	15	1	1
Other types, average	7	0	1
Parsley Patch, Sesame, 1 tsp	16	1	1
Salt-free blends, average	10	0	1
All-purpose, 1 tsp	6	0	1

Seasonings & Flavorings
	C	F	Cb
Accent Flavor Enhancer, 1 tsp	10	0	0
Angostura Bitters, 1 tsp	12	0	3
Bacon Bits, average, 1 Tbsp	30	1	0
Bacon Chips (Durkee), 1 Tbsp	45	2	2
Best O'Butter, 1 tsp	10	<1	2
Braggs Liquid Aminos, 1 tsp	5	0	0
Butter Buds, 1 tsp	8	<1	2
Garlic Bread Sprinkle, 1 tsp	8	<1	1
Garlic Salt, 1 tsp	2	0	0
Italian Seasoning, 1 tsp	4	0	1
Lemon Pepper Season., 1 tsp	7	<1	1
Meat Tenderizer, aver., 1 tsp	7	0	1
Molly McButter, 1 tsp	5	1	1
Mrs Dash Blends, 1 tsp	0	0	2
Perc Salt-free Seasoning, 1 tsp	8	0	2
Salad Sprinkles (Lawry's), 1 tsp	16	<1	2
Salad Supreme (McCormick), 1 tsp	10	<1	1
Salt: Regular, Sea Salt, Lite Salt	0	0	0
Seasoning Mixes, aver., 1/4 pkg	70	1	9
Taco Seasoning, aver., 1/4 pkg	30	<1	4
Old El Paso: Chili Season. Mix, 1 T.	15	0.5	3
Cheesy Taco Season. Mix, 1 Tbsp	15	0.5	3
Taco/Burrito Seasoning Mix, 2 tsp	15	0	4
Enchilada Seasoning Mix, 2 tsp	10	0	2
Fajita Seasoning Mix, 1 tsp	10	0	3
Vegit Seasoning Mix, 1 tsp	5	0	1

Condiments, Sauces
Average of Brands & Homemade	C	F	Cb
Apple Sauce:			
Sweetened, 1/4 cup, 2 1/4 oz	45	0	11
Unsweetened, 1/4 cup, 2 oz	27	0	12
Eden; Tree of Life, 1/2 cup	50	0	15
Bac O's (Betty Crocker), 1 tsp, 1/2 oz	60	3	4
Barbecue: Average, 1 Tbsp	25	0	6
Bearnaise Sce, 1/4 cup, 2 1/2 oz	190	19	5
Braggs Liquid Aminos, 1 tsp	5	0	0
Catsup (Ketchup): Reg., 1 Tbsp	15	0	4
Cheese, h/made, 1/4 cup, 2 1/2 oz	150	10	12
Chili Sauce: Heinz, 1 Tbsp	15	0	4
Del Monte, 1 Tbsp	20	0	5
Wolf Hot Dog, 1 Tbsp	15	1	2
Cocktail Sce: 1/4 cup	110	0	15
Cranberry, jellied, 1/4 c., 2 1/2 oz	110	0	27
Escoffier Sauces, 1 Tbsp	20	0	4
Honey Mustard (French's): 1 tsp	5	0	1
Horseradish: 1 tsp	2	0	0
Sauce: Sauceworks, 1 tsp	20	2	0
Ketchup: Regular, 1 Tbsp	16	0	4
Heinz Lite, 1 Tbsp	8	0	2
Mayonnaise: See Page 84			
Mushroom Sauce, 1/2 cup, 2 oz	50	2	5
Mustard, average, 1 tsp	0	0	0
Pizza Sauce, cnd., 1/4 cup, 2 oz	25	0	5
Seafood Cocktail Sce, 1/4 cup	60	0	14
Soy Sauce, all types, av., 1 Tbsp	10	0	1
Sour Cream Sce, 1/2 cup	250	15	22
Spaghetti Sce: 1/2 cup, 4 1/2 oz	135	6	19
Steak Sauce: Heinz/A.1., 1 Tbsp	15	0	3
Lea & Perrins, 1 Tbsp	25	0	6
Str'berry Puree Sce: Unsweet., 2 T.	9	0	2
Sweet & Sour Sauce:			
Contadina, 2 Tbsp	40	1	8
Kikkoman Lite Soy, 1 Tbsp	10	0	1
La Choy, 2 Tbsp, 34g	60	0	14
Tabasco Sauce, 1 Tbsp	2	0	0
Taco Sauce, average, 2 Tbsp	10	0	1
Tartar Sauce: Heinz, 2 Tbsp, 30g	140	14	4
America's Choice, 2 Tbsp, 27g	160	17	1
Hellman's: Regular, 2 Tbsp, 30g	80	7	3
Lowfat, 2 Tbsp, 30g	40	1.5	7
Teriyaki Sauce: Kikkoman, 1 Tbsp	15	0	2
Vinegar: White or wine, 1 fl.oz	4	0	1
White Sauce, 1/2 cup, 5 oz	130	7	12
Worcestershire Sauce, 1 tsp	5	0	1

Pickles ◆ Gravy ◆ Sloppy Joe

Pickles & Relish | C | F | Cb

Average All Brands

	C	F	Cb
Bread & Butter Pickles, 4 sl.,1 oz	20	0	5
Chutney, 2 Tbsp, 1¼ oz	40	0	12
Dill Pickle:			
Slices, 4 slices, 1 oz	3	0	0.5
1 large,			
(3¾"x 1¼" diam.), 2¼ oz	12	0	3
Extra lrg (4"x 1¾" diam.), 5 oz	30	0	6
Halves: Small, 1 oz	3	0	0.5
Large, 2½ oz	8	0	2
Sweet, small, ½ oz	22	0	6
Gherkins, sweet, 1 med., 1 oz	15	0	7
Green Chilies, chopped, 2 Tbsp	5	0	1
Horseradish, 1 Tbsp	10	0	2
Jalapenos, pickled, 2 whole	5	0	1
Jalapeno Relish, 1 Tbsp, ½ oz	5	0	1
Mustard, aver. all brands, 1 tsp	5	0	0.5
Peppers: Hot/Mild, 1 oz	8	0	2
Pickled: Beets, ½ cup, 4 oz	75	0	19
Onions, 1 medium, ¾ oz	10	0	2
Cocktail Onion, 1 onion	2	0	0
Red Cabbage, ½ cup, 3 oz	60	0	13
Pickles:			
Sweet, 2 Tbsp, 1 oz	35	0	0
Large (3" x ¾" diam.), 1¼ oz	40	0	10
Pickle in a Pouch, 1 large	12	0	3
Relishes: Sandwich Spread, 1 tsp	20	1	5
Cranberry-Orange, 1 Tbsp	30	0	7
Hot Dog *(Heinz)*, 1 Tbsp	17	0	28
Sweet Pickle, 1 Tbsp	20	0	5
Sauerkraut, ½ cup, 3½ oz	25	0	5
Sweet Cauliflower	35	0	8

Salsa

Average all types

	C	F	Cb
Regular, no oil, 2 Tbsp	15	0	3.5
w. Oil, homemade, 2 Tbsp	40	3	8
Chef's Kitchen, 2 Tbsp	10	0	2
Del Monte, all flavors, 2 Tbsp	10	0	2
Kaukauma, 2 Tbsp	15	0	3

Pasta Sauces ~ *See Page 81*

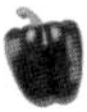

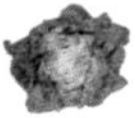

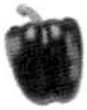

Gravy | C | F | Cb

	C	F	Cb
Homemade Gravy:			
Thin, little fat, 2 Tbsp, 1 oz	20	1	3
Thick, 2 Tbsp, 1¼ oz	50	2	9
¼ cup, 2½ oz	100	4	18
Franco-American (Canned)			
Au Jus Gravy, ¼ cup, 2 oz	10	0	2
Beef/Mushrm; Turkey Gravy, 2 oz	25	1	3
Chicken Gravy, 2 oz	40	4	3
Golden Pork Gravy, 2 oz	45	4	3
Fat Free, Average, 2 oz	25	0	4
Pillsbury (Gravy Mixes)			
Brown; Homestyle, ¼ cup	15	0	3
Chicken, as prep., ¼ cup	20	0	4

Sloppy Joe Sauce

Per Serving

	C	F	Cb
Del Monte: ¼ cup, 67g	50	0	11
Heinz: ½ cup, 125g	70	0.5	14
Hunt's Manwich: ¼ cup, 64g	30	0	6
Libby's: ⅓ cup, 78g	45	0	10

Tomato Products

Whole/Chopped/Crushed/Diced	C	F	Cb
1 cup, 8½ oz	50	0	10
In Aspic, ½ cup	50	0	12
w. Green Chili, 1 cup, 8½ oz	45	<1	11
Stewed, ½ cup	40	2.5	9
Wedges in Tom Juice, 1 cup	70	0.5	15
Salsa, average, 1 Tbsp	15	0	3.5
Tomato Ketchup:			
Regular, 1 Tbsp	16	0	4
Green *(Heinz)*, 1 Tbsp	20	0	5
Tomato Paste, 2 Tbsp	25	0	5
Regular, 6 oz, ¾ cup	150	0	34
Tomato Puree, ½ cup	50	0	10
Tomato Sauce:			
Regular, ½ cup	40	0	9
Spanish Style, ½ cup	40	0	9
w. Mushrooms, ½ cup	40	0	9
w. Onions, ½ cup	50	0	11
Tomato Seasoning, 3 tsp	20	0	4
Sundried Tomatoes:			
Natural, 5-6 pces, 0.4 oz	22	0	5
In Oil, drained, 6 pces, ½ cup	60	4	5

Sauce Mixes

	C	F	Cb
Knorr (Mix)			
Made As Directed: *Per 1/4 Cup, 2 oz*			
Au Jus	8	0.2	1
Bearnaise	170	17	5
Classic Brown Gravy	25	1	3
Demi-Glace	30	1	4
Hollandaise	170	18	5
Hunter; Lyonnaise	25	0.3	4
Mushroom Sauce	60	3	5
Napoli Sauce	100	3	17
Pepper Sauce	20	1	3
McCormick			
Grillmates:			
Marinade, aver. all flavors, 2 tsp	15	0	2
Sauce Blend Seasoning Mixes:			
Lemon Herb Chicken, 1 Tbsp	30	0	5
Chicken Fried Rice, 1 Tbsp	35	0	6
Stir Fry Chicken, 1 Tbsp	20	0	4
Chicken Teriyaki, 1 1/3 Tbsp	40	1	5

Marinades

	C	F	Cb
KC Masterpiece: *Per 1 Tbsp*			
Garlic & Herb	30	1.5	4
Honey & Teriyaki	35	0.5	7
Original BBQ	40	1.5	7
Lawry's 30 Minute: *Per 1 Tbsp*			
Hawaiian; Dijon & Honey	20	0	3.5
Carribean Jerk; Teriyaki	25	0	4
Mediterranean; Lemon Pepper	10	0	2
Mesquite	5	0	1
Thai Ginger; Herb & Garlic	10	0	2

Pizza & Enchilada Sauce

Per 1/4 Cup

	C	F	Cb
Pizza Squeeze *(Contadina)*	35	1.5	6
Progresso Pizza Sauce	10	0	2
Ragu: Pizza Sauce	30	1	4
Pizza Quick; average all types	40	1.5	6
Enchilada Sauce *(Old El Paso)*	10	0	2

Brands

	C	F	Cb
Amy's: *Per 1/2 Cup*			
Family Marinara	50	1	8
Garlic Mushroom	120	7	10
Tomato Basil	80	3	11

Brands (Cont)

	C	F	Cb
Barilla: *Per 1/2 Cup*			
Arrabbiata; Siciliana	80	3.5	9
Marinara; Ortolana	80	4	10
Mushr. & Garlic; Pepperonata	70	2	12
Puttanesca	80	2.5	13
Classico: *Per 1/2 Cup*			
Florentine Spinach & Cheese	80	4.5	8
Italian Sausage & Fennel	90	5	7
Mushroom & Olive	50	1	8
Roasted Peppers & Onions/Garlic	60	2	9
Spicy Red Pepper	60	2.5	6
Sun Dried Tomato; 4 Cheese	80	4	8
Tomato & Basil	50	1	8
Contadina: *Per 1/2 Cup*			
Alfredo Sauce	360	32	10
Lite	160	10	10
Garden Vegetable Sauce	40	0	9
Marinara Sauce	80	4	9
Mushroom Alfredo	200	14	12
Mushroom Marinara Sauce	70	2.5	11
Pesto with Basil, Red. Fat	460	26	22
Pesto w. Sundried Tomato	380	30	20
Roasted Garlic Marinara	60	2	10
Del Monte: *Per 1/2 Cup*			
Chunky: Average all varieties	60	1.5	11
D'Italia Pasta: Four Cheese	60	2	8
Other varieties	50	1.5	9
Spaghetti Sauce: Traditional	60	0.5	15
Garlic & Onion	60	1.5	11
w. Mushroom/Meat	70	1.5	14
Dominick's: *Per 1/2 Cup*			
All Natural: Garlic & Onion	80	4	10
Marinara	80	4	10
Mushr. & Olive; Tomato & Basil	80	1	8
Italian Classics: Four Cheese	80	2.5	12
Portabella Mushroom	60	2	9
Puttanesca	70	3	8
Spicy Roasted Garlic	70	2	10
Sun Ripened Tomatoes	80	4	8
Tomato Basil	50	1	8
Estee: Spaghetti Sce, 1/4 cup, 4 oz	60	2	13
Frank Sinatra: *Per 1/4 Cup*			
Alfredo	160	14	4
Pesto	160	14	3

Brands (Cont)

	C	F	Cb
Five Brothers: Per 1/2 Cup			
Alfredo w. Mushrooms	160	12	6
Creamy Alfredo/Pesto	200	18	4
Fresh/Summer Tomato Basil	60	1.5	10
Grilled Summer Vegetable	80	5	12
Marinara w. Burgundy Wine	80	3	12
Mushroom & Garlic	90	3	13
Oven Roasted Garlic & Onion	70	1.5	10
Imported Romano & Garlic	90	4	10
Garden Valley: Per 1/2 Cup			
Chunky Vege. Primavera	35	0.5	12
Four Cheese	35	1	8
Millina's Finest; Roasted Garlic	50	0	12
Sundried Tomato; Tom. Mushroom	50	0	11
Sweet Tomato Basil	60	0	13
Hagerty Foods: Per 4 oz			
Asparagus Garlic	95	7	9
Caponata	60	3.5	8
Healthy Choice: Per 1/2 Cup			
Four Cheese Creamy Alfredo	45	3	3
Garlic & Herbs	50	0	10
Marinara w. Burgundy	50	0.5	11
Mushroom Alfredo	45	3	3
Roasted Garlic & Romano	60	1	11
Sundried Tomato & Herb	60	0.5	12
Traditional Pasta Sauce	50	0	11
Super Chunky:			
Tomato, Mushroom Garlic	45	0	10
Vegetable Primavera	45	0	9
Hy Top: Per 1/2 Cup, 125g			
Spaghetti Sauce: All flavors	90	4	11
Mama Coco's: Per 1/2 Cup			
Basil & Garlic	70	4	9
Marinara	100	7	8
Mushroom	110	8	8
Newman's Own: Per 1/2 Cup			
Bombolina	100	5	12
Other flavors	60	2	9
Prego: Per 1/2 Cup			
Extra Chunky: Garden Comb.	90	2	16
Garlic Supreme	120	3	23
Mushroom & Green Pepper	120	4.5	18
Mushroom Supreme	120	4.5	21
Zesty Mushroom	120	4	20
Tomato, Onion & Garlic	110	3.5	19

	C	F	Cb
Prego (Cont): Per 1/2 Cup			
Regular:			
Diced Onion & Garlic	110	3	19
Flavored w. Meat	140	6	21
Fresh Mushroom; Traditional	150	5	23
Hamburger	120	4	17
Italian Sausage & Garlic	120	5	16
Mushroom & Garlic	110	2	20
Mushroom/Tomato Parmesan	120	3.5	19
Pepperoni	120	4.5	18
Roast Red Pepper/Herb & Garlic	110	3.5	17
Roast Garlic Parmesan	120	1.5	23
Savory Chicken	130	5	17
Three Cheese	100	2	18
Pasta Bake: Per 1/8 Jar			
3-Cheese Marinara	100	4.5	11
Hearty Meat Sauce	120	6	12
Tomato, Garlic & Basil	80	3.5	11
Mushroom w. Garlic & Onion	90	3	13
Progresso: Per 1/2 Cup, 4 1/4 oz			
Pasta Sauces: Alfredo (Authentic)	200	15	7
Creamy Clam	110	6	8
Lobster	100	7	6
Marinara (Authentic)	100	4	12
Pizza	40	0	8
Red Clam	60	1	8
White Clam (Authentic)	150	10	5
White Clam, regular	140	10	5
Ragu: Per 1/2 Cup			
Cheese Creations:			
Creamy Tomato Romano	120	5	14
Classic Alfredo	240	24	6
Four Cheese	240	22	4
Light Parmesan Alfredo	160	12	4
Mushroom Green Pepper	110	3.5	18
Roasted Garlic Parmesan	240	22	6
Tom. Garlic Onion; Super Mushr.	120	3.5	19
Rinaldi			
Meat/Mushroom, 1/2 c.	90	4	11
Seeds of Change: Per 1/2 Cup			
Average all varieties	50	0.5	9
Sutter Home: Per 1/2 Cup			
Italian Style Pasta Sauce	80	2	12
Sicilian Style; Spicy Mediterranean	80	2	12
Marinara Pasta Sauce	70	2	14

Brands (Cont)

Taj: *Per 1/2 Cup*

	C	F	Cb
Bombay Curry Simmer Sauce	90	5	10
Calcutta Masala Simmer Sauce	100	5	13
Kashmir Tandoori Marinade Sce	50	3	5
Seasoning Mixes: *Per 2 tsp*			
Meat Loaf; Sloppy Joe's	30	0	4
Beef Stew	15	0	3
Chili	40	1	6
Chicken/Taco Seasoning	25	0	4
Spaghetti Sauce: Italian Style, 1 T.	25	0	5

Simpone's: *Per 1/2 Cup*

	C	F	Cb
Spaghetti Sauce: Classic	50	2.5	8
Mom's	70	3.5	8

Tomaso's: *Per 1/2 Cup*

	C	F	Cb
Basil & Fresh Garlic; Spicy Eggplant	60	3	7
Black Olive Fresh Basil	40	2	5
Xtra Garlic	55	2	8
Fresh Mushroom & Artichoke	50	2	7
Sugo Rosa	105	7.5	8

Tree of Life: *Per 1/2 Cup*

	C	F	Cb
Pasta Sauce Plus: All varieties	45	0	9
Organic: Classic Tomato	40	0	8
Average other varieties	30	0	7

Other Sauces

Bookbinders: *Per 1/2 Cup*

	C	F	Cb
White Clam Sauce	300	30	4
Bullseye: BBQ, 1 Tbsp	25	0	6
Estee: Barbecue Sauce, 1 Tbsp	18	<1	3
Steak Sauce, 1 Tbsp	14	<1	3

French's Grill & Glaze

	C	F	Cb
Honey Mustard, 1 Tbsp	90	1	18
Teriyaki, 2 Tbsp	60	0	13

Green Giant

	C	F	Cb
Sloppy Joe S'wich Sce, 1/4 c., 2.5 oz	50	0	11
Sloppy Joe Sauce & Meat	200	11	11

Heinz: *Per 1 Tbsp: Approx. 1/2 oz*

	C	F	Cb
Barbecue Sauces: All flavors	35	0	9
Chili Sauce	15	0	4
Horseradish Sauce	70	7	13
Mustard: Pourable/Mild	8	<1	5
Spicy Brown	13	1	6
Seafood Cocktail Sauce	20	0	10
Steak Sauce 57	15	0	4

Other Sauces (Cont)

Heinz (Cont): *Per 1 Tbsp: Approx. 1/2 oz*

	C	F	Cb
Tartar Sauce	70	7	2
Tomato Ketchup	16	0	26
Worcestershire Sauce	8	0	11

Hunt's BBQ: Original, 36g, 2 T. 50 0 13

	C	F	Cb
Hunt's BBQ: Original, 36g, 2 T.	50	0	13
Hickory & Brown Sugar, 38g, 2 Tbsp	70	0	18

Kraft

	C	F	Cb
Sauceworks: Cocktail, 2 Tbsp	30	0.3	6
Horseradish, 1 tsp	20	1.5	0
Sweet 'n Sour, 1 Tbsp	30	0	7
Tartar: 1 Tbsp	50	5	2
Lemon & Herb, 1 Tbsp	75	8	0
Nonfat Tartar, 1 Tbsp	12	0	5
Barbecue Sauces: Average, 2 T.	50	0.5	9
Other Sauces: Mustard, 1 Tbsp	10	0	0
Horseradish: Reg./Cream Style, 1 T.	10	0	0
Sandwich Spread & Burger, 1 Tbsp	50	4	3
Sweet 'n Sour, 1 Tbsp	40	0.5	9

Knudsen: Potato Toppings, 2 T 50 4.5 2

	C	F	Cb
Knudsen: Potato Toppings, 2 T	50	4.5	2

Las Palmas

	C	F	Cb
Red Chile Sauce, 1/4 cup, 2 oz	15	0.5	2
Enchilada Sauces: Green Chile	25	1.5	3
Hot/Original, 1/4 cup, 2 oz	15	0.5	3
Salsa: Mexicana. Mild, 2 Tbsp, 1 oz	5	0	1
Mexicana Hot/Medium, 2 Tbsp	10	0	2

Mr Yoshida's

	C	F	Cb
Original Gourmet, 2 Tbsp, 30ml	90	0	20
Hawaiian Sweet & Sour, 2 Tbsp	35	0	9

Old El Paso

	C	F	Cb
Salsa: Thick 'n Chunky, 2 T., 1 oz	10	0	2
Homestyle; Green Chili; Verde 2 Tbsp, 1 oz	10	0	2
Taco Sce: All varieties, 2 Tbsp, 1 oz	10	0	2
Enchilada Sces: All types, 1/4 c., 2 oz	20	1	3
Grilling Sauces: All types, 2 Tbsp	60	0	14
Tom. & Gr. Chiles/Jalapenos,1/4 c., 2 oz	10	0	2

	C	F	Cb
Open Pit: Honey, 2 Tbsp	40	0	10
Hickory; Original BBQ, 2 Tbsp	50	0.5	11
Thick & Tangy, 2 Tbsp	50	0	12

President's Choice: *Per 2 Tbsp*

	C	F	Cb
Honey Dijon	50	0.5	11
Hot & Spicy	55	0	13
Original BBQ	60	0	12

Quick Guide — Mayonnaise

	C	F	Cb
Regular			
Average All Brands, 1 Tbsp	100	11	0
(*Bestfoods, Kraft*), 1 Tbsp	100	11	0
½ cup, 4 oz	800	88	0
Light/Reduced Fat			
Kraft; Best Foods, 1 Tbsp	50	5	1
½ cup, 4 oz	400	40	8
Hain, 1 Tbsp	60	6	2
Hellman's; Estee, 1 Tbsp	50	5	1
Smart Balance, 1 Tbsp	50	5	2
Smart Beat, 1 Tbsp	40	4	1
Weight Watchers, 1 Tbsp	25	2	1
Fat Free			
Kraft; Weight Watchers, 1 Tbsp	10	0	3
½ cup, 4 oz	80	0	16

Mayonnaise Type Dressing

	C	F	Cb
BAMA Dressing, 1 Tbsp, 0.5 oz	50	4	3
Miracle Whip Salad Dressing:			
Regular, 1 Tbsp, 0.5 oz	70	7	2
Light, 1 Tbsp, 0.5 oz	40	3	3
Free, 1 Tbsp, 0.5 oz	15	0	3
Nayonaise (Nasoya)			
(Tofu Base/Dairy Free/Eggless)			
Regular, 1 Tbsp, 0.5 oz	35	3	1
Fat-Free, 1 Tbsp, 0.5 oz	10	0	2

Quick Guide — Salad Dressings

Average All Brands
Per 2 Tbsp (Approx 1 oz)

	C	F	Cb
Blue Cheese: Regular	150	16	2
Light/Reduced Fat	80	8	1
Caesar: Regular	140	14	2
Light/Reduced Fat	50	5	0.5
French: Regular	130	11	2
Light/Reduced Fat	50	3	4
Fat/Oil-Free	40	0	4
Italian: Regular	130	11	2
Light/Reduced Fat	70	7	2
Fat/Oil-Free	10	0	2
Ranch: Regular	180	18	2
Light/Reduced Fat	90	8	3
Fat-Free	50	0	2
Russian: Regular	130	10	3
Light/Reduced Fat	50	5	2
Fat-Free	30	0	2
Thousand Island: Regular	130	12	5
Light/Reduced Fat	50	4	3
Fat-Free	35	0	3

Brands ~ Salad Dressings

Per 2 Tbsp (Approx 1 oz)

Bernstein's	C	F	Cb
Balsamic	110	11	2
Roasted Garlic Balsamic	45	3.5	3
Cheese: Garlic Italian; Fantastico	110	11	2
Creamy Caesar	120	13	1
Fat Free Cheese & Garlic Italian	10	0	2
French Herb Garden	130	11	2
Restaurant Recipe Italian	130	13	1
Best Foods: Caesar, 2 Tbsp	100	9	6
Chardonnay Vinaigrette	50	4	4
Chunky Blue Cheese	140	15	1
Creamy Caesar	170	18	2
Creamy French	160	16	4
Creamy/Garlic/Spr. Onion Ranch	140	15	1
Creamy Thousand Island	130	13	4
Fat Free Caesar; Dijonnaise	30	0	7
Fat Free Ranch	45	0	4
Fat Free Italian	15	0	4
Rst. Tomato & Balsamic Vinegar	100	9	3

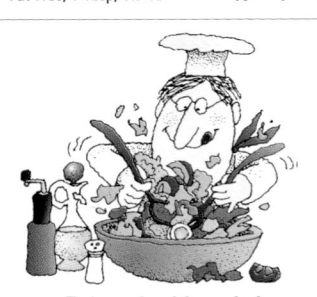

*Enjoy a healthy salad
but don't drown it
in high-fat salad dressings.*

Per 2 Tbsp (Approx 1 oz)	C	F	Cb
est Foods (Cont)			
Citrus Splash:			
Oriental Orange; Ruby Red Ginger	90	7	7
Or. Vinaigrette; Tangy Tangerine	80	7	6
Tangerine Balsamic	80	7	7
rianna's			
lush Vintage	100	6	12
ardini's			
aesar, 2 Tbsp	160	17	1
erb Poppy Seed	35	1	7
esty Garlic	120	13	2
ummer Honey Mustard	150	14	5
arolina's Swamp Stuffs'			
er 2 Tbsp			
lue Tick Dressing	220	16	6
edar Spray	40	3	2
Milk Weed	100	10	2
ure Tar	60	5	2
ed Tide	30	3	2
eaweed Splash	30	2	2
wamp Sauce	20	0	6
adpole Tea	30	2	2
irards: *Per 2 Tbsp*			
aesar	150	16	1
Lite	80	7	2
te Champagne	60	5	2
riental	120	11	6
riginal French	120	13	0
pinach Salad	80	2	14
at Free: Caesar	40	0	9
Raspberry Vinaigrette	40	0	9
Red Wine Vinaigrette	40	0	9
ood Seasons (Mix): *Prepared, 2 T. (Approx 1 oz)*			
lue Cheese, Cheese Garlic	145	16	2
heese Italian, Garlic & Herbs	145	16	2
lassic Dill, 1 pkg	28	0	5
alian; Mild Italian; Zesty Italian	145	16	2
alian Lite; Lite Cheese Italian	55	6	2
anch	115	12	2
ain			
lo Oil Range: Bleu Cheese	28	2	2
Buttermilk	22	0	2
Caesar	12	0	2
French	24	0	6
Italian	4	0	2

Per 2 Tbsp (Approx 1 oz)	C	F	Cb
Hain			
Regular Pourable: Per 2 Tbsp			
Canola: Garden Tomato	120	12	2
Italian; French Mustard	100	10	2
Creamy Caesar: French	120	12	2
Creamy Italian	160	16	0
Garlic & Sour Cream	140	14	0
Poppyseed Rancher's	120	14	0
Savory Herb (No Salt Added)	180	20	0
Thousand Island	100	10	5
Traditional Italian	160	16	0
(No Salt Added)	120	12	2
Mix: Made Up Per 2 Tbsp			
Healthy Sensation			
Blue Cheese, French, 2 Tbsp	40	2	8
Honey Dijon	50	2	10
Italian	15	0	2
Ranch	30	0	6
Thousand Island	40	0	8
Hidden Valley			
B.L.T. Ranch	150	15	3
B.L.T. Ranch Lite	90	7	5
Fat Free: Caesar	30	0	6
Honey & Bacon French	50	0	11
Honey Dijon	35	0	7
Italian Herb & Cheese; Ranch	30	0	6
Italian Parmesan	20	0	4
Red Wine & Herb Vinaigrette	45	0	11
Roasted Garlic Italian	40	0	5
Honey & Bacon French	150	12	10
Original Ranch/w. Bacon	140	14	1
Light Original Ranch	80	7	3
Ranch Caesar Creamy	110	11	1
Ranch Cole Slaw	150	15	5
Ranch Garden Veg./Garlic & Spice	130	13	3
Hollywood			
Caesar; Creamy French	140	14	4
Italian; Creamy Italian	180	18	3
Italian Cheese	160	16	4
Poppy Seed Rancher's	150	16	2
Thousand Island	120	12	6

Per 2 Tbsp (Approx 1 oz)	C	F	Cb
Knott's Berry Farm			
Honey Dijon, 2 Tbsp	130	13	4
Raspberry Vinaigrette	30	2	8
Roasted Garlic Caesar	140	14	3
Sun Dried Tomato Vinaigrette	100	10	3
Kraft			
Regular Dressings: Per 2 Tbsp			
Bacon & Tomato	140	14	2
Buttermilk Ranch	150	16	2
Caesar; Salsa Ranch	130	13	2
Caesar Ranch; Pesto Italian	140	15	1
Catalina French/ with Honey	140	12	8
Chunky Blue Cheese	90	7	5
Coleslaw	150	12	8
Creamy Caesar; Cucumber Ranch	140	15	2
Creamy Garlic; Creamy Italian	110	11	3
French	120	12	4
Honey Dijon	150	15	4
House Italian	120	12	3
Peppercorn Ranch; Ranch	170	18	1
Free	50	0	11
Roka Brand Blue Cheese	90	7	5
Russian	130	10	10
Salsa Zesty Garden	70	6	3
Sour Cream & Onion Ranch	170	18	1
Thousand Island	110	10	5
Thousand Island w. Bacon	120	12	5
Zesty Italian	110	11	2
Kraft Free (Fat Free):			
Blue Cheese, Catalina, French	50	0	12
Honey Dijon, Peppercorn/Ranch	50	0	11
Italian	10	0	2
Red Wine Vinegar	15	0	3
Thousand Island; Sr Cream & Onion	45	0	11
Light Done Right!: Classic Caesar	70	6	3
Italian; Red Wine Vinaigrette	50	4.5	3
Raspberry Vinaigrette	60	4	6
Thousand Island	70	4	17
Special Collection:			
Balsamic Vinaigrette	110	12	1
Creamy Cucumber Dill	120	12	4
Creamy Parmesan Romano	170	18	1
Creamy Roasted Garlic	160	17	2
Greek Vinaigrette	120	13	2
Savory Mayo: Roast Garlic/Onion	100	10	1
Tangy Tomato Bacon	130	11	8

Per 2 Tbsp (Approx 1 oz)	C	F	Cb
Kraft (Cont)			
Taste of Life: Garden Italian	50	4.5	3
Country Ranch; Tomato & Garlic	60	4.5	4
Honey Catalina	80	5	8
Vinaigrette: Caesar Parmesan	60	5	1
Roast Garlic	50	4.5	3
LadyLee (Lucky Stores)			
Fat Free French	120	11	7
Fat Free Italian	10	0	2
Fat Free Ranch/Thousand Island	35	0	8
Lawrey's			
Caesar; Italian, 2 Tbsp	130	13	2
Creamy Caesar	130	14	8
Red Wine Vinaigrette	90	7	7
Manischewitz			
Garlic Ranch, 2 Tbsp	15	0	4
Maple Grove			
Fat Free: Caesar, 2 Tbsp	30	0	6
Honey Dijon	45	0	10
Marzetti			
Regular Dressings:			
Blue Cheese	160	17	0
Buttermilk: Bacon Ranch; Ranch	180	19	1
Blue Cheese	160	18	1
Caesar; Chunky Blue Cheese	150	16	1
California French; Celery Seed	160	13	11
Classic Caesar Ranch	190	20	2
Country French	150	13	7
Creamy Italian	150	16	1
Dijon Honey Mustard	140	13	6
Garden Ranch; Ranch	180	19	1
Honey French/Blue Cheese	160	13	11
Italian w. Olive Oil	120	13	1
Potato Salad Dressing	120	13	7
Red Wine Vinegar & Oil	130	14	2
Slaw	170	16	6
Southern Slaw	100	11	14
Thousand Island	150	15	5
Fat Free Dressings: Italian	15	0	3
California French; Honey French	45	0	11
Honey Dijon	60	0	14
Ranch; Peppercorn Ranch	30	0	7
Slaw; Sweet & Sour	45	0	12
Thousand Island	35	0	9

Per 2 Tbsp (Approx 1 oz)

	C	F	Cb
Marzetti (Cont)			
Light Dressings: Blue Cheese	60	6	4
Buttermilk Ranch	90	9	3
California French	80	6	8
Chunky Blue Cheese	80	7	4
French	40	2	6
Honey French	80	4	12
Italian	60	5	3
Ranch	90	8	7
Red Wine Vinegar & Oil	20	1	3
Slaw	60	7	10
Sweet & Sour	100	6	11
Thousand Island	70	5	6
Newman's Own			
Balsamic Vinaigrette, 2 Tbsp	90	9	3
Creamy Caesar	170	18	1
Family Recipe Italian	120	13	1
Italian Light	20	0	3
Olive Oil & Vinegar, 2 T.	150	16	1
Parmesan & Roasted Garlic	110	11	2
Ranch	180	18	2
Nasoya			
Vegi-Dressing (Tofu Base/Dairy Free):			
Thousand Island	60	4	6
Other flavors	60	5	3
(Nayonaise - See Mayonnaise)			
Pfeiffer			
California French, 2 Tbsp	140	12	9
French	150	13	7
Honey Dijon	140	13	6
Lite Italian	50	5	3
Ranch	180	20	1
Savory Italian	110	12	3
Thousand Island	140	14	4
Pritikin			
Dijon Balsamic; Zesty Italian	30	0	6
Honey Dijon	45	0	11
Honey French Style	40	0	10
Raspberry	35	0	11
Ralph's Chef Express			
Blue Cheese, 2 Tbsp	170	18	1
Lite Ranch	90	8	3

Per 2 Tbsp (Approx 1 oz)

	C	F	Cb
Red Wing			
Chunky Blue Cheese, 2 Tbsp	130	13	3
Creamy Ranch	150	15	2
French Tradit'nal; Spicy Sw. French	130	11	8
Italian Traditional	100	9	4
"K" Dressing	140	14	8
Thousand Island	110	9	8
San-J			
Fat Free: Honey Curry, 2 Tbsp	25	0	6
Tamari Mustard	25	0	5
Thai Peanut (lowfat)	50	2.5	7
S & W			
Light: Oriental Rice Wine, 2 Tbsp	30	0	7
Red Wine Vinegar Herb	40	0	10
Low Calorie Range: Blue Cheese	50	4	4
Creamy Cucumber; Thousand Island	50	4	4
Creamy Italian	20	2	2
French	35	0	6
Italian No-Oil	4	0	0
Russian	50	2	8
Seven Seas			
Regular Dressings			
Chunky Blue	90	7	5
Creamy Caesar	140	15	1
Creamy Italian	110	12	1
Green Goddess	120	13	1
Herbs & Spices	120	12	1
Ranch	150	16	2
Red Wine Vin. & Oil; Viva Italian	110	11	2
Two Cheese Italian	70	7	3
Viva Caesar	120	12	2
Viva Russian	150	16	3
Free (Fat-Free): Italian	10	0	2
Ranch	50	0	12
Red Wine Vinegar	15	0	3
Reduced Calorie:			
Crmy Italian; Red Wine Vin. & Oil	60	5	2
Italian w./Olive Oil	50	5	2
Ranch	100	9	5
Viva Italian	45	4	2
Spike Splashes!			
Original, 2 Tbsp	100	11	1
Salt Free	100	10	2
Fat Free	10	0	2

Per 2 Tbsp (Approx 1 oz) — **C** **F** **Cb**

Spectrum

	C	F	Cb
Fat Free: Creamy Dill	25	0	4
Creamy Garlic	20	0	4
Sweet Onion & Garlic; Tstd Sesame	15	0	3
Lowfat: Blue Cheese Style	35	2	3
Creamy Roasted Pepper	45	2	5
Honey Dijon	35	2	5
Mango Madness	50	2	7
Southwestern Caesar	40	2	3
Zesty Italian	30	2	1

The Spice Hunter
Mix: ~ As Prepared, Per 2 Tbsp

	C	F	Cb
Caesar Salad, 2 Tbsp	150	13	1
Chinese Salad	140	12	2
Garlic & Herb	140	13	2

Tree of Life

	C	F	Cb
House Dressing: Cafe Venice	120	12	2
Maison Caesar	70	6	1
Shanghai Palace	80	7	3
Lowfat Free: Blue Cheese	15	1	2
Fat Free: Honey French	35	0	8
Italian Garlic	20	0	4
Oriental Ginger	15	0	3

Walden Farms
Fat Free, Calorie Free Range

	C	F	Cb
Average All Types, 2 Tbsp	0	0	0

Weight Watchers
Salad Celebrations Dressings

	C	F	Cb
Fat Free: Caesar (Single), 0.75 oz	5	0	1
Caesar, 2 Tbsp	10	0	1
Creamy Italian (8 oz), 2 Tbsp	30	0	7
French Style, 2 Tbsp	40	0	9
Honey Dijon, 2 Tbsp	45	0	11
Italian (8 oz), 2 Tbsp	10	0	2
Ranch Style, 2 Tbsp	35	0	7
Ranch (Single), 0.75 oz	25	0	6

Wishbone

	C	F	Cb
Vinaigrette: Berry	50	4.5	2
Roast Garlic	60	5	3
Sun-dried Tomato	50	5	2
Robusto Italian	90	8	4
Russian: Regular	110	6	15
Thousand Island: Regular	130	12	7
Lite	80	5	8
Thousand Island	35	0	9

Per 2 Tbsp (Approx 1 oz) — **C** **F** **Cb**

Wishbone (Cont)

	C	F	Cb
Chunky Blue Cheese: Regular	170	17	2
Lite	80	8	3
Caesar	110	10	2
Italian	35	2	5
Classic House Italian	140	14	2
Classic Lite Olive Oil	40	4	2
Creamy Caesar	180	18	1
Creamy Italian	110	12	4
Fat Free: Caesar	25	0	5
Honey Dijon	45	0	10
Italian	15	0	2
Parmesan - Onion	45	0	9
Ranch	40	0	9
Red Wine Vinaigrette	40	0	7
French: Lite	60	3	8
Fat-Free	12	0	2
Sweet 'N Spicy; Red French	140	12	6
Lite	35	0	8
Italian: Regular	80	8	3
Lite	15	0.5	3
Italian Cream Lite	50	4	4
Olive Oil Vinaigrette	60	5	4
Parmesan - Onion	110	10	4
Ranch: Regular	160	17	2
Lite	100	8	5
Just Too Good!: Blue Cheese	45	2	6
Classic Caesar, 2 Tbsp	40	2	5
Creamy Caesar	40	2	7
Country Italian	30	2	3
Honey Dijon	50	2	8
Italian	35	2	5
Ranch	40	2	5
Thousand Island	60	2	9

HELP! THE DOOR'S JAMMED! — WORSE! THE LIFT'S FALLING! — WORSE STILL, I'M ON A HIGH FIBER DIET!!

Quick Guide — Cooked Cereals

Food	C	F	Cb
Buckwheat Groats, roasted:			
Dry, 1/2 cup, 3 oz	280	2	60
Cooked, 1 cup, 7 oz	180	1	39
Bulgar: Dry, 1/2 cup, 2 1/2 oz	240	1	53
Cooked, 1 cup 6 1/2 oz	150	<1	34
Corn/Hominy Grits:			
Dry, 1/4 cup, 1.4 oz	145	<1	33
3 Tbsp, 1 oz	110	<1	25
Cooked, 3/4 cup, 6 1/2 oz	110	<1	25
Instant, 1 pkt, 0.8 oz	80	<1	18
w. Imitation Bacon Bits, 1 oz	100	<1	22
Cream of Rice, ckd, 3/4 c, 6 oz	90	0	20
Cream of Wheat:			
Regular, ckd, 3/4 cup, 6 oz	180	<1	37
Quick, ckd, 3/4 cup, 6 oz	95	<1	20
Instant, ckd, 3/4 cup, 6 oz	110	<1	23
Farina: Cooked, 3/4 cup, 6 oz	85	0	18
Millet, dry, 1/4 cup, 1 oz	100	0	20
Oat Bran: Raw, 1/3 cup, 1 oz	75	2	14
Cooked, 1/2 cup	45	<1	8
Oatmeal: Dry, 1/3 cup, 1 oz	110	0	19
Regular, ckd, 3/4 cup, 6 oz	110	2	19
1 cup, 8 oz	145	3	25
Instant: Regular, aver., 1 oz	100	2	18
Flavored, average	150	2	32
Quaker: *See Brands*			
Wheat Hearts, 1 oz dry, 3/4 c. ckd	110	1	21

Brans, Wheatgerm, Add-Ons

Food	C	F	Cb
Bran: Wheat, unprocessed,			
1 Tbsp, 3g	10	0	3
Rice Bran, raw, 1 Tbsp, 5g	16	1	2.5
1/3 cup, 1 oz	90	6	14
Oat Bran, 1 Tbsp, 5g	15	<1	3
1/3 cup, 1 oz	75	2	15
Wheat Germ, 1 Tbsp, 1/4 oz	25	1	3.5
1/4 cup, 1 oz	105	3	15
Fruit: Dried, average, 1 oz	80	0	21
Banana, 1/2 medium	50	0	23
Prunes in Syrup, 5, 3 oz	90	0	24
Honey: 1 Tbsp, 3/4 oz	65	0	17
Lecithin Granules, 1 Tbsp, 10g	50	5	1
Nuts: Almonds, 6 (1/4 oz)	40	4	5
Bee Pollen Granules, 1 T., 8g	25	1	2
Psyllium Husks, 1 Tbsp, 5g	10	0	1

Quick Guide — Cold Cereals

Average All Brands

Food	C	F	Cb
Bran (processed), 1/3 cup, 1 oz	70	<1	16
Bran Flakes, 3/4 cup, 1 oz	90	<1	21
Corn Flakes, 1 cup, 1 oz	110	<1	24
Granola, 1/4 cup, 1 oz	130	4	21
Oat Bran Cereal, 1/3 cup, 1 oz	110	1	22
Puffed Rice, 1 cup, 1/2 oz	55	0	12
Puffed Wheat, 1 cup, 1/2 oz	55	0	12
Raisin Bran, 1/2 cup, 1 oz	85	<1	20
Rice Crisps, 1 cup, 1 oz	110	1	25
Shredded Wheat, 1 bisc., 3/4 oz	80	<1	18
Sugar-frosted Flakes, 3/4 c, 1 oz	110	<1	26
Wheat Flakes, 1 cup, 1 oz	105	<1	23

Ready-To-Eat

Food	C	F	Cb
Alpen Swiss			
Original, 2 oz	200	3	41
No Added Sugar, 2 oz	200	3	40
Arrowhead			
Amaranth, 1 cup, 1.2oz	130	1	23
Bran Flakes, 1 cup, 1 oz	90	1	21
Corn Flakes, 1 cup, 1.2 oz	130	0	30
Kamut Flakes, 1 cup, 1.1 oz	110	1	25
Maple Buckwheat Flake, 1 c., 1.5 oz	160	1	35
Multi Grain Flakes, 1 cup, 1.2 oz	140	1.5	29
Nature O's, 1 cup, 1.1 oz	130	2	24
Oat Bran Flakes, 1 cup, 1.2 oz	140	2.5	24
Puffed Corn/Rice, aver., 1 c., 0.8 oz	60	0.5	12
Puffed Kamut, 1 cup, 0.6 oz	50	0	11
Puffed Millet/Wheat, 1 cup, 0.5 oz	60	0.5	12
Raisin Bran, 1 cup, 2 oz	190	1.5	40
Rice Flakes, 1 cup, 1.7 oz	80	1	19
Shredded Wheat, 1 cup, 2 oz	200	1	44
Spelt Flakes, 1 cup, 1.1 oz	100	0.5	23
Sweetened Nature O's, 1 c., 1.5 oz	160	2.5	31
Wild Wheat Flakes, 1 cup, 1.5 oz	160	0.5	37
Betty Crocker: Scooby Doo! 25g	80	0	21
Breadshop: Granola, 1/2 c. 1.7 oz	220	7.5	32
Cinnamon Grins, 3/4 cup, 1 oz	110	0.5	25
Crispy Rice'n Corn Flakes, 3/4 c., 1 oz	110	0	26
Health Nuggets, 1/2 cup	170	1	38
Kamut 'n Honey, 1/2 cup	120	3	23
Puffs 'n Honey, 3/4 cup, 1 oz	120	3	21

Ready-To-Eat (Cont)

Barbara's Bakery	C	F	Cb
Breakfast O's, 1 cup, 1 oz	120	2	22
Brown Rice Crisps, 1 cup, 1 oz	120	1	26
Cinnamon Puffins, 3/4 cup, 1 oz	100	1	26
Corn Flakes, all types, 1 cup, 1 oz	110	0	26
Fruity Punch, 1 cup, 1 oz	110	0.5	26
Organic Ultra Minis, 3/4 cup, 2 oz	190	1	46
Shredded Oats, 1 1/4 cup, 2 oz	220	2.5	46
Shredded Puffins, 3/4 cup, 1 oz	90	1	23
Shredded Spoonfuls, 3/4 cup	120	1.5	23
Shredded Wheat, 2 bisc., 1.4 oz	140	1	31
Stars: Cocoa/Honey Crunch, 1 c., 1oz	110	0.5	26
Toasted O's, average, 3/4 cup	120	2	24
Cap'n Crunch: All types, 3/4 cup	110	2	22
Chex: Corn, 1 1/4 cup, 1 oz	110	0	26
Wheat, 3/4 cup, 1.8 oz	190	1	41
Country Inn			
Green Gables Inn, 1/2 cup, 1.8 oz	210	7	36
Greyfield Inn, 3/4 cup, 1.8 oz	210	5	39
Inn at Ormsby Hill, 1 cup, 2.1 oz	220	2.5	48
Dr McDougall's			
Oatmeal & Wheat, 1 cup, 2.4 oz	220	2	57
Oatmeal & 4 Grains, 1 cup, 2.3 oz	210	1.5	52
Dominick's: Corn Flakes, 1 1/4 cup	120	0	27
Crispy Corn & Rice, 1 1/4 cup, 1 oz	120	0	26
Crispy Rice, 1 1/4 cup, 1 oz	130	0	28
Frosted Flakes, 3/4 cup, 1 oz	120	0	28
Fruit Rings, 3/4 cup, 1 oz	100	1	23
Tasteeos, 1 1/4 cup, 1 oz	120	2	24
Erewhon, Per 1 oz: Crisp Brn Rice	110	1	24
Aztec; Raisin Bran; Super O's	100	0	24
Fruit 'n Wheat	100	1	21
Wheat Flakes	100	0	22
Estee: Corn Flakes, 1 oz pkg	90	0	21
Raisin Bran, 1 oz pkg	90	1	24
Familia: Muesli, 1/2 cup, 2.1 oz	210	3	45
No Added Sugar, 1/2 cup	200	3	41
Glenny's: Maple Frosted Corn, 1 oz	110	0	20
Oat/Rice Mini Puffs, 1 oz	110	0	21

General Mills	C	F	Cb
Basic 4, 1 cup, 1 oz	100	1.5	21
Body Buddies; Boo Berry 1 c, 1 oz	120	1	26
Cheerios: Regular, 1 cup, 1 oz	110	2	22
Apple Cinnamon, 3/4 c., 1 oz	120	2	25
Frosted; Team, 1 cup, 1 oz	120	1	25
Honey Nut, 1 cup, 1 oz	120	1.5	24
Multi-Grain, 1 cup, 1 oz	110	1	24
Chex: Corn, 1 cup, 1 oz	110	0	26
Honey Nut, 3/4 cup, 1 oz	120	0.5	26
Multi-Bran, 1 cup, 2 oz	200	1.5	49
Rice, 1 1/4 cup, 1 oz	120	0	27
Wheat, 1 cup, 2 oz	180	1	41
Cinnamon Grahams, 3/4 c., 1 oz	120	1	26
Cinnamon Tst Crunch, 3/4 c., 1 oz	130	3.5	24
Cocoa Puffs, 1 cup, 1 oz	120	1	27
Cookie Crisp; Count Choc, 1 c., 1 oz	120	1	26
Count Chocula, 1 cup, 1 oz	120	1	26
Country Corn Flakes, 1 c., 1 oz	120	0	26
Crispy Wheaties 'N Rais., 1 c., 2 oz	190	1	45
Fiber One, 1/2 cup, 1 oz	60	1	24
Frankenberry, 1 cup, 1 oz	120	1	27
French Toast Crunch, 3/4 c., 1 oz	120	1.5	26
Golden Grahams, 3/4 cup, 1 oz	120	1	26
Grand Slams, 1 cup, 1 oz	120	1	27
Honey Nut Clusters, 1 cup, 2 oz	210	2	47
Jurrasic Park Crunch, 1 cup, 1 oz	120	1	26
Kaboom, 1 1/4 cup, 1 oz	120	1.5	24
Kix, 1 1/3 cup, 1 oz	120	0.5	26
Berry Berry, 3/4 cup, 1 oz	120	1.5	26
Lucky Charms, 1 cup, 1 oz	120	1	25
NesQuik Choc Puff, 3/4 cup, 1 oz	120	2	25
Oatmeal Crisp Almond, 1 c., 2 oz	220	5	41
Apple Cinn.; Raisin, 1 cup, 2 oz	210	2	44
Raisin Nut Bran, 3/4 cup, 2 oz	200	4	41
Reese's P'nut Butter Puffs, 3/4 cup	130	3	24
Sunrise, 1/2 cup, 1 oz	110	0.5	26
Total Corn Flakes, 1 1/3 cup, 1 oz	110	0	26
Total Raisin Bran, 1 cup, 2 oz	180	1	43
Total Whole Grain, 3/4 cup, 1 oz	110	1	24
Trix, 1 cup, 1 oz	120	1.5	26
Vanilla Almond Oat, 1 1/4 c., 2 oz	200	1	44
Wheaties: 1 cup, 1 oz	110	1	24
Energy Crunch, 1 cup, 1.95 oz	210	3	42
Honey Frosted, 3/4 cup, 1 oz	110	0	27
Raisin Bran, 1 cup, 2 oz	180	1	44

Ready-To-Eat (Cont)

	C	F	Cb
Hansen's Natural *Per 1/2 cup, 2 oz*			
Orange & Chocolate Cereal	230	9	35
Strawb. & Yogurt Cereal	230	9	30
Roasted Nut Crunch Cereal	230	6	39
Tropical Cluster Cereal	210	5	36
Health Valley			
98% Fat Free Granola, 2/3 cup	180	1	43
Amaranth Flakes, 3/4 cup	100	0	24
Bran Cereal (w. Fruit), 3/4 cup	160	0	40
Corn Bran Flakes, 3/4 cup	100	0	24
Fiber 7 Flakes (100% Orig.), 3/4 c.	100	0	24
Golden Flax, 1/4 cup	190	3	38
Granola O's, all types, 3/4 cup	120	0	26
Healthy Crunches & Flakes, 3/4 cup	130	0	31
Healthy Fiber Flakes, 3/4 cup	100	0	23
Hot Cups: Apple; 10 Grain, 1 pkt	220	2.5	42
Maple; Banana, 1 pkt	240	2.5	44
Oat Bran Flakes, all types, 3/4 c.	105	0	26
Oat Bran/10 Bran O's, 3/4 cup	100	0	23
Puffed: Honey Sweetened, 1 cup	110	0	28
Raisin Bran Flakes, 1 1/4 cup	190	0	47
Real Oat Bran, 1/2 cup	200	3	34
Healthy Choice			
M/grain Raisin & Almond, 3/4 c., 1 oz	100	1	22
Flakes, 1 cup, 1.1 oz	100	0	26
Heartland			
Granola: Lowfat, 1/2 cup, 2 oz	210	3	40
Original; Raisin, 1/2 cup, 2 1/4 oz	300	11	41
Kashi			
Breakfast Pilaf, 1/2 c., ckd, 5 oz	170	3	30
GoLEAN Crunch!, 1 cup, 1.8 oz	190	3	36
Honey Puffed Kashi, 1 cup, 1 oz	120	1	25
Kashi Go, 1/2 cup, 5 oz	270	3	59
Kashi GoLEAN, 3/4 cup, 1.4 oz	120	1	28
Kashi Good Friends, 3/4 cup, 1 oz	90	1	24
Kashi Medley, 1/2 cup, 1 oz	100	1	20
Kashi Pillows, 3/4 cup, 2 oz	200	1	45
Puffed Kashi, 1 cup, 0.9 oz	70	0.5	13
Keebler			
Apple Cinnamon, 1/4 cup	120	6	19
Peanut Butter, 1/4 cup, 1 oz	150	7	18

	C	F	Cb
Kellogg's			
Apple Jacks, 1 cup, 1 oz	120	0	30
All-Bran, 1/2 cup, 1 oz	80	1	24
Bran Buds, 1/3 cup, 1 oz	80	0.5	16
with Extra Fiber, 1/2 cup, 1 oz	50	1	20
Apple Cinn. Rice Krispies, 3/4 c.	110	0	26
Apple Cinn. Squares, 3/4 c., 2 oz	180	1	44
Apple Raisin Crisp, 1/2 cup, 1 oz	90	0	23
Cinnamon Mini Buns, 3/4 cup	120	0.5	27
Complete Oatbran Flakes, 3/4 cup	110	0.5	23
Wheatbran Flakes, 3/4 cup	90	0.5	23
Cocoa Krispies, 3/4 cup	120	1	27
Common Sense O/Bran, 3/4 cup	110	1	23
Corn Flakes, 1 cup, 1 oz	110	0	24
Honey Flakes, 1 cup, 1 oz	120	1	26
Corn Pops, 1 cup, 1 oz	120	0	28
Cracklin' Oat Bran, 3/4 cup, 2 oz	190	7	35
Crispix, 1 cup, 1 oz	110	0	25
Double Dip Crunch, 3 3/4 cup	110	0	26
Froot Loops: 1 cup	120	1	28
other types, 1 cup, 1 oz	120	1	28
Frosted: Flakes, 3/4 cup, 1 oz	120	0	28
Mini-Wheats: 3/4 cup, 1.8 oz	180	1	42
Bite Size, 1 cup, 1.8 oz	200	1	48
Fruity Marshmallow Krispies, 3/4 c.	110	0	25
Healthy Choice:			
Lowfat Granola, 1 cup, 2.2 oz	220	3	48
Müeslix, 2/3 cup, 2 oz	200	3	41
Just Right, 1 cup, 2 oz	210	2	48
Low Fat Granola: 1/2 cup, 2 oz	190	3	39
w. Raisins, 2/3 cup, 2 oz	220	3	47
Mini Wheats:			
Raisin Squares, 3/4 cup, 1.8 oz	180	1	42
Strawberry Squares, 3/4 c., 1.8 oz	170	1	40
Frosted, 3/4 cup, 1.8 oz	180	1	41
Frosted Bite Size, 1 cup, 2 oz	200	1	48
Müeslix: Apple & Almond, 3/4 c.	200	5	39
Raisin & Almond, 2/3 cup	200	3	40
Nut & Honey Crunch, 1 1/4 c., 2 oz	220	2.5	46
Nutri-Grain: Almond, 1 1/4 c., 2 oz	180	3	38
Golden Wheat, 3/4 cup, 1 oz	100	1	23
Twists, 1 bar, 1.3 oz	140	3	26
Pokèmon, 1 cup, 1 oz	110	0.5	25
Pop Tarts: Lowfat, each, average	190	3	39
Toaster Pastries, average, 1 oz	210	6	37
Mini Pastries, aver., 1 pouch	170	7	31
Pastry Swirls, 2.2 oz	260	11	37
Snak Stix, 1 pastry, 1.8 oz	190	4	37

Breakfast Cereals (Cont)

Kellogg's (Cont)

	C	F	Cb
Product 19, 1 cup, 1 oz	100	0	25
Raisin Bran, 1 cup, 2 oz	190	1.5	45
Raisin Bran Crunch, 1cup, 1.9 oz	190	1	44
Rice Krispies: 1 1/4 cup	120	0	29
Treats, 3/4 cup	120	1.5	26
Bars: Original, 1 bar	90	2	18
Caramel/Peanut Butter, (1)	110	4	19
Double Choc Chunk, (1)	100	4.5	15
Scotcheroos, (1)	120	5	18
Smacks, 3/4 cup, 1 oz	100	0	24
Smart Start: Soy Protein, 1 cup	200	1.5	40
Original, 1 cup, 1.8 oz	180	0.5	43
Special K, 1 cup, 1.1 oz	110	0	23
Special K Red Berries, 1 cup, 1 oz	150	0	25
Special K Plus, 1 cup	210	2	47
Wheat Chex, 1 cup	170	1	38

Nabisco

	C	F	Cb
100% Bran, 1/3 cup, 1 oz	70	1	21
Cocoa Blasts, 1 cup	130	1	29
Cream of Wheat: All types, 1 pkg	150	1.5	32
Fruit Wheats, 1/2 cup, 1 oz	90	0	23
Shredded Wheat: 1 biscuit	80	0.5	19
Spoon size, 2/3 cup	90	1	23
Shredded Wheat'n Bran, 2/3 cup	90	0	23
Shredd. Wheat w. Oatbran, 1 oz	100	1	22
Toaster Pastry, 1.7 oz ea., average	190	5	34
Team Flakes, 3/4 cup	110	0	24

Nature's Path:

	C	F	Cb
Corn Flakes, 3/4 c.	115	0.5	26
Heritage: all varieties, 3/4 c., 1 oz	115	0	24
Heritage Muesli, 1/2 cup, 2 oz	215	3	41
Honey'd Raisin Bran, 3/4 cup, 1 oz	110	0	25
Millet Rice, 3/4 cup, 1 oz	120	1	25
Multigrain, 2/3 cup, 1 oz	110	0.5	24

New Morning

	C	F	Cb
Bran Flakes; Crispy Rice, 1 c., 1 oz	110	1	23
Cocoa Crispy Rice, 1 cup, 2.1 oz	210	1.5	45
Corn/Honey Frost. Flakes, 1 c., 1 oz	120	1	25
Ginky O's; Orig. Otios, 1 c., 1 oz	120	1	25
Granola Clusters, 3/4 c., 1.9 oz	200	2	42
Otiola: Blueberry, 1 cup, 1.9 oz	200	1.5	41
Otios: Cocoa, 1 cup, 1.76 oz	170	1.5	21
Apple Cinnamon, 1 cup, 1 oz	90	1.5	22
Honey Almond, 1 cup, 1 oz	100	1	21
Original, 1 cup, 1 oz	120	1	21
Raisin Bran, 1 cup, 30g	90	0.5	21
Ultimate Oat Bran Flakes, 1 c., 28g	110	1	21

Post

	C	F	Cb
Alpha Bits, 1 cup	110	1	2.
Blueberry Morning, 1 cup	220	3	4.
Cranberry Almond Crunch, 1 cup	220	3	4.
Cocoa Pebbles, 7/8 cup	115	1	2.
Great Grains, 2/3 cup, 1.8 oz	200	6	3.
Fruit & Fibre, 1 cup, 2 oz	210	3	4.
Fruity Pebbles, 1 1/4 cup	130	1.5	2.
Grape Nut 'O's, 1 cup, 1.1 oz	120	0	2.
Grape Nuts; Raisin, 1/2 cup, 2 oz	200	1	4.
Honey Bunches of Oats, 3/4 cup	120	1.5	2.
Honeycomb, 1 cup	90	0.5	2.
Natural Bran Flakes, 2/3 cup	90	0	2.
Oreo O's, 3/4 cup	110	2.5	2.
Raisin Bran, 2/3 cup, 1.4 oz	120	1	3.
Shredded Wheat: Frosted, 1 cup	190	1	4.
Big Biscuit, 2 biscuits	160	1	3.
Honey Nut, 1 cup, 1.8 oz	200	1.5	4.
Spoon Size, 1 cup	170	1	4.
Toasties Corn Flakes, 1 cup	90	0	2.
Waffle Crisp, 1 cup	130	3	2.

Quaker

	C	F	Cb
Breakfast/Cereal Bars: each	130	3	2.
Ready to Eat: Oat Bran, 1 1/4 cup	210	3	4.
100% Natural Granola, 1/2 cup	220	9	3.
Lowfat, 2/3 cup	210	3	4.
w. Raisins, 1/2 cup	230	9	3.
Cap'n Crunch: Regular, 3/4 c., 1 oz	110	2	2.
Crunch Berries, 3/4 cup, 1 oz	110	2	2.
Peanut Butter Crunch, 1 oz	110	3	2.
Crunchy Corn Bran, 1 cup, 1 oz	90	1	2.
Honey Graham Oh's, 3/4 cup	110	2	2.
Life, all types, 1 oz	120	1.5	2.
Oatmeal Squares, 1 cup, 1.8 oz	230	3	4.
Oats Honey & Raisin, 1/2 c., 1.8 oz	230	9	3.
Lowfat, 1 cup, 1.8 oz	210	3	4.
Puffed Rice, 1 cup, 1/2 oz	50	0	1.
Puffed Wheat, 1 cup, 1/2 oz	55	0	1.
Quisp, 1 cup, 1 oz	110	1.5	2.
Shredded Wheat, 3 bisc.	220	1.5	5.
Toasted Oatmeal, 1 cup	190	2.5	3.
Unprocessed Bran, 1/3 cup	30	0	1.
Bagged: Cocoa Blasts, 1 cup	130	1	2.
Apple Zaps; Fruity O's, 1 cup	120	1	2.
Frosted Flakers, 3/4 cup	120	0	2.
Frosted/Honey Nut Oats, 1 cup	110	1	2.
Frosted Oats/ Sweet Crunch, 1 cup	110	1.5	2.
Fruitangy Oh's, 1 cup	120	1	2.

Quaker (Cont)

	C	F	Cb
Jagged (Cont): Rice Crisps, 1 cup	110	0	26
Honey Crisp Corn Flakes, 3/4 cup	110	0	27
Honey Dipps, 1 1/4 cup	130	1.5	28
Grits: *Per Packet*			
Regular: All types, aver., 1/4 cup	130	0.5	31
Instant: All types, average	100	1	22
Quick'n Hearty *(Microwave Oatmeal): Per Pkt*			
Regular, 1 oz	110	2	19
App.Spice; Cinnamon Dble Raisin	170	2	35
Br.Sugar Cinnamon; Honey Bran	150	2	30
Instant Quaker Oatmeal: *Per Pkt*			
Oatmeal: Regular, 1 oz	100	2	19
Baked Apple, 1.4 oz	150	1.5	31
Cinn. Roll; Fr. Vanilla, 1 1/2 oz	160	2	33
Cookie Blast, average, 1 1/2 oz	160	2.5	32
Honey Nut, 1 1/2 oz	170	3.5	31
Maple/Br.Sug; Rais./Spice	160	2	33
Raisin/Date/Walnut, 1 1/4 oz	140	2	27
Dinosaur Eggs, 1.76 oz pkt	190	3.5	38
Kid's Choice: 1 pkt, aver., 1 1/2 oz	160	2.5	32
Nutrition For Women, 1 pkt	170	2	33
Sea Adventures, 1 pkt, 1 1/2 oz	190	4	37
Treasure Hunt, 1.65 oz	170	2	36
Quaker/Hot: Multigrain, 1/2 cup	130	1.5	29
Oat Bran, 1/2 cup	150	3	25
Whole Wheat Hot Nat. 1/2 cup	130	1	30
Oats: Quick; Old Fash., Steel, 1/2 c.	150	3	27

Sun Country Granola

	C	F	Cb
Almond, 1/2 c.	270	9	38
w. Raisins & Dates, 1/2 cup	260	8	43

Ralston

	C	F	Cb
Bran Flakes, 3/4 c., 1 oz	110	1	24
Chex Multi Bran, 1 1/4 cup, 2 oz	220	2	46
Cocoa Crispy Rice, 1 c., 1 3/4 oz	200	1	45
Cookie Crisp, 1 cup	120	2	25
Frosted Flakes, 3/4 cup, 1 oz	120	0	28
Hot Ralston, 1/2 cup, 1.5 oz	150	1	31
Muesli: Blueberry, 1 cup, 2 oz	200	3	41
Cranberry, 3/4 cup, 2 oz	200	3	40
Strawberry, 1 cup, 2 oz	210	3	41
Raisin Bran, 3/4 cup, 2 oz	190	1	41
Sun Flakes, 3/4 cup	110	1	30
Tasteeos, 1 1/4 cup, 1 oz	130	3	22
Stone-Buhr: Bran, 1/4 c., 0.5 oz	65	0	14
Grain, 1/3 cup, 1 1/2 oz	140	2	31
Uncle Sam: Wheat/Flaxseed, 1 c.	190	5	38

Grains & Flours

Per 1/2 Cup (8 level Tbsp)

	C	F	Cb
Amaranth, 1/2 cup, 3 1/2 oz	350	6	60
Arrowroot, 1/2cup, 2 1/4 oz	230	0	57
Barley: Regular, 1/2 cup, 3 1/4 oz	325	2	56
Pearled, raw, 3 1/2 oz	350	1	78
Flakes, 1/2 cup, 1 1/2 oz	150	0.5	33
Buckwheat: Regular, 1/2 c., 3 oz	290	3	61
Groats, roasted, dry, 3 oz	285	2	60
Roasted, cooked, 3 1/2 oz	90	0.5	19
Flour, whole-groat	200	2	42
Bulgur: Dry, 1/2 cup, 2 1/2 oz	240	1	54
Cooked, 1/2 cup, 4 oz	75	0.5	17
Carob Flour, 1/2 cup, 1.8 oz	95	0.5	25
Corn kernels (blue/yellow), 3 oz	300	4	66
Corn Bran, 1/2 cup, 1.4 oz	85	0.5	32
Corn Flour/Masa, 2 oz	210	2	44
Corn Grits: Dry, 1/2 cup, 2 3/4 oz	290	1	62
Cooked, 1/2 cup, 4 1/4 oz	75	0.5	16
Corn Germ, toasted	245	13	21
Cornmeal: Average All Types			
3 Tbsp, 1 oz	100	0.5	22
1/2 oz, 2.2 oz	220	2	46
Mixes: same as above	220	2	46
Cornstarch: 1 Tbsp, 8g	30	0	7
Cooked, 1/2 cup, 2 1/4 oz	230	0	57
Couscous: Dry, 3 1/4 oz	345	0	72
Cooked, 4.1 oz	60	0	12
Farina: Dry, 3 oz	325	0	70
Cooked, 4.1 oz	60	0	13
Flax Seeds, 2 oz	280	20	22
Garbanzo (Chick Pea), 1/2 c., 2 oz	200	3	35
Kuzu Root Starch, 1 Tbsp, 10g	35	0	8
Matzo Meal, 1/2 cup	260	1	55
Millet: raw, 1/2 cup, 3 1/2 oz	375	4	76
Cooked, 1/2 cup, 4 1/4 oz	145	1	29
Oat Bran: Raw, 1/2 cup, 1.7 oz	115	2	31
Cooked, 1/2 cup, 4 oz	115	1	33
Oats, rolled/oatmeal:			
Dry/Groats, 1/2 cup, 1.5 oz	155	3	28
Cooked, 1/2 cup, 4.2 oz	75	1	13
Polenta: See Cornmeal			
Made Up, 1/2 cup, 5 oz	220	2	24
Potato flour, 1/2 cup, 3.2 oz	315	0	72
Psyllium Husks, 1 Tbsp (5g)	10	0	2
Quinoa, 1/2 cup, 3 oz	320	5	53
Eden, 1/2 cup, 3 oz	340	5	62
Rice ~ *See Next Page*			

Grains & Flours (Cont)

	C	F	Cb
Rice Bran, 1/3 cup, 1 oz	90	6	14
Rice Flour, 1/2 cup, 2 3/4 oz	290	2	63
Rice Polish, 1/2 cup	220	7	39
Rye Grains:			
1/2 cup, 3 oz	280	2	59
Flakes, 1/2 cup, 1 1/2 oz	150	0.5	32
Flour, dark, 2 1/4 oz	210	2	44
Medium light, 1.8 oz	185	1	40
Semolina, 1/2 cup, 3 oz	305	1	61
Sorghum, 1/2 cup, 3.4 oz	325	3	72
Soybean Flakes, 1/2 cup, 1 1/2 oz	190	8	14
Soy Flour, 1/2 cup, 2 oz	250	11	18
Tapioca, pearl, Dry: 1/2 c., 2.7 oz	260	0	67
3 Tbsp, 1 oz	100	0	26
Teff (Seed) Flour, 2 oz	200	0.5	41
Tortilla Flour Mix, 1/2 cup, 2 oz	225	12	37
Triticale, 1/2 cup, 3.4 oz	325	2	70
flour, whole-grain, 1/2 cup	220	1	47
Wheat: Average, 1/2 cup, 3 1/2 oz	320	2	28
Wheat Bran, unproc., 1/2 c., 1 oz	65	1	20
Wheat Flakes, 1/2 cup, 1 1/2 oz	160	0.5	32
Wheat Germ: Crude, 2 oz	200	8	29
toasted, 1/2 cup, 2 oz	215	12	28
Wheat Flour: Whole grain, 2.1 oz	205	1	44
White, all types, 1/2 c., 2.2 oz	220	0.5	46

Also See *Arrowhead Mills Cereals* ~ Page 88

Brown Rice

Average Short or Long Grain

	C	F	Cb
Raw/Dry: 1/2 cup, 3 1/2 oz	350	2.5	73
1 cup, 7 oz	700	5	144
Cooked: Hot, 1/2 cup, 3 1/2 oz	110	0.5	23
1 cup, 7 oz	220	1.5	46
Cold, 1/2 cup, 2 1/2 oz	90	0.5	19

White Rice

	C	F	Cb
Raw: Short/Med. Grain, 1 c., 7 oz	720	1	156
Long Grain, 1 cup, 6 1/2 oz	670	1	144
Glutinous, 1 cup, 6 1/2 oz	680	1	150
Cooked (Boiled/Steamed):			
Short/Medium Grain:			
Hot, 1/2 cup, 3 1/4 oz	120	0	27
1 cup, 6 1/2 oz	240	0.5	54
Cold, 1/2 cup, 2 3/4 oz	90	0	20
Long Grain: Hot, 1/2 c., 2 3/4 oz	100	0	22
1 cup, 5 1/2 oz	200	0.5	44
Cold, 1/2 cup, 2 1/2 oz	80	0	20
Glutinous/Sticky, ckd 1 c., 6 oz	170	0.5	36
Parboiled, ckd, hot, 1/2 c., 3 oz	90	0	20
Precook./Instant: Dry, 1/2 c., 3 1/2 oz	370	0	80
Cooked, hot, 1/2 c., 3 oz	90	0	20
Wild Rice: Raw, 1 cup, 5 1/2 oz	570	13	120
Cooked, hot, 1 cup, 5 3/4 oz	165	0.5	35

Rice Dishes

	C	F	Cb
Chinese Fried Rice: 1/2 c., 2 1/2 oz	160	5	21
1 cup, 5 oz	320	13	42
2 cups, 10 oz	640	26	84
Mexican Rice: 1 cup	500	12	90
Taco Bell, 1 serving	190	10	23
Taco John's, 1 serving	250	18	44
Taco Time, 1 serving	160	2	30
Rice-A-Roni ~ See Page 68			
Rice Pilaf: Restaurant, 1 cup	270	7.5	43
Boston Market, 2/3 cup	180	5	32
Denny's, 1 serving	85	1	17
Sizzler, side serving	260	5	47
Rice w. Raisins/Pinenuts, 1 cup	400	11	70
Risotto, 1 cup	420	18	65
Saffron Rice, 1 cup	370	12	66
Spanish Rice, 1 cup	390	9	72
El Pollo Loco, 1 serving	130	3	20
Sticky Thai Rice, plain, 1 cup	170	0.5	36
Sushi Rice, 1 Tbsp	25	0	

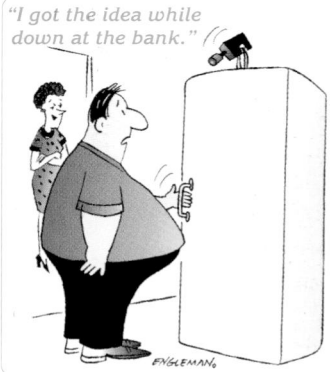

"I got the idea while down at the bank."

ENGLEMAN

Macaroni includes all shapes and sizes;
(e.g. spaghetti, fettuccine, shells, tubes, ziti,
twists, sheets, cannelloni, manicotti, elbows).
All regular macaroni products have
the same cals/fat/carb. on a weight basis.
1oz Dry = approx. 2¹⁄₂ -3 oz cooked.

Dry Spaghetti/Macaroni

	C	F	Cb
oz quantity	105	0.5	21
b box/pkg., 16 oz	1680	7	336
bows, 1 cup, 3³⁄₄ oz	395	2	77
ells, small, 1 cup, 3¹⁄₄ oz	340	2	66
irals, 1 cup, 3 oz	315	2	61

Cooked Spaghetti/Macaroni

	C	F	Cb
ain, All Types (no added fat):			
Firm/Al Dente (8-10 mins.), 1 oz	42	0.5	8.5
Medium (11-13mins.), 1 oz	37	0.5	7.5
Tender (14-20mins.), 1 oz	32	0.5	7
(Longer cooking increases water absorbed)			
aghetti, ¹⁄₂ cup, 2 ¹⁄₂ oz	90	0.5	18
Medium serving, 1 cup, 5 oz	185	1	37
Large (restaurant), 2 c., 10 oz	370	2	74
bows/Spirals, 1 cup, 5 oz	185	1	38
all Shells, 1 cup, 4 oz	150	0.5	31
otein-fortified: Dry, 1 oz	107	0.5	21
Cooked, 1 cup, 5 oz	230	0.5	44
inach/Vegetable: Dry, 1 oz	105	0.5	21
Cooked, 1 cup, 5 oz	180	0.5	37
hole-wheat: Dry, 1 oz	100	0.5	21
Cooked, 1 cup, 5 oz	175	0.5	37

Fresh Pasta (Refrigerated)

	C	F	Cb
ain/Spinach/Tomato, average:			
As purchased, 4 oz	325	2.5	64
Cooked, 1 cup, 5 oz	190	1	38
ome-made, without egg:			
Cooked, 1 cup, 5 oz	175	1	35
uitoni			
ngel Hair, 1¹⁄₄ cup, 3 oz	230	2.5	43
ttuccine/Linguini: 1¹⁄₄ cup, 3 oz	240	2.5	45
Spinach, 1¹⁄₄ cup, 3 oz	260	4	43
avioli: Beef, 1¹⁄₄ cup, 3.6 oz	330	9	46

Buitoni (Cont):	C	F	Cb
Ravioli: Chk., Herb Parm., 1¹⁄₄ c., 3.6oz	310	9	44
Dblestuff. Mozz. Herb, 1¹⁄₂ c., 4 oz	360	12	44
Four Cheese, 1 cup, 3 oz	290	9	38
Light, 1 cup, 3 oz	230	4	37
Garden Vegetable, 1 cup, 3 oz	250	5	39
Mini Beef, 1 cup, 3.5 oz	270	5	44
Rst Chick. & Garlic, 1 c., 4.5 oz	330	11	45
Tortellini: Chse & Rst Garlic 1 c., 3 oz	270	8	38
Chkn & Prosciutto, 1 c., 3.6 oz	360	13	45
Herb Chicken, ³⁄₄ cup, 3 oz	260	7	40
Mozzarella & Herb, 1 c., 3.6 oz	320	9	45
Mushroom & Chse, 1 c., 3.6 oz	290	6	46
Sundried Tomato, 1 cup, 3.6 oz	320	10	46
Sweet Italian Saus., 1 c., 3.6 oz	320	8	49
Three Cheese, ³⁄₄ cup, 3 oz	250	6	39

Noodles

	C	F	Cb
Plain/Egg: Dry, 1 oz	108	1	20
1 cup, 1¹⁄₃ oz	145	1.5	28
Cooked, 1 oz	38	0.5	7
¹⁄₂ cup, 2³⁄₄ oz	105	1	20
1 cup, 5¹⁄₂ oz	210	2	40
Stir-Fried: 1 cup, 5¹⁄₂ oz	270	9	40
2 cup serving, 11 oz	540	18	80
Yolk Free: Cooked, Per Cup			
'No Yolks' (Foulds)	210	2	40
Passover Gold (Manischewitz)	200	0	42
Chinese: Cellophane/Rice, dry, 1 oz	100	0	25
Chow Mein/hard, dry, 1 oz	150	5	17
Ramen Noodles ~ See Page 66			
Japanese: Soba, dry, 1 oz	95	0.5	21
cooked, 1 cup, 4 oz	110	0.5	24
Somen, dry, 1 oz	100	0.5	22
cooked, 1 cup, 6 oz	225	0.5	49
Japanese Style Pan Fried:			
Maruchan's Yaki-Sobu, 1 c., 5.6 oz	260	3	50
Udon (Chikara), aver., 7.5 oz pkt	250	1	52
Stir Fry/Yakisoba, 1 serve, 3.5 oz	220	2	44

Egg Roll Skins/Won Ton

	C	F	Cb
Egg Roll Skins:			
(Golden Dragon) 1 pce, 1 oz	80	0	18
(Wung Hung) 4 skins, 4 oz	300	0	64
Won Ton Wrappers:			
(Dynasty) 10 wrappers, 2.1 oz	170	1	36
Egg Roll/Spring Roll Wrapper:			
(Dynasty) 3 wrappers, 2.1 oz	170	1	36

Breads

Note: All breads have similar calories on a weight basis. However, volume may vary. For example, 1 oz of bread may equal 1 slice regular bread or 2 slices of a lighter bread. It is best to weigh bread used and calculate on 1 oz bread = 70 calories.

Quick Guide

Bread

Average All Varieties:

	C	F	Cb
Thin slice (1/4") 1 oz	70	1	13
Extra thin slice 3/4 oz	55	<1	10
Light thin slice, 0.6 oz	40	<1	7.5
Toasting slice, 1.2 oz	85	1	16
Thick slice (3/8"), 1.5 oz	105	1.5	20
Large thick (1/2"), 2 oz	140	2	26
1-lb Loaf, 16 oz	1120	6	208

Toast has same calories as bread used.

	C	F	Cb
1 thin slice + 1 tsp of fat	105	5	13
1 thick slice (3/8") +2 tsp fat	175	10	20

Breads

	C	F	Cb
Batard (8 oz), 1/4, 2 oz slice	140	0.5	28
Boule, 1/2" thick, 2 oz slice	130	0	29
Bran style, 1 oz slice	70	1	14
Buttermilk, average, 1 oz slice	80	2	13
Caraway Rye, 1 oz slice	70	0	15
Challah, 1 oz slice	85	2	14
Corn Bread, aver., 1 pce., 3 oz	180	7	36
Cracked Wheat Sourdough, 11/2 oz	130	0.5	27
Croutons, 2 Tbsp	35	1	6
Dark Bread, 1 oz slice	70	1	14
Date & Nut, 1 oz slice	90	1	14
'Enriched' Breads, aver., 1 oz sl.	75	1	18
5-Grain Honey Whole Wheat, 1 slice, 11/2 oz	110	1	23
Foccacia: Plain, 2 oz portion	150	4	23
Cheese & Garlic, 2 oz	170	8	21
Pesto, 2 oz	170	6	21
Tomato & Olive, 2 oz	120	2	23
French Stick, 1 oz slice	70	1	15
French Toast, 1 slice, 21/4 oz	160	7	18
Sticks (Aunt Jemima), 1 pce, 1 oz	75	3	12
Garlic Bread, 1 pce. w. fat, 1 oz	125	6	14
Garlic Toast, (Pepp.Farm), 1.4 oz sl.	160	10	15
Italian Bread, 1 oz slice	75	1	15
Light Bread, aver., 0.8 oz slice	40	<1	7.5
1 oz slice	70	1	13
Melba Toast, 2 pces	25	0	6

Breads

	C	F	Cb
MultiGrain: 1 slice, 1 oz	75	1	14
Fat Free, 1 oz	70	0	15
Nut/Health Nut, 1 oz slice	85	2	15
Oatmeal/Oatbran Bread, 1 oz sl.	70	1	13
Party Breads (Pepp. Farm): Rye, 1 sl.	15	<1	3
Dijon; Pumpernickel, 1 sl.	18	<1	3.5
Pita Bread, aver. all types, 2 oz	150	2	30
Mini/Pocket, 1 oz	75	1	15
Poppyseed (Vienna), 0.8 oz sl.	55	1	10
Pumpernickel, 1 oz slice	75	1	15
Cocktail size, 0.4 oz	30	<1	6
Raisin Bread, 1 oz slice	80	1	14
Raisin Walnut, 2 oz slice	160	3.5	29
Roman Meal, 1 oz slice	70	1	14
Country Potato & Oat, 11/2 oz	110	1.5	20
Rye: Average, 1 thin slice, 1 oz	75	1	13
1 thick slice, 2 oz	150	2	25
Cocktail size, 0.4 oz	25	<1	4
Sandwich Bread, 1 oz slice	70	1	13
Sandwich Pockets: Reg., 2 oz	150	1	30
Sourdough, 1 oz slice	70	1	12
Sourdough, 1 oz slice	70	1	12
Turkish/Middle Eastern, 1 oz sl.	80	1.5	16

Bread Rolls & Buns

	C	F	Cb
Brown 'n Serve, average, 1 oz	80	2	15
Dinner Rolls: 1 small, 1 oz	85	2	15
1 medium (3" diam),11/2 oz	130	3	23
English Muffins, aver., 2 oz	140	2	27
Frankfurter/Hot Dog: 11/4 oz	100	2	19
11/2 oz size	120	2	23
French: 1 medium, 1.3 oz	110	1	24
1 large, 3 oz	240	2	52
Hamburger: Regular, 11/2 oz	120	2	23
Large, 3 oz	240	4	46
Hoagie/Submarine, 43/4 oz	400	8	77
Kaiser Roll, 2 oz size	170	3	18
Onion Roll, 2 oz size	170	2	24
Parker House Roll, 0.7 oz size	65	1	12
Party Roll, 0.6 oz	55	1	10
Sandwich Roll, 1.6 oz size	120	2	23
Soft Pretzel Bun (J & J), 3 oz	235	3	50
Sourdough Roll, 11/4 oz	100	1	18
Sweet Rolls, 1 oz	100	2	20
w. Icing, average	160	6	20
Wheat Roll: Small, 1 oz	75	0.5	14
Medium, 11/2 oz	110	1	20

Quick Guide

	C	F	Cb

Bagels

Average All Brands

Plain/Onion:

	C	F	Cb
1 mini/bagelette, 1 oz	80	<1	15
1 small bagel, 2 oz	160	1.5	30
1 medium bagel, 3 oz	240	2	45
1 large bagel, 4 oz	320	3	60
Bagel Chips (New York Style), 4 slices, 3/4 oz	90	2	17
Pizza Bagel, 6 oz each	380	7	60
Bagel Bites (Ore-Ida), 4 pces	190	7	25
Bagel Crisps (Burns Ricker), 1 oz	150	9	28

Bagel Brands

	C	F	Cb
Amy's Kitchen, aver., 3 1/2 oz	235	2	50
Awrey's, 2.7 oz each	190	0.5	42
Cosco Bakery: Plain, 4 oz	300	1	61
Everything, 4 oz	330	3.5	62
Lenders, all flavors, 3.6 oz	280	3	55
Oroweat: Oatmeal, 3.4 oz	270	4	49
Multi-Grain, 3.4 oz	260	1.5	51
Sara Lee: Mini, average, 1 oz	80	0	15
Toaster Size, all types, 2.2 oz	160	0.5	33
(5g) 3.4 oz Size: Egg	260	2	50
Other flavors, 3.4 oz	260	1	55
(13g) 4 oz Size:			
Apple Cinnamon	310	1.5	64
Banana Walnut	350	7	61
Chocolate Chip	320	3.5	61
Cranberry Orange	310	1.5	64
Honey & Oat	310	2	61
New York Style, 4 1/2 oz	330	1	69
Sun Dried Tomato Basil	300	1.5	61
The Works	330	3.5	62
Western: All flavors, aver., 3 oz	230	1	47

Bagels ~ see *Einstein Bros Bagels,* Pp 197
Bagel Sandwiches ~ See Pp 166

Bagel Spreads

	C	F	Cb
Cream Cheese: Plain, 1 oz	80	8	2
Reduced Fat, 1 oz	60	5	2
Flavors: Lox, 1 oz	75	6	1
Raisin Walnut, 1 oz	90	6	8
Strawberry, 1 oz	60	3	7
Sundried Tomato, 1 oz	80	7	2
Vegetable, 1 oz	60	6	1

Bread Products

	C	F	Cb
Bread Crumbs, dry:			
Plain or seasoned, 1 oz	110	1	20
1 rounded Tbsp, 10g	35	<1	6
1 cup, 3 1/2 oz	390	5	73
Corn Flake Crumbs, 1 oz	110	1	20
Graham Cracker Crumbs, 1 oz	115	1	21
Keebler, 1 cup, 4 1/4 oz	520	14	84
Bread Dough: Frozen, 1 oz	75	<1	14
Refrigerated, French, 1" slice	60	1	13
Wheat/White, 1" slice	80	2	14
Breadsticks: Boboli, 1.75 oz	130	2	22
Stella D'oro: Sesame, (1)	50	2	7
Plain/Onion/Wheat, 1 pce.	40	1	7
Keebler/Lance, 2 sticks	30	<1	6
Salt Sticks, plain, 1 oz	110	1	20
Croutons: Aver. all brands, 1 oz	100	3	17
2 Tbsp, 10g	35	1	6
Coating Mixes:			
Seasoned, average, 1 oz	110	3	20
Featherweight, 1.4 oz pkg	72	<1	17
Pretzels: See Snacks ~ Page 126			
Stuffing: Average, dry mix, 1 oz	110	1	10
Made-up, 1/2 cup, 4 oz	180	9	11

Croissants ~ *See Page 106*

Rice Cakes

Average All Types/Brands:

	C	F	Cb
Regular size, 1 cake, 9g	35	0	7.5
Hain, Mini, average, 3g each	12	<1	2
Lundberg, all types, 15g each	60	<1	14
Quaker: Large, all flavors, 13g each	50	0	11
Crispy Mini's, average, 15g	70	2	12

Taco Shells

	C	F	Cb
Regular size, all types, each	55	3	6
Super Size, each	90	4	11
Mini Size, 1 taco	25	1.5	2
Salad Shell, flour (Azteca), 1.4 oz	180	11	19
Tortilla (Soft Taco), each	85	2	15
Corn Tortilla: 6", 1.2 oz each	45	0.5	9
Flour Tortilla: each, 1.75 oz	160	3	28
Lowfat	110	1.5	22
Burritos, 1 tortilla, 2.3 oz	190	5	32
Lowfat	110	1.5	22
Tostada Shells, each	55	3	6

Crispbreads • Crackers, Cookies

Crispbreads

Per Crispbread/Cracker

	C	F	Cb
Ak-Mak: Sesame, 5 crackers, 1 oz	35	0	7
Finn Crisp: Original, rye,1	35	0	7
Other types,1	19	0	3
Kavli Norwegian: Thin,1	17	0	3
Thick,1	20	0	3
Malsovit, Meal Wafers.1	75	4	7
New York Flatbread Crisps, 1	35	0	7
Ry-Krisp: Natural, 1 crispbread	20	0	3
Seasoned,1	30	0	3
Sesame,1	25	1	3
Ryvita: Dark/Light, 1 piece	26	0	4
WASA: Breakfast; Sesame	50	0	9
Extra Crisp; Light Rye	25	0	5
Hearty Rye	45	0	9
Organic Rye	25	0	7
Sourdough Flatbread, 3	50	0	11
Sourdough Rye	35	0	7

Matzos

Manischewitz

	C	F	Cb
American Matzos, 1 board, 1 oz	115	2	22
Passover Matzos, 1 board, 1.1 oz	130	2	27
Passover Egg Matzos, 1.1 oz	130	2	27
Egg 'n Onion Matzo, 1 oz	112	1	23
Thin Salted Tea Matzos, 0.9 oz	100	0	21
Unsalted; Whole Wheat, 1 oz	110	0	24
Dietetic Matzo Thins, 0.83 oz	90	0	19
Crackers: Miniatures, 1 cracker	9	0	20
Passover Egg Matzo, 1 cracker	11	0	20
Matzo Meal, 1 cup, 4³/4 oz	515	2	110
Matzo Farfel, 1 cup, 2.7 oz	180	0.5	60
Grape Matzo, 1 oz each	110	0	25

World's Biggest Cookie!

Paul "Cookie" James

Quick Guide

Crackers

Average All Brands: Per Cracker

	C	F	Cb
Cheese Crackers:			
Plain, 1" square	5	0	0.5
Small, octagonal	10	0	1
Round (2" diam.)	15	0	1.5
Sandwich (Peanut Butter)	35	1	4
Graham, 2¹/2" square,1 cracker	30	0.5	5
Melba Toast, plain, 1 piece	20	0	4
Oyster & Soup crackers, ¹/4 oz	60	2	10
(40 small oysters/20 lge hexagons)			
Rice Crackers: 1 small	9	0	2
Rice Snax (*Amsnack*), ¹/2 oz	60	1	12
Saltines, 1 cracker	25	1	4.5
Snack-type, 1 round cracker	15	0	3
Soda, 1 cracker, ¹/2 oz	60	2	10
Water (*Carr's*), regular, 1 cracker	32	0	7
Bite-size, 1 cracker	13	0	2
Wheat, thin, 1 cracker	9	0	1
Zweiback Toast, 1 piece	30	0	5

Quick Guide

Cookies

Average All Brands: Per Cookie

	C	F	Cb
Biscotti: Almond, 2.5 oz	55	2	8
Chocolate Chip Cookies:			
Small/Thin 0.5 oz	55	3	8
Regular, 1 oz	110	6	15
Large, 2.5 oz (*Mrs Field's*)	280	14	40
Jumbo, 4 oz	450	22	64
Oatmeal/Oatmeal Raisin:			
Small/Thin 0.5 oz	50	1.5	8
Regular, 1 oz	95	3.5	15
Large, 2.5 oz (*Mrs Field's*)	240	9	38
Jumbo, 4 oz	380	14	60
Peanut Butter:			
Small/Thin 0.5 oz	60	3	7
Regular, 1 oz	125	6.5	15
Large, 2.5 oz (*Mrs Field's*)	310	16	38
Jumbo, 4 oz	500	25	58
Lowfat Cookies			
Choc Chip (Lowfat), 1 oz (1)	100	1	22
Oatmeal Raisin (Fat-free), 1 oz (1)	90	0	20
Peanut Butter (Lowfat), 1 oz (1)	105	2	20

Brands	C	F	Cb
Per Cookie/Cracker (Unless Indicated)			
Archway			
Apple/Date-filled Oatmeal	100	3	16
Apricot/Strawb.-filled Oatmeal	100	3.5	16
Aunt Bea's Pound Cake Cookie	100	4	16
Coconut Macaroon	100	6	12
Chocolate Chip: Drop	100	3.5	16
Ice Box	120	6	15
N' Toffee	130	6	18
Fat-Free: Oatmeal Raisin (1)	110	0	25
Cinnamon Honey Heart (3)	110	0	25
Devil's Food Cookie (1)	70	0	16
Frosty Lemon/Orange	110	4.5	17
Fruit & Honey Bar	100	3.5	18
Ginger Snaps: Regular (5)	150	5	23
Reduced Fat (5)	140	3.5	25
Iced (5)	150	5	23
Lemon Snaps (5)	150	7	20
Molasses	100	3	18
Oatmeal: Regular; Raisin	110	3.5	17
Iced	120	5	18
Old Fashioned Peanut Butter	120	6	15
Old Fashioned Windmill	90	3.5	14
Peanut Butter Choc	150	7	17
Peanut Jumble	110	6	13
Pecan Icebox	120	6	15
Ruth's Golden Oatmeal	120	5	18
Sugar Cookies (1)	100	3	16
Austin: *Per Serving*			
Big Munch Wafer Bar, each	200	2.5	24
Cheese/Toast/Wheat Crackers, w. filling			
all types, average	200	2.5	29
Reduced Fat	170	1.5	25
Sandwich Cookies, all types	240	2	36
Snackers Crackers, all types	130	1	32
Zoo Animal Crackers, all types	125	1	20
Zoo Animal Pretzels	200	0	40
Bakery Wagon			
Iced Molasses, lowfat	90	1.5	18
Iced Oatmeal	120	4.5	18
Lemon Heaven	120	3.5	20
Peanut Butter	130	6	15
Sugarless Molasses	120	3	21
Fat-Free: Cobbler	70	0	16

	C	F	Cb
Barbara's Bakery			
Animal Cookies, each	16	0.6	2
Cheese Bites, all types, 26 crackers	120	1.5	24
Coconut Almond, 1 bar, 1 oz	120	4.5	20
Crisp Cookies, all types (1)	80	4	11
Espresso Bean; Lemon Yog., 1 bar	120	3.5	22
Fat Free: Mini, all types, each	18	0	4
Fig Bars, average	60	1	15
Rite Lite Rounds, 5 crackers	55	0.5	12
Roasted Peanut, 1 bar, 1 oz	130	4.5	20
Snackimals, 1 cookie	15	0.5	2
Wafer Crisps	60	1	12
Wheatines, all types, 1 large square	50	1.5	10
Breadshop: Animal Cookies	8	0	1.5
Bremner: Wafers, all varieties (1)	10	0.3	2
Breton: Low Sodium Wheat (3)	70	3	8
Vivant Vegetarian (3)	60	2.5	9
Cape Cod: Choc Chip Cranberry	140	6	20
Carr's: Cheddar (3)	80	4	8
Croissant (3)	70	3	10
Wholewheat Crackers (2)	80	3.5	11
Cheeze-It: Heads & Tails (31), 1 oz	140	6	18
Dare: Breton Wheat (3)	60	3	8
Delicious: Butter Finger (3)	130	6	18
Land O' Lakes (3)	120	6	15
Raisinets Oatmeal (3)	140	4.5	22
Skippy Peanut Butter (3)	150	10	13
Dominick's			
Grahams: Cinnamon (8)	140	5	22
Fudge (3)	140	7	19
Honey (8)	150	6	22
Lowfat (9)	120	1.5	25
Saltine Crackers (5)	60	2	10
Sugar Wafers (5)	140	7	25
Unsalted Tops (5)	70	2	10
Cookies: Choc Chip: Chewy (1)	100	5	14
Chunky (1)	80	4.5	10
Reduced Fat (3)	150	6	23
Old Fashioned: Assort.; Oatmeal	80	3.5	11
Pecan Shortbread	100	6	11
Sandwich Cremes: Chocolate	70	2.5	11
Vanilla	80	3	13
Striped Shortbread (3)	160	4	21
Vanilla Wafers (6)	160	6	23
Dr Soy: Average (2)	85	2	5

Per Cookie/Cracker (Unless Indicated)

Entenmann's	C	F	Cb
Chocolate Brownie (2)	150		21
No Fat, 2 cookies	100	0	24
Original Choc Chip (3)	150	7	20
Soft Baked: Choc Chip	100	5	13
Gourmet English Toffee	100	5	13
Milk Choc Chip	100	5	13
Oatmeal Raisin, Fat Free (2)	100	0	23
White Choc Macadamia Nut (1)	100	6	12

Estee	C	F	Cb
Chocolate Chip; Fudge Cookies	38	2	5
Coconut Cookies, Oatmeal Raisin	35	1.5	5
Fig Bars, each	50	0.5	11
Sandwich Cookies	55	2	6
Shortbread; Vanilla; Lemon	35	1.5	5

Famous Amos: Butter Shorties	C	F	Cb
Famous Amos: Butter Shorties	80	4.5	10
Chocolate Chip (1)	32	1.5	5
4 cookies, 1 oz	130	7	19
with Pecans (1)	35	2	4.5
Choc Cake Sandwich (3)	150	7	23
Choc Chip & Pecans (4), 1 oz	140	8	18
Chocolate Chunk	80	4	10
Oatmeal Raisin (4), 1 oz	135	5	20
Pecan Shorties	90	5	10
Vanilla Sandwich (3)	160	6	23
Lowfat: Iced Lemon (7), 1.1 oz	130	1.5	25
Iced Gingersnaps (7), 1.1 oz	120	1.5	25

Frookie	C	F	Cb
Cookies: Average all types	45	2	7
Animal Frackers	10	0.3	1.5
Apple Cinnamon Oatbran	45	2	7
Fruitins: Apple: Fig	60	1	12
Large Frooks: All types	120	4	18

Grandma's	C	F	Cb
Choc Chip; Nutty Fudge	190	9	25
Fudge Choc Chip; Oatmeal Raisin	170	7	26
Old Time Molasses	160	4	29
Peanut Butter varieties, aver.	190	9	23
Cookie Bits: Average, (9)	150	7	22
Sandwich: Fudge (3)	180	5	31
Fudge Vanilla (3)	120	4	21
Vanilla (3)	180	5	32
Peanut Butter (5)	210	10	28
Rich & Chewy, 1 pkt	270	12	39
Sugar Wafers (3)	160	7	23
Tiny Bites (12)	280	12	39

Hain	C	F	Cb
Cheese Bites (22)	120	1.5	23
Cookie Jar Bits (Rice Cakes):			
Average all flavors, 17 bits	60	0.5	12
Mini Rice Cakes: Plain (8)	60	0	13
Oyster Crackers, Fat-Free (36)	60	0	13
Veg/Rice/Sesame Crackers (11)	140	6	19
98% Fat-Free, all types (11)	110	0	23

Health Valley	C	F	Cb
Graham: Amaranth: Oat Bran	15	0	3
Original Amaranth/Oat Bran	20	0.5	4
Healthy Pizza, all flavors (6)	50	0	
Lowfat, all flavors (6)	60	1.5	10
Original Rice Bran	18	0.5	
Whole Wheat, all flavors	10	0	
Cookies (each): Raisin Oatmeal	35	0	
Apple Spice; Hawaiian Fruit	35	0	
Apricot Delight; Date Delight	35	0	
Healthy Biscotti, all flavors	60	1.5	12
Healthy Choc./Chips, all flavors	35	0	
Jumbo, all flavors	80	0	19
Raspberry Fruit Center	70	0	
Tarts: All types, 1 tart	150	0	

Hy-Top	C	F	Cb
Assorted Cookies (5), 1 oz	120	4	
Assorted Sandwich Creme, aver.	80	3	
Chewy-a-riffic	90	3.5	
Chip-a-riffic (3)	170	9	2
Chocolate Chip (5), 1 oz	110	5	1
Cookie Time Assortment	80	3	1
Honey Cinnamon Grahams (2)	120	4	2
Oatmeal	80	3.5	1
Iced Oatmeal	70	3	1
Pecan-a-riffic	100	5	1
Sugar	80	3	1
Vanilla Wafers (8), 1 oz	130	5	2

Jewel	C	F	Cb
Jewel: Animal Crackers (9)	140	3.5	2
Chip-A-Riffic (3)	180	9	2
Choc/Vanilla Sandwich Creme (2)	130	5	2
Chocolate Chip: Regular (3)	170	9	2
Chewy (1)	90	3.5	1
Chunky (1)	80	4.5	1
Choc Chunk, 1 1/2 oz	200	9	2
Chocolate Sandwich Creme (2)	120	5	2
Cinnamon Grahams (8)	140	5	2
Cookie Jar Assortment (3)	150	9	2
Duplex Sandwich Creme (2)	120	5	2

Per Cookie/Cracker (Unless Indicated)

Jewel (Cont)

	C	F	Cb
Fudge Creme Wafer (3)	150	8	18
Fudge Marshmallow	110	4	18
Oatmeal; Oatmeal Old Fashioned	80	3.5	11
Peanut Butter (2)	140	5	21
Peanut Butter Chip, 1½ oz	210	12	21
'nut Butter Fudge Wafer (2)	140	8	14
Saltine Crackers; Unsalted Tops (5)	60	1.5	11
Striped Shortbread (3)	170	8	20
Sugar Wafers (5)	140	7	20
Unsalted Top Crackers (5)	70	2	10
White Choc Macadamia, 1½ oz	200	10	26

Keebler

Crackers:

	C	F	Cb
Club: Orig.; 50% Red. Sodium (4)	70	3	9
33% Reduced Fat (5)	70	2	12
Grahams: Regular (8), 1 oz	130	3.5	23
Lowfat varieties (9), 1 oz	115	1.5	24
Snackin' (21), 1 oz	120	3.5	22
Munch'ems, average (40), 1 oz	140	5	20
Sandwich, 1 pkt, 1.3 oz	190	10	23
Max Stix, average (20)	130	5	18
Toasted: Reduced Fat (5)	60	2	10
Regular varieties (5)	80	3.5	10
Town House: Regular (5)	80	4.5	9
Reduced Fat (6)	70	2	11
Wheatables: Reduced Fat (13)	130	4	21
Other varieties (12)	140	6	20

Cookies: Classic Collection (1)

	C	F	Cb
Classic Collection (1)	80	3.5	12
Chips Deluxe: Soft & Chewy (1)	80	3.5	11
Peanut Butter Cup; Rainbow (1)	80	4.5	9
Chocolate Lovers; Coconut (1)	90	5	11
Crunchy Walnut; Chips Deluxe (1)	90	6	9
Mini's (4)	150	8	19
Cookie Stix (5)	140	6	22
Country Style Oatmeal (2)	120	6	15
Danish Wedding (4)	120	5	20
E.L. Fudge Sandwich (2)	120	6	17
Fudge Shoppe: S'mores (3)	160	8	22
Deluxe Grahams, Reg.(3)	140	7	19
Double Fudge 'n Caramel (2)	140	7	20
Fudge Sticks (3)	150	8	20
Fudge Stripes (3)	160	8	21
Reduced Fat (3)	140	5	21
Grasshopper (4)	150	7	20
Mini's (4)	150	7	20

Keebler (Cont)

	C	F	Cb
Ginger Snaps (5)	150	6	24
Golden Fruit (1)	80	2	14
Iced Animal, (6)	150	5	24
Krisp Kreem, (5)	140	7	19
Lemon Coolers (5)	140	5	23
Sandies: 25% Red. Fat (2)	80	3	11
Regular varieties, average (2)	80	5	9
Soft Batch, 0.5 oz all types, each	80	3.5	10
Choc Chunk types, 1 oz	130	7	17
Homestyle Oatmeal Raisin, 1 oz	130	4.5	20
Vienna Fingers: Regular (2)	140	6	21
Reduced Fat (2)	130	4.5	22
Wafers: Golden Vanilla Wafers (8)	150	7	20
Reduced Fat (8)	130	3.5	25
Rainbow (artif. flavored) (8)	130	5	20
Sugar: Vanilla (3)	130	6	19
Peanut Butter (4)	160	9	18

Kraft

	C	F	Cb
White Cheddar Chse Nips (27), 1 oz	150	7	19

Lance

	C	F	Cb
Big Town, 1 pkg	250	11	38
Chocolate Chip, each	130	6	18
Dunking Sticks, each	180	10	22
Fig Bar, each	180	3.5	34
Fat Free: Apple/Cranberry, ea.	160	0	38
Oatmeal, each	130	6	18
Creme, each	240	10	35
Apple Bar, each	190	6	32
Peanut Butter, each	140	8	14
Peanut Butter Creme Wafer, 1 pkg	230	12	26

Lenell

	C	F	Cb
Almonettes (2)	80	4	10
Deluxe Assortment (2)	90	5	11
Icebox Pinwheels (2)	90	5	11
Jelly Stars (3)	100	5	13
Peanut Butter (3)	100	5	13

Lil' Dutch Maid

	C	F	Cb
Butter; Chip Delight (2)	80	3	11
Coconut Macaroons (2)	130	5	20
Creme: Chocolate/Duplex (2)	90	3	13
Strawberry/Vanilla, (2)	90	4	13
Oatmeal (2)	70	3	11
Iced Oatmeal (2)	80	3	11
Sugar (2)	80	4	10

Per Cookie/Cracker (Unless Indicated)

Little Debbie	C	F	Cb
Apple Flips	150	5	24
Chse Crackers w. P'nut Butter (4)	140	8	16
German Choc Cookie Rings	140	8	18
Ginger Cookies	90	3	15
Marshmallow Pies, each	160	6	27
Nutty Bar (2), 2 oz	310	18	32
Toasty Crackers w. P'nut Butter (4)	140	7	16
Yo-Yo's	130	6	21
Peanut Clusters, each	190	11	23
Figaroos, each, 1.5 oz	150	3.5	31
Peanut Butter & Jelly Sandwich	130	5	22
Lotte			
Chocolate (13), 1 oz	190	10	13
Koala Vanilla (13)	190	11	15
Koala Yummies (13), 1 oz	200	11	13
Peanut Butter (13)	190	10	11
Strawberry (13)	190	10	14
Lu Marie Lu			
Le Petit Beurre (4)	150	4	25
Le Petit Ecolier (2)	130	6	17
Le Truffe (2)	170	9	20
Pim's, Orange (2)	90	2.5	17
Mrs Fields' Cookies			
Per 1 Cookie, 2.5 oz			
Butter; Butter Toffee	290	12	40
Chewy Fudge	300	14	40
Coconut Macadamia	280	13	39
Debra's Special; Milk Choc	280	12	39
Milk Choc w. Walnuts	320	17	37
Milk Choc Macadamia	320	18	38
Oatmeal Raisin	240	9	39
Peanut Butter	310	16	34
Pumpkin Harvest	270	14	31
Semi-Sweet Chocolate	280	14	40
with Pecans	300	16	37
with Walnuts	310	16	38
Triple Chocolate	300	14	41
White Chunk Macadamia	310	17	37
Nibblers: *Per 2 Cookies, 1 oz*			
Debra's Special	100	4.5	13
Milk Choc w/Walnuts	120	6	14
Milk Chocolate; Peanut Butter	110	6	15
White Chunk Macadamia	120	7	13

Per Cookie/Cracker (Unless Indicated)

Mrs Fields' Cookies (Cont)	C	F	Cb
Nibblers (10 oz ctn): *Per Cookies, 1.23 oz*			
Oatmeal Raisin w. Nuts	150	7	21
Milk Chocolate Chip	150	8	21
Semi Sweet Chocolate Chip	150	7	22
White Chunk Macadamia	160	8	21
Manischewitz			
Matzo Boards ~ See Page 98			
Biscotti: Toffee Crunch Macaroons	50	2.5	7
Choc. Chip Cappucino	70	2.5	10
Chocolate Macaroons, each	45	2	8
Matzo Cracker, Miniatures	9	0	2
Whole Wheat Crackers	9	0	2
Marie Lu: Original Biscuit (1)	170	6	25
Matt's: Choc Chip	140	6	19
Oatmeal Raisin	120	4	20
Peanut Butter	140	6.5	18
Mother's			
1.2.3. Cookies (1)	10	0.5	2
ABC Cinnamon Grahams (1)	12	0.5	1.5
ABC Sugar Cookies (1)	12	0.5	1.5
Almond Shortbread	60	4	6
Butter Cookies; Wafers, all types	25	1	4
Checkerboard Wafers	20	1	4
Chocolate Chip: Cookies	80	4	10
Cookies (bag) (1)	30	1	5
Cookie Parade Assortment, each	35	1.5	5
Chocolate Chip Parade	35	1.5	5
Angel Cookies	60	3	5
Circus Animal Cookies	25	1	4
Cocodas Coconut	30	2	4
Dinosaur Grrrahams	65	1.5	11
Double Fudge	90	4.5	12
English Tea/Taffy Sandwich	90	3.5	14
Flaky Flix Fudge/Vanilla	70	3.5	9
Gaucho Peanut Butter S'wich	95	5	11
Iced Raisin; Macaroon	80	4	11
Marias	55	2	9
Oatmeal Cookies: Regular	55	2.5	8
Butterscotch Chip	60	2.5	8
Iced; Chocolate Chip	65	2	11
Oatmeal Raisin Cookies	30	2	4
Oatmeal Walnut Choc. Chip	65	3	8
Peanut Butter	75	4.5	8
Striped Shortbread Cookies	55	2.5	7

Cookies (Cont) ◆ Refrigerated

Per Cookie/Cracker (Unless Indicated)

Mother's (Cont)	C	F	Cb
Sugar Cookies	70	3	10
Sugared Lemon	75	4	9
Taffy	90	4	13
Wallops, all types	80	1.5	15
Walnut Fudge	65	3.5	8
Zoo Pals	10	0.5	1

Nabisco: *Per Cookie/Cracker, Unless Indicated*

Crackers: Cheese Nips (29), 1 oz	140	6	20
Air Crisps: Ritz, 1 oz (23)	140	5	22
Potato varieties, 1 oz (22)	120	3.5	21
Pretzel Original, 1 oz (23)	110	1	22
Wheat Thins, 1 oz (23)	130	4.5	21
Bacon Flavored Thins (7), 1/2 oz	80	4	9
Better Cheddars: Reg; Low Salt	70	3	11
Chicken in a Biskit (12), 1.1 oz	160	9	19
Garden Crisps (7), 1/2 oz	60	2	10
Oysterettes (19), 1/2 oz	60	2.5	10
Ritz; Wheatsworth; Stoneground (1)	16	1	2
Mini Ritz (33), 1 oz	150	8	18
Ritz Bits S'wiches: Chse (13), 1.1 oz	170	10	17
Xtreme Cheese (13), 1 oz	160	10	16
Royal Lunch (1)	50	2	8
Snackwell's Red. Fat Fr. Onion (32)	120	2	24
Sociables (7)	80	4	9
Swiss (7), 1/2 oz	70	3.5	10
Tid Bit, cheese (16), 1/2 oz	70	4	8
Triscuit Thin Crisps (14)	130	5	20
Triscuit Wafers: All types	20	1	1
Uneeda, Unsalted Tops	30	1	5
Vegetable Thins (7), 1/2 oz	80	4.5	9
Waverly (7)	70	3.5	10
Wheat/Oat Thins: (8), 1/2 oz	70	2	10
Big Wheat Thins (10)	140	6	20
Ranch (14)	150	7	19
Wings! 1 pkg, 1.8 oz	240	11	34
Cookies: Barnum's Animal Cracker	12	0.5	2
Biscos: Sugar Wafers	17	1	2
Waffle Cremes	35	2	4
Brown Edge Wafers	28	1	4
Bugs Bunny Graham Cookies	12	0.5	5
Café Creme: Vanilla Fudge (2)	200	10	27
Vanilla; Cappuccino (2)	160	8	22
Cameo Creme Sandwich	65	2.5	10
Choc Cherry Bar, 1 bar	130	2	26
Chocolate Chip Bite Size	10	0.5	2
Chocolate Chip Honey Grahams	5	0.2	1

Nabisco (Cont):	C	F	Cb
Chocolate Snaps	17	0.5	3
Chocolate Wafers (Red. Fat)	14	0.2	3
Chips Ahoy: Chewy	60	3	8
Choc. Chip; Sprinkled; Red. Fat	50	2	7
Chunky	80	4	10
Mini	12	0.5	2
Soft Cookies (2-Pack), 1 cookie, 39g	160	7	26
Other types, average	95	5	11
Cookie Break; Van. Crm. S'wich	53	2	8
Famous Chocolate Wafers	28	1	5
Fig Newtons, each	55	1	11
Fat Free, each	35	0	11
Grahams	15	0.5	3
Honey Maid: Grahams, all types (2)	30	0.5	6
Low Fat Cinnamon Grahams (2)	28	0.4	6
Ideal Bars: Chocolate & Peanut	90	5	10
Lorna Doone: Shortbread	35	2	4
Marshmallow Puffs; Mystic Mint	90	4	14
Marshmallow Twirls	140	6	20
Newtons: Tropical; Strawb., aver (2)	90	1	21
Cobblers, all varieties	50	0	12
Nilla Wafers: Regular; Cinnamon	15	0.5	3
Reduced Fat (1)	15	0.3	3
Nutter Butter: Chocolate	65	4	9
Bites, each	15	0.6	2
Peanut Butter Sandwich	65	3	10
Soft Cookies (2-Pack), 1 cookie, 39g	170	8	22
Oatmeal Crunch	15	0.5	3
Old Fash. Ginger Snaps	30	0.6	5
Oreo: Regular, 3 cookies	160	7	23
Reduced Fat, 3 cookies	130	3.5	25
Chocolate Creme, 2 cookies	150	7	20
Double Stuf, 2 cookies	140	7	19
Fudge-Covered, 1 cookie	110	6	14
Mini Oreos, 9 pieces, 1 oz	140	6	19
Pecanz	90	5	9
Pinwheels: Choc./Marshmallow	130	5	21
Snackwell's: Coconut Creme (2)	110	4	19
Lemon Creme (3)	130	6	24
Reduced Fat Vanilla Creme	65	1.5	10
Shortbread Creme (3)	130	5	21
Teddy Grahams Snacks: All types	5	0.1	1
Pepperidge Farm			
American Collection: Sante Fe	120	4.5	18
Average other flavors	140	7	16
Biscotti: Figaro	110	4	14
Caruso; La Scala; Tosca	90	3	13

Pepperidge Farm (Cont)	C	F	Cb
Chocolate Chunk Minis (4)	150	8	20
Fruit Cookies: Cherry Cobbler	70	2.5	11
Average other flavors	50	2	7
Distinctive: Bordeaux; Pirouette	35	2	5
Brussels	50	2.5	7
Brussels Mint; Milano	65	3	7
Chantilly Hazelnut Raspberry	80	3	12
Chessman; Toy Chest Butter	40	1.5	6
Double Choc. Milano	75	4	8
Endless Choc. Milano	180	10	21
Geneva	55	3	6
Hazelnut Milano	65	3.5	8
Lido	90	4.5	11
Linzer Strawberry Filled	100	4	15
Milk Choc. Bordeaux	60	3	7
Milk Choc. Milano	170	9	21
Mint/Orange Milano	70	4	8
Goldfish: Plain, 55 pces, 30g	140	6	19
Chocolate (19)	140	5	22
Choc. Chunk; Van.; Cinnamon (19)	150	7	21
Flavor Blasted (51), 1.1. oz	150	8	17
Giant: Cheddar (14)	140	6	19
Flavor Blasted, average (31)	145	7	19
Graham Snacks, average (38)	140	5	22
International: Esprits Noir	90	5	10
Chocolat A L'Orange; Medaillon	75	3	12
Nantucket: Choc Chunk Minis (4)	150	8	20
Double Choc Chunk (1)	140	7	18
Old Fashioned: Hazelnut	55	2.5	7
Brownie; Butterscotch Oatmeal	55	3	6
Chocolate Chip; Irish Oatmeal	45	2.5	6
Gingerman; Molasses Crisps	30	1	5
Lemon Nut Crunch	60	3	6
Oatmeal Raisin	55	2	8
Pecan Shortbread	70	4.5	7
Shortbread	70	3.5	8
Sugar	45	2	7
Sausalito: Choc Macadamia (4)	160	9	18
Soft Baked: Caramel; Choc Chunk	130	6	15
Choc. Macadamia/Walnut	130	6	16
Oatmeal Raisin	110	4	17
Spritzers, all flavors (5)	140	7	21
Vanilla Raspberry Tart	60	1.5	12

President's Choice	C	F	Cb
Animal Crackers (14)	150	5	2
Butter Pecan (2)	190	13	1
Choc Chip varieties (2)	160	9	1
Family Arrowroot (5)	140	4	2
Grandma's Butter First (2)	180	10	2
Peanut Butter First (3)	160	9	1
Peanut Butter Persuasion (2)	160	8	1
Raisins First (2)	120	6	1
Temptations: all types (2)	150	7	2

Pirouline	C	F	Cb
Pirouline, 8 rolls, 1 oz	130	3.5	1

Salerno	C	F	Cb
Almond Windmill (2)	120	4.5	1
Bonnie Shortbread (4)	160	7	2
Butter Cookies: Original (6)	160	7	2
Reduced Fat (6)	150	5	2
Coconut Bar (4)	150	8	1
Creme Wafer Sugar-free (5)	190	13	1
Dinosaur Graham	70	2.5	1
Farm Animal Crackers (13)	140	5	2
Grahams: Cinnamon (2)	130	3.5	2
Chocolate (2)	130	3	2
Iced Oatmeal (2)	120	5	1
Mini Butter: Flavored (25)	150	6	2
Angel/Chocolate Creme (9)	140	6	2
Mini Dinosaur (15)	140	5	2
Mint Creme Patties (2)	130	7	1
Oyster Crackers: Regular (42)	60	1.5	1
Fat-Free (42)	60	0	1
Royal Crispy Stix (3)	150	8	1
Royal Stripes (3)	180	8	2
Saltine Crackers: Regular (5)	60	1.5	1
Fat-Free (5)	50	0	1
Unsalted Tops (5)	60	1.5	1
Santa's Favorites, aniseed (6)	150	5	2
Scooter Pie Choc Marshmallow	140	5	2
Sugar Wafers, assorted (5)	180	11	2
Vanilla Wafers (7)	130	5	2

Sesame Street	C	F	Cb
Grahams, all types, 1 oz	140	5	2

Sinful	C	F	Cb
Chocolate Chip (2)	150	7	1
All Butter Raisin & Oatmeal (2)	130	6	1
Butter w. Soft Creme Raspberry (1)	70	3	1
Choc w. Vanilla Creme (2)	120	5	1

Cookies (Cont) ⬩ Refrigerated

Snackwell's	C	F	Cb
Caramel Delights	70	2	13
Chocolate Chip (2)	20	0.5	3
Choc/Creme Sandwich; Oatmeal	55	1.5	10
Coconut Creme (2)	110	4	19
Streusel Squares	150	3	31

Stella D'Oro	C	F	Cb
Angel Bars	80	5	7
Almond Toast Cookie	55	1	10
Anginetti (4)	140	4	23
Anisette Sponge (2)	90	1	19
Anisette Toast (3)	130	1	27
Apple Pastry	80	3	14
Breakfast Treats	100	3	16
Biscotti (Hazelnut)	100	3.5	15
Castelets, regular/chocolate	70	3	9
Dutch Apple Bars	110	3	19
Egg Biscuits, Low Sodium	40	1	7
Egg Jumbo	50	1	9
Fruit Delight Apple Cinnamon	70	0	17
Golden Bars; Love Cookies	110	4	16
Kichel, low sodium	7	0.4	0.5
Lady Stella Assortment (3)	130	5	19
Margherite, chocolate/vanilla	70	2.5	11
Peach Apricot/Prune Pastry	90	4	14
Swiss Fudge	70	3	9

Sunshine	C	F	Cb
Crackers: *Per Cracker, Unless Indicated*			
Cheez-It Crackers	6	0.3	0.5
Big Cheez-It	12	1	1
Cheez-It Juniors (44), 1 oz	140	7	13
Heads & Tails, 1 pkt, 1.5 oz	210	9	28
Hi-Ho Crackers	17	0.5	2
Reduced Fat	14	0.5	2
Krispy: Regular	12	0.3	2
Oyster & Soup, 17 crackers	60	1.5	11
Reduced Fat	10	0	2
Party Mix, 1 pkt, 1.7 oz	230	9	32
Reduced Fat, 1/2 cup, 1 oz	130	3	21

Weight Watchers	C	F	Cb
Apple Raisin Bars, each	70	2	14
Chocolate Chip (2)	140	5	22
Choc. S'wich Cookies (2)	140	3.5	23
Fruit Filled, 1 bar	70	0	16
Oatmeal Raisin (2)	120	2	22
Vanilla Sandwich Cookies	140	3	25

Thaw, Bake & Serve	C	F	Cb
Big Country: Aver. all types (1)	100	4	15
Cookietree: *Per Cookie*			
Buttersugar; Cinn. Apple Oatmeal	120	5	17
Choc. varieties; Pecan/Macadam.	130	7	17
Cookie w. *M&M's*	120	6	17
Fat Free varieties, average	125	0	28
Peanut Butter/Chocolate	130	7	17
Raisin Oatmeal	110	3.5	18
Guiltless Indulgence (1.3 oz Cookie)			
Fat Free varieties, aver.	120	0	28
Lowfat Fudge/Choc., aver.	130	2	28
Grands!: *Per Biscuit*			
Blueberry; Golden Corn	210	9	28
Butter Tastin'; Buttermilk	200	10	24
Reduced Fat	190	7	27
Cinn. Raisin; Extra Fluffy; Wheat	200	8	28
Extra Rich	220	12	25
Flaky; Homestyle	200	10	25
Southern Style	200	10	24
Hungry Jack: Aver. all types (1)	100	4.5	14
Jewel			
Buttermilk Biscuits (2)	100	1.5	20
Old Fashioned Biscuits (2)	100	1.5	20
Pillsbury Cookies: *Per 1 oz*			
Buttermilk; Country, each	50	1	3
M & Ms	130	6	17
Choc. Chip/Dbl Choc Chip Chunk	140	7	17
Choc. Chip. Reduced Fat	110	4	18
Chocolate Chip w. Walnuts	130	7	16
Holiday, all types (2), 1 oz	130	7	16
Oatmeal Choc. Chip; Reeses	125	6	16
Peanut Butter	120	6	16
SnackWells, Choc. Chip, Red. Fat	110	3	18
SnackWells, Chocolate Fudge	90	1.5	18
Sugar (2), 1 oz	130	5	20
Tender Layer Buttermilk	160	4.5	9
One Step Pan Cookies	130	6	19
Toll House (*Nestlé*)			
Choc Chip	140	6	20
Reduced Fat Choc Chip	130	3.5	23
Choc. Chip White; Chunk	150	6	22
Peanut Butter Choc Chip	150	7	20
Sugar	120	5	18

Cakes, Pastries, Croissants

Ready-to-Eat C F Cb

	C	F	Cb
Angel Food:			
Plain, no oil, 2 oz	120	0	25
Plain with oil, 2 oz	160	1.5	25
w. Cream Frosting	230	7	37
Apple Fritters, 3 oz	360	22	38
Apple Pie: See Pies/Tarts Page 107			
Baklava, 1½" square, 1½ oz	110	6	13
Banana w. Butter Cream, 3 oz	300	13	40
Black Forest, 3 oz	230	10	34
Brownie, 3.5 oz	420	25	52
Bundt, 3 oz	300	17	35
Carrot Cake: Plain, 3 oz	230	8	41
w. Cream Cheese Frosting	380	21	42
Cheesecake: Small serving, 3 oz	260	18	24
Large serving, 5 oz	430	30	40
w. Lowfat Cheese/fruit, 3 oz	150	8	30
Cheesecake Factory: 1 sl., 7 oz	700	48	56
Lite, 1 slice, 7 oz	570	28	60
Denny's Cheesecake, 1 slice	470	27	48
Cherry Cobbler, 5 oz	350	10	62
Chocolate Cake: Plain, 2 oz	220	11	40
w. Chocolate Frosting, 3 oz	320	15	42
& Cream Filling, 3½ oz	360	21	43
Cinnamon Crumb Cake, 4 oz	450	23	57
Cinnamon Roll, Large, 6 oz	630	27	87
Coffee Cake, 2½ oz	230	7	38
Cream Cheese Crumb, 4 oz	410	20	52
Cream Puff (custard fill), 4½ oz	300	18	26
Creme Horns, each	190	13	19
Croissants: See Next Column			
Cupcake: Plain, 1½ oz	140	6	25
w. Frosting	170	7	30
Danish Pastry: Small, 2 oz	220	10	25
Large, 4 oz	440	20	51
Date Nut Roll, ½" slice	80	2	12
Devil's Food, w. Frosting, 3 oz	460	25	55
Donut Holes, 1¼" balls, 2 oz (5)	220	10	30
Donuts: See Page 108			
Eclair, Choc., Cust. fill, 3½ oz	240	14	23
Fig Bars, average, each	150	3	30
Fig Cake, ½ piece	110	2	21
Fruit Cake, Dark/Light, 1½ oz	165	7	26
Fudge Nut Brownie, each	340	13	56
Gingerbread: From mix, 3" sq.	200	6	37
Honey Bun, each	330	13	47
Key Lime Pie, 4.5 oz	440	22	54
Kolacky, Apricot/Rasp., ½ oz (1)	60	3.5	8

Ready-to-Eat (Cont) C F Cb

	C	F	Cb
Lemon Cake, 2½ oz piece	220	9	40
Lemon Poppy Seed Creme, 3 oz	310	15	40
Mississippi Mud Pie, 4 oz	380	24	37
Mud Cake, 1 piece, 3½ oz	350	16	48
Orange Creme (Ring), 3 oz	300	15	40
Pineapple Upside Down, 2½ oz	230	9	37
Peach Melba, 3½ oz	300	8	52
Strawberry Creme, 3 oz	290	14	40
Strudel Bites, ¾ oz	85	4	12
Pecan Twirls, 1 piece	110	5	16
Pecan Pie, 3 oz	330	13	51
Pies & Tarts: See Page 109			
Pound Cake, 3 oz	420	27	42
Sponge: Plain, 2½ oz	190	3	36
w. Cream & Strawberry	325	8	38
w. Chocolate Icing	300	12	38
Raisin Bun, 1 bun, 2¼ oz	180	2	37
Strudel, fruit, average, 3 oz	280	8	45
Sweet Roll, average, 1½ oz	155	7	24
Swiss Rolls, each	170	9	23
Tarts: See Page 109			
Tiramisu, 1 piece, 5 oz	400	29	30
Toaster Strudel, 2 oz	190	10	26
Turnovers, fruit, average, 3 oz	270	12	36

Croissants

	C	F	Cb
Average All Brands			
Plain/All Butter:			
Petite, 1 oz	120	7	14
1 Medium, 1½ oz	180	10	21
1 Large, 2½ oz	300	18	35
Sweet: *Per Croissant, 3½ oz*			
Almond Croissant	420	25	39
Apple Croissant	250	10	30
Chocolate Croissant	400	24	36
Sandwich (Ham/Cheese), 5 oz ~ See Page 160			
Au Bon Pain: See Page 170			
Burger King: Croissan'wich–See Page 178			
Dunkin' Donuts: Plain	290	18	26
Almond	350	22	34
Chocolate	400	25	37
Sara Lee:			
All Butter, 1½ oz	180	9	19
All Butter Petite, 1 oz	120	6	13

Quick Guide C F Cb

Muffins: Ready-to-Eat

Average All Types:

	C	F	Cb
Small, 1 oz	80	3	12
Medium, 2 oz	160	6	24
Large, 3 oz	240	9	36
Extra Large, 4 oz	320	12	48
Jumbo, 6 oz	480	18	60
Super Jumbo, 8 oz	640	24	96
English Muffin, 2 oz	150	2	29

Brands ~ Ready-to-Eat

	C	F	Cb
Awreys: Blueberry, 2.25 oz	210	9	29
Raisin Bran, 2.5 oz muffin	190	7	30
Carl's: Blueberry Muffin	340	14	49
Bran Muffin	370	13	61
Dunkin' Donuts: See Page 194			
Hostess: Mini, average, each	55	3	7
Blueberry; Raspberry, each, 4 oz	440	19	62
Jewel: English Muffin, 2 oz	130	1	25
McDonald's: Apple Bran, 4 oz	300	3	61
Oroweat:			
Cinnamon Raisin, 2.4 oz	170	1	35
Extra Crisp; Sourdough, 2 oz	130	0.5	26
Health Nut, 2.3 oz	170	3	30
Otis Spunkmeyer: Per Whole Muffin (4 oz)			
Banana Nut, 4 oz	480	24	60
Cheese Streudel	440	20	60
Wild Blueberry	420	22	48
Our Daily Muffin: Each, 3 oz	120	0	31
Pepperidge Farm: Average	150	3	28
Ralphs: Banana, 4.5 oz muffin	470	21	62
Blueberry, 4.5 oz	410	16	60
Bran & Raisin, 5 oz	380	8	78
Sara Lee: Blueberry	220	11	27
Corn	260	14	30
Snackwell's: Blueberry, 1/6 pkt	120	0	28
Weight Watchers: Per Muffin			
Chocolate Chocolate Chip	190	2	39
English Muffin Sandwich	210	5	28
Fat Free, average, all flavors	165	0	39
Low Fat, average, all flavors	175	3	37

Muffin Mixes C F Cb

Prepared: Per Muffin

	C	F	Cb
Betty Crocker: Banana Nut	150	5	24
Cinnamon Streusel	170	7	22
Lemon Poppyseed	190	7	30
Twice the Blueberry	140	4	25
Fat Free, all flavors	120	0	26
Duncan Hines: Blueberry, reg.	120	3	21
Bakery Style: Blueberry	190	6	32
Cinnamon Swirl	200	7	32
Cranberry Orange Nut	200	8	29
Pecan Crunch	220	11	27
Cinnamon Topp. Oatbran Honey	140	5	21
Oat Bran Blueberry	110	4	17
Oatmeal & Apples/Walnuts	210	9	30
Pillsbury: Blueberry Lowfat	160	2	34
Cinnamon	160	4	27
Other varieties	180	5	30
Robin Hood: Blueberry; Corn	160	6	24
Other flavors	170	8	23
Sweet Rewards: Fat Free	120	0	28

Sweet Rolls & Buns

	C	F	Cb
Cinnabon			
Classic Cinnabon, 1 serving	730	24	114
Caramel Pecanbon, 1 serving	1100	56	141
Minibon, 1 serving	300	11	45
Entenmann's: Cinn. Bun, 2.15 oz	230	10	32
Reduced Fat, 2.15 oz	160	3	32
Pecan Danish Ring, 1/6, 2 oz	250	15	25
Twist: Raspberry, 1/8, 2 oz	220	11	27
Nonfat, 1/8, 2 oz	140	0	32
Cinnamon Danish, 1/8, 2 oz	240	13	29
Lemon Danish, 1/8, 2 oz	210	11	27
Walnut Danish Ring, 1/8, 2 oz	240	15	25
Hostess: Honey Bun: Glazed	320	19	34
Iced/Frosted, 3.4 oz	410	24	42
Jewel Bake Shop			
Cinnamon Swirl Bread, 1 oz sl.	160	2.5	30
Gourmet Cinn. Rolls, 6 oz roll	640	29	88
Little Debbie: Pecan Spinwheels, 1 oz	110	4	16
Mickey: Cinnamon Pastry, 4 oz	200	5.5	35
Cinnamon Nut, 2 1/2 oz	230	8	37
Raisin Cinnamon, 2 1/2 oz	200	4.5	35
Pillsbury: Cinnamon Roll, 1.5 oz	150	5	23
Reduced Fat, 1.5 oz	140	3.5	24

Donuts

Quick Guide

	C	F	Cb
Donuts			
Average All Brands			
Plain, 1¾ oz	210	12	25
Sugared, 1¾ oz	220	11	27
Glazed, 2 oz	250	12	34
Chocolate Iced, 2 oz	260	14	29

Brands

	C	F	Cb
Buttercrumb			
Cinnamon, 1 cake, 1.6 oz	170	6	28
Dolly Madison Donuts			
Regular, 1¾ oz	270	12	40
Gem varieties, ½ oz each	65	3	8
Powdered Mini, ½ oz each	60	3	8
Dunkin' Donuts: *See Fast-Foods Section ~ Page 194*			
Dutch Mill: Plain, 1¾ oz	210	12	25
Sugared, 1¾ oz	220	11	27
Glazed, 2 oz	250	12	34
Double-Dipped Chocolate, 2 oz	280	17	31
Entenmann's Donuts			
Cinnamon Powdered, 1¾ oz	240	15	24
Frosted Devil's Food, 2.4 oz	310	19	34
Glazed Buttermilk, 2¼ oz	270	13	35
Light, 2 oz	190	7	31
Light Fantastic Fudge, 2 oz	210	9	40
Milk Chocolatey, 2.4 oz	310	19	35
Rich, Frosted, 3 pces, 2 oz	280	18	26
Hostess Donuts			
Cinnamon Sweet Roll, 2 oz	220	7	36
Regular: Plain, 1 oz	140	7	15
Chocolate Frosted, 1½ oz	180	11	19
Pwd Sugar/Cinnamon, 1½ oz	210	10	25
Old Fashioned; Glazed, 1½oz	180	9	23
Blueberry, 1½ oz	210	13	21
Hostess O's, Raspberry, 2 oz	230	10	34
Donettes: Frosted, ½ oz	77	4.5	8
Crumb; ½ oz	57	2.5	8
Powdered, ½ oz	84	4	12
Jewel: Cinnamon Spiced, 2 oz	230	15	24
Krispy Kreme: *See Fast-Foods Section ~ Page 206*			
Little Debbie Donuts			
Donut Sticks, 1.6 oz pkg	210	13	21
3 oz pkg	390	23	39

Brands (Cont)

	C	F	Cb
Mickey			
Egg Fluff, 2, 1.65 oz	210	11	25
French Twirl, 2, 1.65 oz	240	16	21
Jumbo, aver. all types, 1, 1.5 oz	190	11	21
Mini, 2, 1 oz	130	8	15
Sara Lee Donuts			
Choc. Frosted Mini, ¾ oz each	100	5.5	13
Powdered Mini, ½ oz each	85	4.5	9
Glazed, ½ oz each	110	5	14
Reduced Fat, ½ oz each	55	2.5	8
Tastykake Donuts			
Plain, 1½ oz	190	10	22
Cinnamon, 1½ oz	180	8	26
Frosted Rich, 2 oz	260	16	28
Honey Wheat, 2 oz	210	8	32
Powdered Sugar, 1½ oz	180	9	24
Van De Kamp's Donuts			
Old Fashioned: Plain	270	11	40
Chocolate, 2.4 oz	340	22	34
Powdered, 2 oz	240	11	35
Assorted, 2¼ oz	280	17	32
Mini Donuts: Chocolate, 4, 2 oz	290	17	32
Crumb, 4	220	8	35
Powdered, 4	250	12	33
Lowfat: Maple Buttermilk, 1	200	2	43
Chocolate Buttermilk, 1	200	2	43
Double Chocolate, 1	190	2.5	41
Powdered, 1	150	1.5	32
Zingers			
Devil's/Vanilla Food, 2 cakes	280	8	50

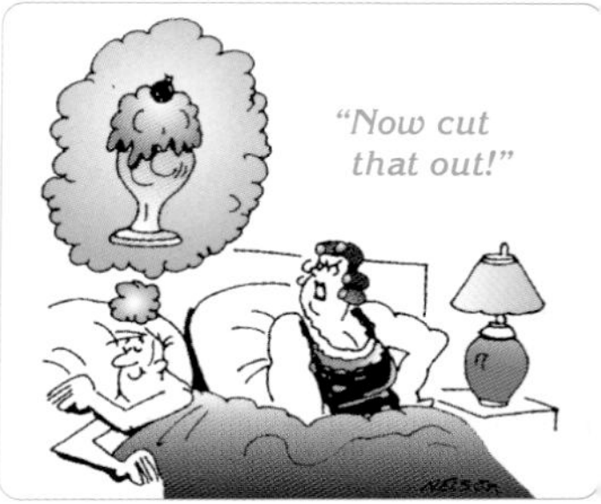

"Now cut that out!"

108

Quick Guide ⒸⒻℂⓑ

Pies ~ *Average All Brands*
1/8 of 9" Pie, 4 oz Serving

	C	F	Cb
Apple; Blueberry; Cherry	290	13	46
Boston Cream Pie	330	14	55
Chocolate Pie	300	18	35
Custard; Coconut Custard	250	13	27
Lemon Chiffon Pie	360	14	50
Lemon Meringue	270	11	42
Mince Pie	300	13	46
Pecan Pie	470	24	52
Pumpkin Pie	240	13	28
Strawberry Pie	230	9	37

Brands *Per Serving*

	C	F	Cb
Denny's: Apple Pie	470	24	64
Cherry Pie	630	25	100
Chocolate Peanut Butter	655	39	64
Chocolate Silk Pie	650	43	60
Dutch Apple Pie	440	19	55
Hershey's Choc Chunks N' Chips	600	36	58
Oreo® Cookies & Creme	690	30	73
Pumpkin Pie	235	7	38
Entenmann's			
Homestyle Apple, 1/6 pkg, 4.3 oz	340	12	56
Hostess: Fruit; Cherry, 4.5 oz pie	470	22	65
Lemon, 4.5 oz pie	500	24	66
Long John Silver: Per Serving			
Chocolate Crème Pie	280	17	29
Double Lemon Pie	350	18	41
Pineapple Cream Cheesecake	310	17	36
Marie Callender's			
Per 1/5 Pie: Apple	865	49	92
Blueberry	885	57	76
Boysenberry	860	57	82
Cherry	900	58	87
Banana Cream	630	28	67
Chocolate Cream	535	29	66
Coconut Cream	650	32	64
Per 1/4 Pie: Fresh Strawberry	615	28	89
Mince	885	59	97
Lemon Meringue	550	23	76
Pumpkin	615	28	80
Tastykake: Fruit, average	310	11	50
French Apple	360	12	61
Coconut Creme	390	20	47

Pastry & Pie Crusts ⒸⒻℂⓑ

	C	F	Cb
Pie Crust: Baked, 9" diameter shell			
1 Pie Shell, 61/2 oz	900	60	79
2-crust Pie, 9", 111/4 oz	1500	93	137
Betty Crocker, 9", 1/8 shell	110	8	9
Boboli, thin Pizza Crust, 1/5, 2 oz	160	4	24
Jewel, 1/8 of 9" crust	130	8	13
Keebler Graham Cracker, 1/8 of 9"	110	5	14
Mrs Smith's Deep Dish, 9" (1/8)	110	7	11
Nabisco Oreo, 1/6 of 9" crust	140	7	18
Pet-Ritz, all types, 1/8, 3/4 oz	90	5	11
Pillsbury (All Ready), 1/8 pie, 1 oz	120	7	13
Piecrust Sticks, 8 oz	960	64	90
Choux Pastry, raw, 1 oz	60	4	3
Filo Pastry: 4 sheets, 21/2 oz	210	2.5	40
Athens: 1/8 pkg, 2 oz	180	1	35
Mini Dough Shells, 2, 8g	45	2	1
Pepp. Farm, 2 sheets, 11/2oz	120	1	25
Flaky Pastry, 1 sheet, 6 oz	780	72	18
Puff *(Pepp.Farm)*, 1/2 sheet, 4.5 oz	510	33	42
1/6 sheet, 11/2 oz	170	11	14
Bake & Fill Shell, 1.7 oz	190	13	16
Pizza Crust, 1/8 whole	90	1	16
***Bisquick* Baking Mix:**			
Original, 1/3 cup, 11/2 oz	170	6	25
Reduced Fat, 1/3 cup, 11/2 oz	150	2.5	28

Pie Filling

Canned: *Average All Brands ~ Per 4 oz*

	C	F	Cb
Apple, 4 oz	120	0	28
1 Can, 21 oz	600	0	145
Apricot, 4 oz	150	0	36
Blackberry, Blueberry, Cherry	120	0	28
Chocolate, Coconut, 4 oz	140	3	33
Lemon, 4 oz	200	2	47
Mincemeat, 4 oz	190	1	45
Peach, Strawberry	120	0	28
Pumpkin, 4 oz	170	0	40
Raisin, 4 oz	130	0	30
Raspberrry, Black/Red, 4 oz	190	0	45
Strawberry, 4 oz	120	0	28

Cakes & Pastries - Packaged

Cakes & Pastries	C	F	Cb
Amy's: Apple Pie, 8 oz	280	12	42
Banquet: Crm Pies, aver., 1/3 pie	350	21	42
Eli's Frozen Cheesecakes: *Per 1/8 Pkg, 3 oz*			
Cookies N Creme; Choc. Caramel	320	23	11
Keylime; Original, average	320	22	26
Entenmann's			
All Butter Loaf, 1/6 loaf, 2 oz	210	9	30
Banana Cake, 1/8 cake, 2.5 oz	290	15	39
Brownie: Ultimate Fudge, 1	220	13	27
Light: Fudge,1/10 strip, 1.4 oz	110	0	27
Lemon; Coffee, 1/8 strip, 1.9 oz	130	0	29
Cheese Coffee, 1/8 cake, 1.7 oz	160	7	21
Cheese-Filled Crumb Coffee 1/8 cake, 2 oz	200	9	25
Chocolate Fudge, 1/6 cake, 3 oz	310	14	46
Creme-Filled: Choc Cupcakes, 1	160	0	39
Golden Cakes, 1 cake, 2.3 oz	280	15	34
Crumb Coffee, 1/10 cake, 2 oz	250	12	33
Golden Loaf, (Light) 1/8, 1.7 oz	130	0	28
Louisiana Crunch, 1/9, 3 oz	330	14	48
Marshmallow Ice Devil's Food, 1/8	300	14	42
Mocha Cake, 1/6 cake, 3 oz	340	17	45
New York Crumb Coffee, 1/10, 2 oz	250	12	33
Ultimate Choc Crumb, 1/9, 2 oz	250	13	34
Ultimate Crumb, 1/10, 2 oz	250	13	33
Grands!: Blueberry Biscuits, 2 oz	210	9	29
Cinnamon Rolls, 3.5 oz roll	300	7	54
Hostess: Angel Food Cake, 1/8	160	1.5	33
Brownie Bites, each	57	3	7
Carrot Cake, 2 pces, 3.5 oz	300	7	55
Suzy Q's, 2 cakes, 2 oz	230	9	35
Twinkies, 2 pces, 1.5 oz	150	5	25
Per cake: Chocodiles	240	11	33
Chocolicious	190	7	30
Chocolate/Orange Cupcake, aver.	170	6	28
Crumb Coffee	130	5	19
Dessert Cups, each	100	2	17
Ding Dongs; King Dongs	180	9	22
Ho Ho's, each	125	6	17
Honey Bun: Glazed	320	19	34
Iced/Frosted	410	24	42
Light: Brownie	140	2.5	28
Cupcakes; Twinkies	135	1.5	28
Crumb Cakes	90	0.5	19
Snoballs	180	5	31

Jewel Bake Shop	C	F	Cb
Choc Mini Cupcakes, 1 cake	100	12	30
Cinnamon Swirl Bread, 1 oz slice	160	2.5	30
Creme Horns, 1 horn	190	13	19
Elephant Ears, 2.5 oz	340	22	34
Fancy Jelly Roll, 1/6 roll, 2.7 oz	190	2.5	38
French Torpedo Roll, 2.7 oz	170	1	35
Gourmet Cinn. Rolls, 6 oz roll	640	29	88
Key Lime Meringue Pie, 1/6 whole, 5 oz	340	12	55
Kroger			
Angel Food Cake, 1/5, 2 oz	150	0	35
Dessert Shells, 2 shells, 1.65 oz	150	1.5	31
Gourmet Rugala, (18g), 0.6 oz	80	5	8
Little Debbie (Fresh)			
Cakes:			
Coffee, 2, 2 oz	230	7	39
Choc Chip Snack, 2, 2.4 oz	290	14	42
Chocolate Cup, 1.5 oz	180	9	26
Creme-filled Strawb. Cupcake ,1	200	9	29
Devil Cremes, 1.65 oz cake	190	8	29
Devil Squares, 2 cakes, 2.2 oz	270	13	37
Frosted Fudge , 1.5 oz cake	200	10	25
Swiss Cake Rolls, 2 cakes	260	12	39
Zebra Cakes, 2 cakes, 2.6 oz	330	16	45
Fudge Brownies, 2 oz, 1	270	13	39
Honey Buns, 1.75 oz bun	220	13	24
Muffin Loaves, 2 oz loaf	230	11	30
Oatmeal Creme Pies, 1	170	7	26
Pecan Spinwheels, 1 oz roll	110	4	16
Manischewitz			
Cheesecake, 2 oz	250	19	16
Marie Callendar (Frozen)			
Cobbler, all types, 1/4 pie, 4.25 oz	390	19	45
Pepperidge Farm			
Cakes Supreme: *Per 3 oz Slice*			
Lemon Mousse	290	12	35
Chocolate Mousse	250	10	34
Boston Creme	260	9	32
Cream Cakes Supreme:			
Cream Cheese Carrot, 1/9, 3 oz	320	20	38
Pineap./Strawb. Cr., 2.7 oz slice	240	10	38
Old Fashioned Cakes: *Per 3 oz Slice*			
Butter Pound	290	13	39
Deluxe Carrot	310	16	39
Turnovers: All types, aver., 3 oz	290	15	48

epperidge Farm (Cont)	C	F	Cb
ayer Cakes: *Per 3 oz Slice*			
hocolate Fudge	300	16	37
evil's Food; Coconut; Golden	290	14	40
erman Choc. 1/8 cake, 2.5 oz	250	13	31
trawberry Stripe, 1/8	250	11	35
anilla	290	13	41
ruit Squares: *Single, 2.5 oz*			
Apple; Blueberry; Cherry	210	10	27

ich's			
hocolate Eclairs (Frozen), 57g ea.	190	9	24

ara Lee (Frozen)			
akes: *Per Serving*			
ll Butter Pound, 1/6, 2.7 oz	320	16	38
Reduced Fat, 1/4, 2.7 oz	280	11	42
ll Butter; Chocolate, 1/4, 2.7 oz	320	16	40
anana Sundae, 1/10, 3 oz	270	14	32
utter Streusel Coffee, 1/6, 2 oz	220	12	25
arrot Cake Bites, 1 pce, 1/2 oz	80	5	7
hoc Layer, 1/8, 3 oz slice	340	17	46
ble Choc Layer, 1/8, 2.8 oz	260	13	33
ree & Light, 1/4, 2.7 oz	200	4	39
olden Butter, 1/4, 2.7 oz	300	13	41
ecan Coffee, 1/6, 2 oz	230	12	24
ed, White, Blueb. 1/10, 3 oz	210	8	31
trawberry, 1/4, 2.7 oz	290	11	44
Dessert Cakes: *Per 1/6 Whole*			
arrot, 3.2oz	320	17	39
anana, 2.3 oz	230	8	37
ayer Cakes: *Per 1/8 Whole*			
trawberry Shortcake, 2.5 oz	180	7	27
ther flavors, average, 3 oz	260	13	32
heesecake: *Per Serving*			
herry/Strawberry, aver., 4.75 oz	340	12	53
hocolate Chip, 4.3 oz	410	21	47
eanut Butter Cup, 3.5 oz	380	22	34
ew York Style: Classic, 1/6	500	30	50
Mixed Berry Swirl, 1/6	490	28	52
Choc Chip Cookie Crumble, 1/6	520	27	61
riginal: 1/5 whole, 4.3 oz	350	18	39
Classics: Choc. Mousse, 1/5	400	25	37
French, 1/5, 4.7 oz	410	25	41
Strawberry, 1/6 whole	320	14	43
Bars: 1 bar, 2.75 oz	190	14	14
Bites:			
Choc-Dipped Orig., 5 pces	480	33	40
Tstd Almond, 5 pces	450	29	42

Sara Lee (Cont)	C	F	Cb
Cheesecake Singles: *Per Slice*			
Caramel Choc Pecan, 110g	400	25	37
Strawberry Drizzle, 113g	380	20	46
Cream Pies (9"): *Per Serving*			
Choc. Silk; Coconut Crm, 1/5, 5 oz	500	32	49
Lemon Meringue, 1/6, 5 oz	350	11	59
Homestyle Pies (9"): *Per 41/2 oz (1/8 of Pie)*			
Apple; Cherry	340	16	46
Blueberry; Dutch Apple	355	15	53
Mince/Raspberry, averge	390	18	52
Peach	330	13	50
Pecan	520	24	70
Pumpkin	260	11	37
Individual Slices: *Per Slice*			
Apple/Cherry Pie, 4 oz	300	11	47
Carrot; Cookies N Cream, 3.5 oz	335	20	40
Lemon Icebox Pie, 3.5 oz	260	10	41
Southern Pecan Pie, 4 oz	470	23	62
Strawberry Swirl Ch'cake, 3.5 oz	300	17	31
Round Danish: *Per 1/6 Whole*			
Butter Streusel/Pecan	225	12	24
Cheese	180	6	28
Raspberry	200	8	27
Deluxe Cinnamon Roll	320	15	41
Weight Watchers: *Per Serving*			
Brownie à la Mode	190	4	34
Chocolate Mousse	190	5	31
Chocolate Eclair	150	4	25
Choc. Chip Cookie Dough Sundae	180	4	33
Choc. Raspberry Royale	190	3	39
Double Fudge Brownie Parfait	190	2.5	39
Double Fudge Cake	190	4.5	36
French Style Cheesecake	180	5	28
Mississippi Mud Pie	160	5	24
New York Style Cheesecake	150	5	21
Strawberry Parfait Royale	180	2	35
Triple Chocolate Eclair	160	5	25

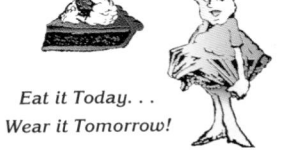

Eat it Today. . .
Wear it Tomorrow!

Cakes & Dessert Mixes

Made As Directed	C	F	Cb
Betty Crocker			
Cakes (Super Moist): *Per 1/12 Cake (Prep'd)*			
Chocolate Chip	270	13	34
Peanut Butter Choc; White	240	10	35
Other flavors, average	250	11	34
Per 1/10 Cake (Prepared):			
Carrot	320	13	42
Cherry; Sour Cream	280	12	43
Strawberry Swirl	290	12	43
Light: White	210	3.5	43
Devil's Food; Yellow	230	4.5	43
If using No Cholesterol Recipe, deduct 40 calories; and 4 grams fat.			
Angel Food Cakes: 1/12 mix	140	0	32
Brownie Mixes: *Per 1/20 Pkg (Prep'd)*			
Chocolate Chunk	180	9	24
Dark Chocolate	170	7	25
Fudge	170	7	23
Original Supreme	160	6	27
Peanut Butter; Walnut	180	9	23
Turtle (Caramel & Pecan)	170	8	23
Classic Dessert:			
Boston Cream Pie (1/10)	200	4.5	38
Choc. Pudding Cake (1/8)	170	3.5	33
Date Bar, 1/12 mix, dry	160	7	23
Gingerbread (1/8)	230	7	38
Golden Pound (1/8)	290	13	38
Lemon Chiffon (1/16)	140	3	26
Lemon Pudding (1/8)	180	4	33
Pineapple Upside Down (1/6)	400	15	63
Creamy Chilled:			
Banana Cream (1/9)	250	11	35
Chocolate French Silk (1/8)	270	11	39
Coconut Cream (1/8)	290	13	38
Cookies & Cream (1/6)	380	16	53
Sunkist Lemon Supreme (1/9)	320	13	52
Stir 'n Bake Mixes: *Per 1/6 Pkg*			
Carrot Cake w. Crm Chse Frosting	250	7	46
Chocolate Brownies	220	8	35
Coffee	200	6	36
Devil's Food Cake w. Choc. Frost.	240	8	42
Supreme Dessert Bars: *Per Bar*			
Caramel Oatmeal; Choc. Chunk	180	9	24
Strawberry Swirl Cheesecake	180	19	24
Sunkist Lemon	140	4	23
Other varieties, average	170	8	24

Made As Directed	C	F	Cb
Aunt Jemima			
Coffee Cake, 1/8 cake	170	5	30
Duncan Hines			
Angel Food, 1/12 Whole	140	0	30
Other flavors, average, 1/12	190	5	34
Cookies: All flavors, 1 cookie	65	3	8
Estee			
Brownie, 1 pce, 2"x 2"	50	2	12
All cakes, 1/5 cake	200	4	38
Choc. Chip Cookie, 1 cookie	45	2.5	6
Jell-O-No Bake: *Prepared As Directed*			
Cheesecakes:			
Cherry/Strawberry, 1/8 pkg	340	13	52
Peanut Butter Cup, 1/8 pkg	380	23	44
Real/Homestyle, 1/6 pkg	360	17	48
Cookies & Creme, 1/6 pkg	390	8	29
Double Layer Lemon, 1/8 pkg	260	13	35
Manischewitz			
Apple Cake w. real apple, (1/6)	260	10	43
Nancy's			
Petite Desserts, 1 tartlets, 0.6 oz	80	4.5	9.5
Pillsbury			
Moist Supreme: *Per 1/12 Cake (Prepared)*			
Angel Food	140	0	31
Devil's Food	270	14	33
French Vanilla; German Choc.	250	11	34
Funfetti	240	9	38
Other flavors, average 1/12	260	12	35
Streusel Coffee: 1/16 Cake	260	11	37
Bundt: Hot Fudge, 1/12	350	20	39
Chocolate Caramel Nut, 1/16	290	18	28
Strawberry Cream Cheese, 1/16	300	17	34
Deluxe Brownies: *Per 2" Square*			
Fudge, 1/16	150	6	22
Fudge, 1/16	190	9	24
Thick 'n Fudgy: Cheesecake Swirl	170	9	21
Double Choc.	150	6	23
Chocolate Chunk	160	7	22
Deluxe Bar Mixes: *Per Serving*			
Apple Streusel	150	6	23
Chips Ahoy	150	5	25
Fudge Swirl Cookie	180	8	25
Lemon Cheesecake	190	10	22
Other flavors, average	175	7	26

Frostings ♦ Baking Ingredients

Cakes & Dessert Mixes (Cont)

Robin Hood	C	F	Cb
Devil's Food, 1/5 cake	310	17	36
Yellow 1/5 cake	280	13	37

Sweet Rewards

Fat Free, all flavors (1/8)	170	0	40
Reduced Fat, all flavors (1/12)	200	5	37
Brownie Mix: Supreme, 1 pce	150	4	27
Lowfat Fudge, 1/18 pkg	130	2.5	27

Snackwell's

Brownie: Devil's Food (1/12)	150	2.5	28
Fudge (1/12)	150	2.5	29
Cakes: Devil's Food, 1/6 cake	200	4	38
White; Yellow, 1/6 cake	210	4.5	39
Cookies: Choc. Chip, 1 oz (1/18)	110	3	19
Chocolate Fudge, 1 oz (1/18)	90	1.5	18
Streusel Squares, 1.5 oz piece	150	3	31

Cake Frostings

Betty Crocker
Ready-to-Spread:

Creamy Deluxe, all flav., 2 Tbsp	140	5	24
Whipped Deluxe, 2 Tbsp	100	5	15
Sweet Rewards: Red. Fat, 2 Tbsp	125	2	25
Frost. Mixes: C'nut Pecan, 2 T. prep	160	8	21

Duncan Hines: *Per 2 Tbsp, 1.2 oz*

Coconut Pecan	150	9	18

Pillsbury: *Per 2 Tbsp (approx. 1/12 Tub)*

Caramel Pecan	150	8	19
Cream Cheese; Lemon	150	6	24
Chocolate; Choc. Fudge/Mocha	140	6	21
Coconut Pecan	160	10	17
Dark Choc	130	6	20
All other flavors	150	6	25
Decorators, Choc., 1 Tbsp	70	2	11

Sweet Rewards

Average all flavors, 1 Tbsp	120	2.5	24

Baking Ingredients

Almond Paste:	C	F	Cb
(Marzipan), 1 oz	125	7	12
Baking Powder: Regular, 1 tsp	3	0	0.5
Cream of Tartar, 1 tsp	2	0	0.5
Bisquick Baking Mix:			
Original, 1/3 cup, 1 1/2 oz	170	6	25
Reduced Fat, 1/3 cup, 1 1/2 oz	150	2.5	28
Butter/Margarine: 1/2 cup, 4 oz	820	91	0
Butterscotch/Rasp. Chips, 2 T., 1 oz	160	8	20
Carob Flour, 1/2 cup	90	<1	26
Chocolate Baking Bars: *Average All Brands*			
Unsweetened, 1 oz	150	15	8
Grated, 1 cup, 4 1/2 oz	680	68	36
Semi-sweet, 1 oz	160	8	18
Bitter-sweet/White Baking 1 oz	160	9	17
Chocolate Baking Chips: *Average All Brands*			
Milk Choc./Semi Sweet 1 oz	160	8	20
1/4 cup, 1 1/2 oz	240	12	30
1 cup, 6 oz	960	48	120
Cocoa Powder, Baking: Nestle, 1 T.	15	1	3
1/3 cup, 1 oz	80	4	12
Hershey's, 1 Tbsp	20	0.5	3
1/3 cup, 1 oz	115	3.5	21
Coconut, dried: Unsweet., 1 oz	190	18	7
Sweetened/flaked, 1 oz	135	9	14
1/2 cup, 1.3 oz	175	12	18
Toasted *(Baker's),* 1 oz	170	13	17
Creamed, 1 oz	195	19	19
Coconut Cream *(Coco Lopez),* 2 T.	120	5	5
Cornstarch, 1 Tbsp	30	0	7
Flour: All Purpose, 1 cup, 5 oz	400	0	84
Flavor Extracts: *Average All Brands*			
Imitation, 1 tsp	15	0	3.5
Pure Extract, 1 tsp	20	0	4
Almond, Vanilla, 1 tsp	10	0	3
Fruit Pectin: Swtnd, 1 Tbsp, 1/2 oz	35	0	10
Unsweetened, 1 Tbsp	2	0	0.5
Gelatin, dry, 1/4 oz pkg	30	0	0
Lemon/Orange Peel, 1/4 cup	30	0	4
Rennin, 1 pkg (11g)	12	0	3
Sprinkles: All types, 1 Tbsp, 1/2 oz	70	3	10
Vinegar, aver. all types, 1 oz	4	0	2
Whey, sweet, dry, 1 oz	90	<1	20
Yeast: Active, dry, 1/4 oz pkg	15	0	2
Fleischmann's, 0.6 oz pkg	15	0	2
Bakers, compressed, 1 oz	25	0	3
Brewers; Torula, 1 oz	80	<1	11

Puddings, Desserts, Gelatin

Ready-To-Serve

	C	F	Cb
Del Monte Pudding Snacks: Each			
Average all flavors	130	4	24
Fat Free Vanilla	90	0	20
Dr McDougall's: Rice Pudd., 3 oz	310	1.5	69
Hunt's Snack Pack: Per 3.5 oz Cup			
Puddin' Cakes: Choc Brownie	180	7	27
German Choc Cake	160	3.5	30
Puddin Pie: Lemon Meringue	130	2.5	20
Apple; Choc Mud	170	7	26
Imagine Foods: Natural Pudding (Cups)			
Chocolate, 1/2 cup, 3.7 oz	160	3	34
Banana; B'scotch; Lemon, 1/2 pkg	140	3	30
Jell-O Pudding Snacks (6 Pack)			
Choc./Caramel, 4 oz (113g) each	150	4.5	27
Fat Free, 4 oz snack	100	0	23
Chocolate/Vanilla; Van. Swirls	160	5	27
Cheesecake Snacks, aver., 4 oz	150	4.5	25
Jell-O Pudding Pops: Regular	80	2	12
Deluxe Chocolate covered	200	10	27
Jewel: Chef's Kitchen			
Rice Pudding, 1/2 cup, 4.5 oz	230	8	35
Tapioca Pudding, 1/2 cup, 4.5 oz	170	8	35
Jolly Rancher: Per 3.5 oz Cup			
Regular, all flavors	100	0	25
Sugar-Free, all flavors	10	0	1
Kozy Shack: Banana; Van., 4 oz	130	3	22
Lite, 4 oz	110	1	22
Rice Pudding, 4 oz cup	140	3	24
Creme Caramel Flan, 1 cup, 4 oz	150	4	25
Choc./Tapioca Pudding, 4 oz	140	3	25
Manischewitz: Choc., 1/2 cup	110	0.5	26
Passover Gold Noodle, 1/2 cup	140	2	28
President's Choice			
Key Lime Pie (36oz) 1/8 pie, 4.5 oz	440	22	54
Mississippi Mud Pie (36oz) 1/9, 4 oz	380	24	37
Swiss Miss Pudding Snacks			
Swirls, Choc. Pudd. Snacks, 31/2 oz	150	5	23
Tapioca: 1 pudding cup, 31/2 oz	120	3.5	21
Fat Free varieties, 31/2 oz	90	0	20
Weight Watchers (Frozen)			
Chocolate Mousse, 23/4 oz	190	5	31
Instant Pudding: Per 1/2 Cup			
Regular: average all flavors	170	4	30
Reduced Calorie: D-Zerta	70	<1	12
Estee	70	0	12
Jell-O, sugar-free	80	2	11
Royal, sugar-free	100	2	17

Homemade Puddings

	C	F	Cb
Apple Tapioca, 1/2 cup			
Bread Pudding, 1/2 cup	250	8	40
Blancmange, 1/2 cup	140	5	19
Chocolate, 1/2 cup	190	6	30
Corn Pudding, 1/2 cup	135	4	21
Crème Brûlée, 1/2 cup	400	35	16
Plum Pudding, 2 oz	170	3	32
Rennin Dessert, 1/2 cup	115	4	16
Rice with Raisins, 1/2 cup	200	4	38
Sponge Pudding, 31/2 oz	340	16	45
Tapioca Cream, 1/2 cup	110	4	15
Trifle, 1/2 cup	180	7	26

Custards

	C	F	Cb
Custard Mix			
Jell-O (Americana) Golden Egg:			
Dry, 1/6 pkg	80	0	19
Prep. w. 2% milk, 1/2 cup	140	2.5	19
Jello Flan, w. 2% milk, 1/2 cup	140	2.5	20
Royal-Flan: Prep. w 2% milk, 1/2 c.	130	2.5	18
Homemade Custard			
Baked, plain, 1/2 cup, 41/2 oz	150	7	16
w. skim milk, artif. sweetened	70	3	4
Boiled, 1/2 cup	165	7	18

Meringues

	C	F	Cb
Meringue Swirl, 1 oz	50	0	8
Meringue Shell, 1 oz Shell	100	0	16
(Add extra calories/fat/carbohydrate for fillings)			

Jell-O • Gel Snacks

	C	F	Cb
Gelatin Mix:			
Average Of Brands (Jell-O, Royal)			
Regular, all flavors, 1/2 cup	80	0	18
Sugar Free/Low Cal., 1/2 cup	8	0	0
Creme Gelatin/Parfait: Per 1/2 Cup			
Winky: Strawberry (109g)	110	1.5	22
Rainbow (130g)	100	1	24
Reser's: Dessert Parfait (110g)	100	2	19
Mrs Crockett's Kitchen: Str. Parfait	160	4	26
Gel Snack Cups, Del Monte/Jell-O	70	0	17

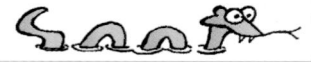

Quick Guide

C **F** **Cb**

Pancakes

Plain: *Average All Types*

	C	F	Cb
Small (3" diam.), $^3/_4$ oz	50	2.5	6
Medium (4" diam.), $1^1/_4$ oz	80	3	11
Large (5" diam.), $2^1/_2$ oz	160	6	21

Add Extra for Syrups/Butter

	C	F	Cb
Pancake Syrup: Regular, 1 Tbsp	50	0	13
$^1/_4$ cup	200	0	52
Lite, 1 Tbsp	25	0	6
$^1/_4$ cup	100	0	24
Butter/Margarine: Regular, 1 T.	100	11	0
Whipped, 1 Tbsp	70	7.5	0

Restaurant Style Pancakes

Denny's

	C	F	Cb
Hot Cakes, Plain, 3	490	7	95
w. Syrup & Butter	725	17	130
Original Grand Slam Breakfast	795	50	45
w. Syrup & Margarine	1030	60	101
Maple Flav. Syrup, 1 serving	145	0	36
Whipped Margarine, $^1/_2$ oz	90	10	0

Hardees

	C	F	Cb
3 Pancakes (no fat)	280	2	56
w. Sausage Pattie	430	16	56
w. 2 Bacon Strips	350	10	56

IHOP (International House of Pancakes)

Pancakes (Syrup/Butter extra):

	C	F	Cb
Buttermilk, 1 (2 oz)	110	3	17
Short Stack, 3	330	9	51
Full Stack, 5	550	15	85
Buckwheat, 1 (2 oz)	110	4	15
Country Griddle, 1 (2 oz)	120	3.5	19
Harvest Grain 'N Nut, ($2^1/_4$ oz)	180	9	20
Crepes (Egg Pancakes), 1 (2 oz)	120	6	14
Waffles (Plain): Regular, 1 (3 oz)	310	15	37
Belgian: Regular, 1 (4 oz)	390	19	48
Crepe: Egg, 1 (2 oz)	120	6	14

McDonalds

	C	F	Cb
Hotcakes, Plain (3)	340	8	58
w. Marg. (2 pats) & Syrup (1)	600	17	104

Perkins

	C	F	Cb
Buttermilk, 3, plain	440	12	70
Harvest Grain: Short Stack, Plain, 3	270	2	56
w. lowcal Syrup	295	2	63
5-Stack w. lowcal Syrup	475	3.5	93

Brands

C **F** **Cb**

Aunt Jemima

Frozen: Lowfat, 3

	C	F	Cb
Frozen: Lowfat, 3	130	2	33
Original; Blueberry, 3	200	3	40

Pancake & Waffle Mix:

	C	F	Cb
Original, $^1/_3$ cup, prepared	240	6.5	38
Complete, $^1/_3$ cup	160	2.5	32
Mini Pancakes (13)	240	4	46

Thaw & Pour B'milk Pancake Batter:

	C	F	Cb
$^1/_2$ cup, 4 x 4" pancakes	260	3.5	51

Betty Crocker Pancake Mixes

	C	F	Cb
Complete Original, 3	200	3	40
Complete Buttermilk, 3	200	2.5	40

Bisquick (Shake 'N Pour)

Pancake & Waffle Mixes:

	C	F	Cb
Average, all types, 3	200	3	38

Hungry Jack Pancakes

Mixes: Per $^1/_3$ Cup (prep.)

	C	F	Cb
Buttermilk: Complete, $^1/_3$ cup	160	1.5	32
Original, w. 2% Milk, Oil, Egg	290	13	32
w. Skim Milk, Oil, Egg Whites	220	6	32
Extra Lights: Complete	150	2	30
Microwave: Buttermilk, 3	270	4.5	51
Original, 3 pancakes	270	4.5	51

Northern Pines: Complete Gourmet

	C	F	Cb
3 x 4" pancakes, 3.5 oz	380	7	71

Waffles

	C	F	Cb
Homemade: 7" waffle, $2^1/_2$ oz	245	13	26
From Mix: 7" waffle, $2^1/_2$ oz	205	8	28

Frozen Waffles

Aunt Jemima

	C	F	Cb
Blueberry, 1 waffle	95	3	15
Buttermilk, 1	100	3	17
Dominick's: 1 waffle	58	1	10
Eggo (Kelloggs): Banana Bread, 1	95	3	6
Chocolate Chip, 1 waffle	100	3.5	16
Cinnamon Toast, 1 set	96	3	15
Homestyle, average, 1	95	3.5	15
Nut & Honey, 1	110	4.5	15
Nutri-Grain, 1	85	2.5	14
Special K (fat free), 1	60	0	13
Waf-fulls, all types, 1, 2 oz	160	5	26
Hungry Jack: Blueberry, 1 waffle	105	4	17
Buttermilk; Homestyle, 1	95	3	15
Mini Funfetti, 1	65	2	11

Sugar, Syrups, Jams, Honey

Sugar

	C	**F**	**Cb**
White Sugar, granulated:			
1 level teaspoon, 4g	15	0	4
1 heaping teaspoon, 6g	25	0	6.5
1 cube, 1/2"	24	0	6.5
Single portion, 1 packet	25	0	6.5
1 Tablespoon, 12g	48	0	12
1 ounce, 1 oz	110	0	20
1 cup, 7 oz	770	0	203
1 pound	1760	0	464
Brown Sugar:			
1 Tbsp, 13g	50	0	13
1 ounce, 1 oz	109	0	28
1 cup, not packed, 5 oz	540	0	140
1 cup, packed, 7 3/4 oz	845	0	218
Powdered/Confectioners:			
Sifted, 1 cup, 3 1/2 oz	385	0	98
Unsifted, 1 cup, 4 1/4 oz	460	0	117
Other Sugars			
Glucose, 1 oz	110	0	27
Tablets (Dex 4), 1	15	0	4
Barley/Wheat/Rye Malt,			
1 Tbsp, 3/4 oz	60	0	14
Cinnamon Sugar, 1 tsp	15	0	4
Dextrose, 1 oz	110	0	27
Fructose: 1 tsp	15	0	4
3 Tbsp, 1 oz	110	0	27
Estee, 1 pkg	10	0	2
FruitSource: 1 oz (powder)	110	0	27
Sorbitol, 1 oz	110	0	27
Turbinado Sugar, 2 Tbsp, 1 oz	110	0	27
Unrefined Cane Sugar, 1 oz	110	0	27

Sugar Substitutes

Diabetic Sweet: 1 pkt	0	0	1
Equal: Tablet/Liquid	0	0	0
Granulated, 1 pkg	4	0	1
NutraSweet Spoonful, 1 tsp	2	0	0.5
Nutra Taste, 1 pkt	0	0	0
Sprinkle Sweet, 1 tsp	2	0	0.5
Stevia, 1 pkt	0	0	0
Sugar Delight, 1 pkt	8	0	2
Sugar Like (Bateman's), 1 tsp	4	0	1
Sugar Twin: 1 pkt	3	0	1
Sugar Substitute, 1 tsp	2	0	0
Sweet 'N Low, 1 pkt	0	0	1
Sweet One, 1 pkt	0	0	1
Weight Watchers Sweetener, 1 tsp	4	0	1

Honey, Jam, Preserves

	C	**F**	**Cb**
Average All Brands			
Honey: 1 tsp, 1/4 oz	22	0	5.5
1 Tbsp, 3/4 oz	65	0	17
1 ounce, 1 oz	86	0	23
1 cup, 12 oz	1030	0	269
Single Portion, 1/2 oz pkg	43	0	11
Jams/Jellies/Marmalade/Preserves			
Regular, 1 tsp, 1/4 oz	18	0	5
1 Tbsp, 3/4 oz	55	0	16
1 ounce	75	0	22
Single Portion, 1/2 oz pkg	38	0	11
Apple/Fruit Butters, 1 T., 0.6 oz	20	0	6
Fruit Spreads: Regular, 1 tsp	16	0	4
Low Sugar, 1 tsp	8	0	2
Low Cal. (Featherweight), 1 tsp	4	0	1
Jelly: Regular, average, 1 tsp	18	0	4.5
Imitation, Low Calorie, 1 tsp	4	0	1

Syrups, Molasses

	C	**F**	**Cb**
Syrups: *Average All Types & Brands*			
(Corn/Rice/Maple/Pancake/Sundae/Waffle)			
Includes *Aunt Jemima, Cary's, Karo, Hershey's,*			
Hungry Jack, Log Cabin, Mrs Butterworth's			
Regular/Dark/Light Color:			
1 Tbsp, 1/2 fl.oz	55	0	14
1/4 cup (4 Tbsp)	220	0	55
Single Portion: 1 1/2 oz pkg	170	0	42
Lite: 1Tbsp	25	0	6
1/4 cup (4 Tbsp)	100	0	25
Sugar-Free: *Cary's,* 2 Tbsp, 1 oz	18	0	5
Cozy Cottage, 2 Tbsp, 1 oz	10	0	3
Molasses: Dark/Light: 1 T., 3/4 oz	55	0	14
1 cup, 11 1/2 oz	880	0	224
Blackstrap: 1 Tbsp, 3/4 oz	47	0	11
1 cup, 11 1/2 oz	750	0	208

Icecream Toppings

	C	**F**	**Cb**
Average All Types & Brands			
(Hershey's, Kraft, Smuckers)			
Chocolate, Hot Fudge, 2 Tbsp	140	4	22
Lite Hot Fudge (Smuckers), 2 T.	90	0	23
Fat Free (Hershey's), 2 T.	100	0	23
Butterscotch, Caramel, 2 Tbsp	140	1	30
Pineapple, Strawberry, 2 Tbsp	110	0	24
Smuckers Guilt-Free, all flavors	100	0	24

Quick Guide   **C** **F** **Cb**

Chocolate

Average All Brands

Milk Chocolate, regular:

	C	F	Cb
Plain/Nuts/Fruit, average, 1 oz	150	10	13
1¹/2 oz Bar	225	15	23
2 oz Bar	300	20	30
4 oz Block	600	40	60
8 oz Block	1200	80	120
1 Pound, 16 oz	2400	160	240
Dark/White Chocolate, 1 oz	150	10	16

Chocolate-coated:

	C	F	Cb
Almonds, 5-6, 1 oz	160	11	11
Clusters, nut, 2, 1 oz	160	11	15
Coffee Beans, 1.4 oz	180	10	23
Creme/Cordial Centers, 1 oz	120	4	21
Fudge, 1 oz	125	5	18
Macadamias, 2-3 pces., 1 oz	180	13	11
Mints, 1 med., 11g	45	1	9
Nougat & Caramel, 1 oz	120	4	21
Peanuts, 12 med., 1 oz	160	11	15
Raisins, 30 med., 1 oz	120	4	21

Cooking Chocolate:

	C	F	Cb
Sweet/Semi-sweet, 1 oz	160	8	18
Chips, ¹/4 cup, 2¹/2 oz	210	12	24
Unsweetened, 1 oz	150	15	8
Carob: Plain, 1 oz	160	11	9

"Take two of these and call me in the morning."

Brands & Generic

Per Piece/Serving   **C** **F** **Cb**

	C	F	Cb
Abba Zabba, 2 oz bar	250	5	48
Absolutely Almond, 2.5 oz bar	380	23	40
Aero Bar (Nestlé), 1.45 oz bar	210	13	26
After Dinner Mints, 1 small	45	1	9
After Eight Mint, each	35	1.2	6
Allen Wertz: Simply Sugar Free			
Coffee Time (decaf), 4	45	1.5	8
Coffee Toffee, 6	120	3	23
Other types, 4	120	2.5	24
Almond Joy, 1.76 oz bar	240	13	29
King Size, 2 pces, 1¹/2 oz	220	12	26
Snack, 1, 0.68 oz	90	5	11
Almond Roca, 1 pce	70	5	6
Almonds, sugar-coated, 7, 1 oz	130	5	20
Altoids (C & B), each	3	0	1
Amazin' Fruit, 1 pouch, 8 pces	60	0	15
Andes: Creme de Menthe; Cherry Jubilee			
Choc covered Patty, (3), 1¹/2 oz	180	3	35
Thins, aver. all flav., (8), 1.4 oz	210	13	22
Anthon Berg: Cognac, each	180	8	25
After Dinner Sweet:			
Marzipan w. Madeira, 1.4 oz	175	7.5	26
Marcipan Brod, each	120	7	13
Asteroid (Nestlé), 54g	260	10	40
Baby Ruth, King Size, 3.7 oz bar	495	21	67
2.1 oz bar	280	12	36
Fun size, each	100	4.5	17
Snack, 1 bar, ³/4 oz	100	5	12
Baci (Perugino), each	85	5	8
Bar None, 1.5 oz bar	240	14	23
Barley Sugar, 1 pce., 0.2 oz	23	0	6
Big Hunt, 2 oz	230	3	47
Bit-O-Honey, 1.7 oz	200	3.5	41
Chews, 6 pces, 1.4 oz	170	3	34
Blow Pops, each	50	0	14
Bonus Bar, 2.1 oz bar	290	16	34
Boston Baked Beans, 30 pces, 1 oz	135	5	20
Brach's: Almond Supremes,11	220	15	18
But'rscotch Disks, 3, 0.6 oz	70	0	16
Choc Bridge Mix, 16, 1.4 oz	190	9	25
Circus Peanuts, each	25	0.6	3
Clusters, 3	220	14	19
Double Dip Choc Peanuts, 15	220	14	19
Golden Butter/Internation. Toffee	25	0.6	5
Lemon Drops, 4, 0.6 oz	50	0	13
Malted Milk Balls, 15	190	9	27

Per Piece/Serving	C	F	Cb
Brach's (Cont):			
Milk Maid Caramel, 18	170	5	30
Orange Slices Hi-C, each	50	0	13
Breath Savers, all types, each	10	0	2
Brite Crackers, 1 bag, 1.5 oz	140	0	32
Brock: Candy Corn, (10) 0.7 oz	75	0	18
Gummy Bears; Sour Balls, each	26	0	6
Lemon Drops, each	20	0	5
Orange Slices, each	35	0	9
Spice Drops, each	12	0	3
Starlight Mints, each	20	0	5
Toffee, each	25	0.8	5
Bubble Gum ~ *See 'Gum'*			
Buncha Crunch, 1/2 cup, 1.4 oz	200	10	26
Burnt Peanuts, 40 pces, 40g	190	8	32
Butterfinger: King Size, 3.7 oz bar	480	18	75
2.1 oz bar	270	11	41
Fun size, each	100	3.5	14
Mini, each	20	1	7
Snack, 2, 1.3 oz	170	7	27
Butterfinger B.B's, 1.4 oz bag	190	8	30
Buttermints, 18 pces, 1 1/2 oz	160	0	40
Butterscotch: 5 pces	120	2.5	20
Buttons *(Walgreens)*, 3, 18g	70	0	18
Chips, 1 oz	150	7	36
Discs *(Sathers)*, 3, 0.6 oz	110	0	16
Candy Cane, Medium, 5", 1/2 oz	50	0	12
Candy Corn, 1 oz	110	0	27
4 oz pkt: 24 pces, 1 1/2 oz	150	0	37
Candy Necklaces, 20g each	80	0.5	20
Caramels: each	30	1	6
Chocolate, each	25	0.3	6
Creams, 3 pces, 1 1/4 oz	130	3	23
2.75 oz pkt, 5 pces, 1 1/2 oz	160	3.5	30
Hershey's Classic Caramels:			
Soft 'n Chewy, 3 pces	80	2.5	13
Choc Creme Filled, 3 pces	80	3	13
Caramel Nips, each	30	1	6
Caramel Popcorn, 1 cup, 1 oz	120	1.5	26
Caramel Truffles *(Godiva)*, 1 pce	110	6.5	13
Caramello *(Hershey's)* 1.6 oz bar	220	10	29
Snack, 0.66 oz	90	4	12
Cellas Choc Cherries,.1 pce	55	2	9
Certs: Breath Mints, 1 pce	6	0	2
Sugar-free, 1 piece	7	0	2
Candy Jar Mix *(Jewel)*, 3, 17g	70	0	17
Charleston Chew, 1 bar, 53g	230	7	40
Cherry Sours *(Sathers)*, 11, 1 1/2 oz	150	0	38

Per Piece/Serving	C	F	Cb
Chews, all types, 1 oz	110	1	25
Chocolate Mints *(Hershey's)*, each	20	0.5	4
Chocolate Parfait Nips, each	30	1	5
Chuckles Jelly: each	35	0	9
Jujubes, each	10	0	3
Chunky Bar *(Nestlé)*, 1.4 oz	210	11	24
Cinnamon Bears *(Walgreens)*, 5	150	0	38
Cinn. Buttons *(Walgreens)*, 3 pce	70	0	17
Cinnamon Drops *(Sathers)*, 19 pce	150	0	36
Coconut Stacks, 4, 41g	190	6	33
Coffee Go Coffee/Cappuccino, ea.	18	0.4	4
Coffee Rio-Gold, each	15	0.5	3
Collard & Bowser: Eng. Toffee, 2	80	4	12
Corn Nuts, 1/3 cup, 1 oz	130	4	20
Cote d'Or: Bouchee, each	130	8	12
Chokotoff, each	210	9	30
Nougatti	150	8	14
Bar & Nuts,1.3 oz	220	18	12
Cotton Candy, 1.2 oz	110	0	27
Cracker Jack, 1.25 oz box	150	2.5	29
Crisped Rice: Almond, 1 bar	130	6	18
Choc Chip, 1 bar	115	4	18
Crispy Rice Snacks, 1 bar	70	2.5	10
Crows, 7 oz pkg	150	0	37
Crunch: 5 oz bar	725	38	90
King Size, 2.75 oz bar	400	21	51
1.55 oz bar	230	12	29
Fun size, each	50	2.5	7
Snack, 3, 1 1/2 oz	220	11	28
Crunch Berries Treats, 1.6 oz bar	190	4.5	36
Decadence *(NuBar)* Bar, 1.3 oz	140	2.5	30
Dots, 12 dots	150	0	37
Double Dip Stick, 1 stick	16	0.5	3
Dove: Dark/Milk, 1.3 oz bar	200	12	22
Bar, 6 oz	920	56	104
Miniatures, each	30	2	3
Drops Candy (9)	100	0	24
Dum Dum Pops *(Spangler)*, 1 pop	25	0	6
English Toffee, 1 pce	48	3	5
Eda's Sugar Free, all flav., 5, 1/2 oz	40	0	15
Estee Dietetic Candies:			
Caramels, all flavors, 1 pce.	30	1	6
Chocolate, Dark/Milk, 1/2 bar	200	14	23
Gummy Bears; Gum Drops, 1 pce.	7	0	1.5
Hard Candies: Butterscotch, 2	25	0	6
Assorted Fruit Lollipops, 5	60	0	15
Peppermint, 3	30	0	7
Mint/Toffee, 5	60	0	15

Per Piece/Serving	C	F	Cb
Estee Dietetic Candies (Cont):			
Lollipop	30	0	8
Milk Chocolate, 1/2 bar, 4 oz	230	17	17
Peanut Butter Cups, 1 cup	40	3	3
Fructose Sweetened, 1 cup	40	2	3
Peanut Brittle, 1/3 box, 1.5 oz	240	9	28
5th Avenue: 2.1 oz bar	290	13	40
King Size bar	460	20	64
Snack Size, 0.58 oz	80	3.5	1
Fanny May: Single wrapped pces			
Mint Meltaway Patty, 1.5 oz	250	17	22
Pixie, 1.5 oz	215	12	24
Trinidad, 1.5 oz	205	11	24
Ferrero Rocher: each	75	5	6
3 pces, 1.3 oz	220	15	17
Fifty 50 Snack Bars:			
Peanut Butter, 2	200	14	16
Almond Choc., 7 pce, 1 1/2 oz	210	15	20
Crunch Choc., 7 pce, 1.1 oz	160	11	19
Fruit & Nut Choc., 7 pce, 1 1/2 oz	200	14	21
Milk Choc., 3 pce, 1/2 bar, 43g	210	14	25
Mini bars, 8 bars, 1 oz	140	9	16
Fondant: Choc-coated, 1.2 oz	130	3	28
Mint, 1 oz	105	0	27
Franklin Crunch 'N Munch:			
all varieties, average, 1.25 oz	170	7	30
Fran's: Gold Bar, 1.75 oz	260	14	34
Gold Bites (Almonds), 1	130	7	17
Fruit Crystals (Walgreens), 3 pces	70	0	17
Fruit Drops, each	6	0	1
Fruit Gems (Sunkist), 3, 1.1 oz	105	0	26
Fruit Leathers, average, 0.5 oz	45	0	12
Fruit Pastilles, 1 roll, 1.4 oz	100	0	26
Fruit Rolls, 1 roll	80	0	20
Fruit Roll-Ups, 1/2 oz	50	0	12
Fruit Runts (Walgreens), 1T., 1/4 pkt	60	0	14
Fruit Shapes (Fruitfield), 1 oz (10)	100	0.5	23
Fruit Waves, 0.5 oz	50	0	12
Fudge: Chocolate/Vanilla, 1 oz	115	3	20
with Nuts, 1 oz	120	4	21
Choco. Marshmallow, 1 oz	120	5	18
w. Nuts, 1 oz	125	5.5	18
Peanut Butter, 1 oz	105	2	21
Ghirardelli: Milk/Dark Chocolate,			
1.25 oz bar	185	12	20
w. almonds, 1.5 oz bar	220	14	25
Choc Nuts & Chews, 1 pce	55	3.5	5

Per Piece/Serving	C	F	Cb
Godiva: Hearts, each	45	2	4
Almond Butter Dome, 1 pce	80	6	6
Bouchee au Chocolate, 1 pce	220	13	23
Cordial Assortment, each	60	2.5	9
Gold Ballotin, 1 pce	70	3.5	9
Milk/Dark/IvoryAssortment, each	75	4	8
Nut & Caramel, each	75	4	6
Truffle Amaretto, 1 pce	110	6.5	12
Golden Almond Bar, 1 bar	520	34	40
Golden 111 Bar, 1 bar	500	30	52
Go Lightly: Box Candies, 4	60	0	15
Bags: Assorted Taffy, 6	140	3	36
Vanilla Caramels, 5	150	6	31
Super Free Choc Crunch, 7,1 1/2 oz	180	13	23
Goobers Peanuts, 1 pkg, 1.4 oz	210	13	20
Good & Fruity, 1 box, 1.8 oz	140	1	35
Snack Size, 1 box, 17g	60	0	15
Good & Plenty: 1/5 box, 1.4 oz	130	0	38
Snack Size, 1 box, 17g	60	0	14
GooGoo Cluster, 1 bar, 1.75 oz	240	11	32
GUM: Per Piece			
Bazooka, each	30	0	7
Beechies	6	0	2
Big League Chew	10	0	2
Bubble Gum Balls (Hershey's)	10	0	2
Bubble Yum	25	0	6
Sugarless	10	0	3
Candilicious	30	0	2
Carefree (Sugarless/Regular)	5	0	2
Chiclets	5	0	1
Clorets, stick	10	0	2
Dentyne	6	0	2
Estee, bubble/regular	5	0	2
Extra (Wrigley's),			
Sugar-Free Bubble Gum, 1	5	0	2
Freshen-Up	13	0	2
Hubba Bubba: Regular	23	0	6
Sugar-free, average	14	0	0.5
Ice Breakers, 1 stick	5	0	2
Sonic Boom Bubble Gum	15	0	3
Sticklets	7	0	2
Super Bubble	15	0	4
Trident: Slab	5	0	1
Soft Bubble Gum	9	0	1
Wrigley's, all flavors	10	0	2

Per Piece/Serving	C	F	Cb
Gum Drops: 1 small	15	0	3
1 large, 0.4 oz	40	0	7
6 oz pkt: 4 pces, 1.4 oz	130	0	31
Gummi Bears: 1 bear	17	0	4
8 bears, 1½ oz	140	0	32
Gummi Novelties *(Walgreens)*, 6	150	0	36
Gummi Savers, each	12	0	3
Gummi Sweet Tarts, 1 bug, 1.5 oz	150	0	34
Gummi Watch, 1, 2 oz	105	0	24
Gummi Worms, each	25	0	5
Guylian: No Sugar Added			
Milk Chocolate, 8 squares, 1 oz	126	9	15
Dark Chocolate, 8 squares, 1 oz	117	9	14
Halvah *(Joyvah):*			
Plain/Marble, ½ bar, 2 oz	390	25	18
Choc.coated Sesame, ½ bar, 2 oz	380	23	20
Hard Candy: all flavors, 1 oz	110	0	28
1 regular piece	18	0	5
Heath: Original, 1.4 oz bar	210	13	25
Bites, 1.4 oz	210	12	25
Snack, 0.33 oz	50	3	6
Hershey's:			
Bar: 1.55 oz bar	240	14	25
King Size bar	410	25	38
w. Almonds, 1.45 oz bar	230	14	20
Bites: Almond Joy (7)	90	6	9
Cookies 'n' Creme (7)	90	5	10
York (15), 39g	150	3	31
Milk Choc w. Almond (7)	90	6	8
Cookies 'N Mint: 1.55 oz bar	230	12	27
Snack, 0.6 oz	90	4.5	11
Crunchy Cookie Cups, 1.4 oz	210	12	23
Hugs: w. Almonds (9), 1.4 oz	230	13	22
1 piece	25	1.5	3
Kisses: Milk Choc./Almond (1)	25	1.5	3
Milk Chocolate: 1.55 oz bar	200	12	25
2.6 oz bar	400	23	42
7 oz bar, ⅕ bar	200	12	21
w. Almonds Snack, 0.6 oz	90	6	8
Miniatures, 5 pces, 1.5 oz	230	13	25
Nuggets: Snack, aver. all bars (1)	50	3	6
P'nut Butter Crispy Rice, (1)	230	13	25
Special Dark Choc., 1.45 oz bar	230	13	25
Sweet Escapes:			
1.4 oz bar, aver.	180	7	27
Snack, average all bars (1)	80	3.5	12
Whoppers, 10 pce	100	4	16
Honeycomb: Plain, 1 oz	115	0	27
Choc-coated, 1 oz	125	1	28
Hot Tamales, 1 box, 60g, 2.1 oz	220	0	55
Sathers, 19 pces, 1.4 oz	150	0	36
Ice Blue Mints *(Walgreens)*, 3, 17g	70	0	17
Jawbreakers *(Sathers)*, 3, 17g	70	0	17
Jellies, 3 medium, 1 oz	120	0	30
Jells Raspberry *(Joyva)*, each	70	1	8
Jelly Beans: Small, 22 beans, 1 oz	100	0	24
Regular, 12 beans, 1 oz	100	0	24
1 bean	8	0	2
Jumbo, 1 bean	20	0	5
Jewel, 13 beans, 1.4 oz	140	0	36
Sathers/Walgreens, 17, 40g	150	0	37
Wonderbeans, 33 beans	100	0	24
Jelly Bellys: each	4	0	1
35 pces, 1.4oz	140	0	37
Jelly Rings *(Jewel)*, 3, 1.5 oz	160	0	39
Jolly Rancher: Candy (1)	40	0	9
Fruit Chews (6), 1.4 oz	150	1.5	33
Jolly Jellies, 7 oz	120	0	30
Lollipops, 1 pce, 0.6 oz	60	0	16
Sugar Free, 4 pces, 0.5 oz	35	0	14
Junior Mints: 1.6 oz box	180	3	38
16 pces, 1.4 oz	160	2.5	34
Juicefuls: Red Raspb., (3), 0.6 oz	60	0	15
Assorted Fruits, 1 pce	20	0	5
Jujubes, all types (6), 1.4 oz	3	0	3
Juju Mix *(Sathers)*, 11 pce, 1½ oz	150	0	36
Juju Toys: 6 pce, 1.5 oz	150	0	37
Jujyfruits, 1 box, 0.2 oz	40	0	10
Kit Kat: 1.5 oz bar	215	12	27
2.6 oz bar	365	21	40
Big Kat, 1.95 oz	290	15	35
Bites (15), 1.4 oz	200	10	25
King Size bar, 2.8 oz bar	410	22	48
Multipack, each	80	4	10
Snack, 3 (2 pce bars), 1.65 oz	240	12	30
Wafer Bar, 2 pce, 0.56 oz	80	4	10
Krackel: 2.6 oz bar	390	21	45
Snack size, 0.3 oz	45	2.5	5
Kudos: 1 oz bar, aver. all types	120	5	20
M&M's Milk Choc Minis, 0.8 oz	90	2.5	17
Snickers, 0.8 oz	100	3.5	15
Lance: Popscotch, 1.2 oz pkg	160	6	24
Chocolaty Peanut Bar, 2 oz bar	320	18	30
Peanut Bar, 1.8 oz pkg	260	14	24

Piece/Serving	C	F	Cb
mon Drops, 3, 1/2 oz	50	0	12
Sugar Free *(Walgreens)*, 5, 1/2 oz	35	0	14
monhead, 10, 1/2 oz	60	0	14
:orice: Average all types, 1oz	100	0	25
Bites *(Switzer)*, each	12	0	1
Chews *(Panda)*, each	10	0	2
Tid Bits, each	5	0	1
Twists: Black/Red, aver. 1 pce	30	0	7
American Licorice Co.: Laces, 1	35	0	8
Stick, (1) 0.5 oz	45	0	11
Choco Sticks, (4) 1.4 oz	145	0	35
Red Bites, 1.4 oz	140	0	34
Super Red Ropes, 1 rope, 2 oz	200	0	46
Vines, 1 pce	70	0	17
fesavers:			
Large size, 1 candy	15	0	4
Regular, all flavors, 1 candy	9	0	2
1 Roll (14 candies), 1.14 oz	130	0	32
Creme Savers (1)	23	0	5
Sugar-free Delites: *Per Candy*			
Orchard Fruits; Summer Blend	5	0	2
Butter Toffee; European Collect.	9	0.5	3
Gummi Savers, 1.5 oz roll	140	0	32
Lollipops Fruit, 1 pce, 0.4 oz	45	0	11
ik-m-aid *(Nestlé)*, 1.7 oz	60	0	15
indt: Lindor, Balls, average	73	4	8
Dark Choc Truffles, each	70	6	4
ollipops, each, 0.2 oz	20	0	5
ollipops C Pops *(Glenny's)*, each	35	0	8
lamba, 9 pces, 1 1/2 oz	160	2	36
1&Ms: Plain, 1.7 oz pkg	240	10	34
Milk Chocolate, 1 pce	4	0.2	0.5
20 pces, 0.6 oz	80	4	10
34 pces, 1 oz	135	6.5	17
68 pces, 2 oz	270	13	34
Almond Choc, 1.3 oz pkg	200	11	21
1.5 oz pkg	230	13	25
Caramel, 1/4 cup, 1.5 oz	220	11	28
Crispy, 1.5 oz	200	9	30
King Size, 1/2 pkg, 1.6 oz	240	12	28
1.5 oz pkg	220	11	28
Mini Milk Choc. Candies, 1 tube	180	8	24
1.5 oz pkg	70	3	7
Peanut: 1.7 oz pkg	250	13	30
Fun Size, 0.7 oz pkg	110	5	13
Peanut Butter, 1.6 oz pkg	240	13	27
Fun Size, 0.7 oz pkg	110	6	12

Per Piece/Serving	C	F	Cb
Mars Bar: All varieties, 1.8 oz	240	13	31
Fun size, 1 bar	95	5	12
Marshmallows: Firm/Soft, 1 oz	90	0	23
Regular size, 6 pces, 33g	110	0	26
Mini-Marshmallow, 1/2 c., 30g	100	0	26
Choc-coat. Twists *(Joyva)*, ea.	95	2	10
Kraft: Mini, 1/2 cup	80	0	21
Creme, 2 Tbsp	40	0	10
Jet-Puffed, 5 pces	90	0	23
Funmallows, each	25	0	6
Miniature, 1/2 cup	100	0	25
Teddy Bear, 1/2 cup	50	0	12
Marshmallow Egg, 1 egg	110	0	26
Marzipan, 1 oz	140	7	16
Mauna Loa: Choc., 2.5 oz bar	420	29	36
Choc coated Macadamias, 9	230	17	19
Mega Fruit Gummi, each	10	0	2
Mexican Hats, (9)	100	0	24
Mike & Ike, 1 pce, 2.1 oz	220	0	55
Milk Choc. *(Hershey's):* 1.55 oz bar	240	14	25
Eggs, candy coated (4)	90	4	12
w. Almonds, 1.45 oz bar	230	14	20
Milk Choc. Crisp, 1.45 oz bar	205	11	22
Milk Duds, 7 pces	90	3.5	15
Milk Shake Bar, 1.8 oz	220	7	37
Milky Way: 2 oz bar	270	10	41
Fun size, 1.4 oz each	90	3.5	14
Miniatures, 5, 43g	190	7	30
Snack, 2, 40g	180	7	28
Milky Way Lite, 1.6 oz	170	5	34
Miniatures, 1.4 oz pkg, 5	150	4.5	29
Midnight Bar, 1.75 oz	220	8	36
Mints: uncoated, 1 oz	100	0	23
1 small mint (3/4" diam.)	7	0	2
1 large mint (1 1/2" diam.)	30	0	7
Mon Cheri *(Ferrero)*, 4 pces, 45g	260	18	20
Mounds: 1.9 oz bar	250	13	31
Snack, 0.68 oz	90	5	11
Mr Goodbar:			
King Size, 2.6 oz bar	410	25	37
1.75 oz bar	270	17	25
Snack, 0.3 oz	45	3	4
Necco Candy Wafers, 3, 57g	15	0	4
Neuhaus, average all types	80	5	7
Nibs, all types, 1 pouch, 0.5 oz	45	0	11
Nips *(Pearson)*, all flavors, 2, 14g	60	2	10
Nite Bite, *(Glucose Bar)*	100	3.5	15

Per Piece/Serving	C	F	Cb
Nothing But Nuts Butter Toffee			
3 Tbsp, 1 oz	200	15	9
Nougat, 2 pces, 1 oz	115	1	25
Chocolate Covered, 1 oz	120	4	20
Nougat Nut Cream, 3.5 oz	340	31	50
Now & Later *(Nabisco)*, 1 pkg	270	2.5	63
Nutrageous Bar *(Reese's)*, 3.4 oz	520	30	52
King Size, 3.4 oz bar	480	24	54
Snack, 0.6 oz	90	5	9
Oh Henry! 1.8 oz bar	240	10	32
100 Grand, 1.5 oz bar	200	8	30
Orange *(Lindt)*, 6 block, 40g	190	10	24
Orange Slices: *(Jewel)*, 3, 41g	140	0	36
(Walgreens), 3, 43g	150	0	36
Pastel Mints *(Walgreens)*, 33 pce	150	0	38
Patteez *(Sweet n' Low)*, 1/2 ctn, 5	120	2.5	32
PayDay Bar, 1.85 oz bar	260	13	29
King Size, 3.4 oz	480	24	54
Snack, 0.7 oz	100	5	11
Peanut Bar, 1.6 oz bar	210	14	20
Peanut Butter Bars, 3 pces, 18g	80	1.5	15
Peanut Brittle, 1 oz	130	5	20
Peanut Chews *(Goldenberg's)*, ea.	60	3	21
Peanut Riesen (5), 41g	190	7	28
Peanuts, choc-covered, each	25	1.5	2
Pearson's Mint Patties, 5, 38g	150	2.5	31
Pecan Roll, 1/3 bar, 40g	200	10	26
Peppermints, 7 small, 0.5 oz	50	0	12
Hershey's, 3 pces	60	0	15
Peppermint Twists, 2, 13g	60	0	12
Pez, 1 roll	30	0	6
Planters:			
Choc. Peanuts, 25, 7 oz	220	13	20
Orig. Peanut Bar, 1.6 oz	230	14	22
Popcorn ~ See Snacks Page 123			
Positively Pecan, 2.5 oz bar	390	24	38
Pralines: small, 0.3 oz	38	2	5
1 large piece, 1.4 oz	180	10	24
Pretzels: choc-covered:			
3 minisize, 1.15 oz	150	5.5	23
1 regular, 1 oz	130	4.5	20
Pretzel Flipz *(Nestlé)*, 8, 1 oz	130	5	19
Raisinets, 1 pkg, 1.7 oz	210	8	33
Raspberry Cream, each	80	2.5	5
Red Hot Dollars, 7 pce	100	0	24

Per Piece/Serving	C	F	Cb
Reese's:			
Chocolate Bar, 2.8 oz	420	24	43
Candy (Multipack), each	95	5.5	9
Miniatures, each	40	2.5	4
Peanut Butter Bites (7)	90	6	9
Mini, 1 pce	42	2.5	5
Peanut Butter Cups, 1.8 oz cup	280	17	28
Mini, 1 pce, 0.27 oz	40	2.5	4
Peanut Butter Eggs (1), 0.6 oz	90	5	9
Reese's Pieces (25), 0.7 oz	90	4.5	11
Snack, 2, 34g	190	11	29
Rice Crunchy Bars: 1 bar, 19g			
Average all flavors	60	0	14
Rice Krispies Treats: 1.3 oz bar	150	3.5	29
Chocolate Chip, 1.3 oz bar	160	5	28
Riesen Choc. Chew, 5, 1.4 oz	180	7	29
Ritter Sport: Plain Choc, 50g	260	16	26
w. Hazelnuts, 1/2 pkg, 50g	290	19	24
Robin Eggs: Large, 2 pces	70	2	13
Medium, 4 pces	90	3	15
Mini, 10 pces	70	2.5	13
Rolo, all types (3), 0.64 oz	80	2.5	13
Root Beer Barrels, 3, 0.5 oz	60	0	16
Russell Stover Candy:			
Creams, each	60	2	10
Almond Delight, 2 oz	290	17	32
Caramel Bar, 46g	230	11	20
Jelly Cups (P/Nut Butter), 2, 34g	140	9	14
Mint Dream	160	8	19
Pecan Delight (Sugar Free), 2 oz	260	18	27
Pecan Delight, 2 oz bar	310	20	27
Pecan Roll, 50g	260	18	23
Salt Water Taffy *(Sathers)*, 5, 43g	150	2.5	34
Seashells *(Guylian)* 1 shell	65	4	6
Sesame Crunch, 3 pces	80	4	7
Simply Lite:			
Li'l Bits Chocolatey/P'nut Butter,			
1/2 ctn, 36 pieces	130	5	18
Simply Sugar Free: See *Allen Wertz*			
Sixlets *(Hershey)*, 24 pces	90	3.5	15
Skittles, all flavors, 1.5 oz pkg	170	2	39
1.6 oz pkg, each	60	0.5	14
King Size, 2.17 oz, 1 pack	240	2.5	54
Skor Toffee Bar, 1.4 oz	220	14	23
Smarties Candy Rolls, 1 roll	25	0	6
Snackwell's Raisin Dips, 5 oz	160	5	34

Candy, Chocolate (Cont)

Per Piece/Serving	C	F	Cb
Snickers: Bar: 2.1 oz bar	280	14	35
King Size, 1/2 bar, 1.2 oz	170	8	21
Munch Bar, 1.4 oz bar	230	15	17
Fun Size, each	95	5	12
Miniatures, each	42	2.5	5
Creme Egg, each	170	10	19
Snack, 2, 40g	190	10	24
Sno Caps, 2.3 oz pkg	300	13	48
Soft 'N Chewy Butter Toffee, ea.	32	0.5	7
Soft Drops (9)	100	0	24
Soft Hot Dollars (11)	90	0	23
Sonic Boom Pops (Walgreens), ea.	60	0	14
Sour Brite Crawlers, 13 pces	140	0	31
Sour Punch, all types, 1 pkg	190	9	45
1 straw	20	0	5
Spearmint Leaves: (Jewel), 5, 40g	140	0	35
(Walgreens), 5, 11/2 oz	150	0	38
Spice Drops, 14 pces, 11/2 oz	140	0	36
Spree (Nestlé): Snack, 1, 11/2 oz	50	0	13
Starburst: Candy Canes, 0.5 oz	70	0	18
Fruit Chews, each	20	0.4	4
2 oz pkg	240	4.5	48
Fruit Twist, each	35	0	8
Fruit Twist, 2 oz pkg	190	1	45
Jellybeans, 1.5 oz	150	0	38
Jellybean Egg, 2 oz	200	0	51
Trop. Fruit Chews, 2.7 oz pack	240	5	48
Starlight Mints: 3 pces, 1/2 oz	60	0	16
Suckers (Walgreens), 1 sucker, 11g	45	0	11
Sweet 'N Low: Chews, each	14	0.2	3
Sugar-Free Hard Candy, each	8	0	2
Sweet Escapes: See Hershey's			
Sweet Success Bars, 1 bar	120	4	23
Sweet Tarts (Nestlé), 7, 1/2 oz	50	0	13
Symphony: All types, 1/5 bar, 7 oz	220	14	24
Snack: Chocolate (1), 0.6 oz	100	6	10
w. Almds & Toffee (1), 0.5 oz	80	5	7
Taffy, 1 pce, 1/2 oz	55	0.5	12
3 Musketeers, 2.1 oz bar	260	8	46
Fun size, each	70	2	13
Miniatures, each	25	0.5	5
Snack, 2, 33g	140	4.5	26
Tang-a-Roos: 1 roll	24	0	6
Tarts: (Walgreens), 4 pce, 15g	60	0	15
Tails: (Walgreens), 8 pce, 15g	60	0	15
Tastetations (Hershey's): Pep'mint	20	0	8
Butterscotch; Caramel; Choc	20	0.5	4

Per Piece/Serving	C	F	Cb
Terry's Orange Milk Choc, 1 pce	50	3	5
Tic Tac, all varieties, each	1.5	0	0
Toblerone: 50g (1.76 oz) bar	270	15	32
1 bar, 100g, (3.5 oz)	540	30	63
1/3 bar, 33g	180	10	21
Toffees: Regular, 1 oz	150	9	15
Tongue Torchers (Walgreens), 3	70	0	17
Tootsie Roll Midgies (Walgreens), 6	160	3	33
Tootsie Roll Pops, 1/2 oz pop	50	0	12
Treasures (Nestlé): (4), 1.6 oz	240	16	26
Nestlé Crunch, 3	160	8.5	20
Butterfinger Pieces, 3	180	9	23
Creamy Caramel, 3	180	9	22
Peanut Butter Miniatures, 3	180	12	17
Truffles: Regular, 1 pce, 0.4 oz	60	4	5
Large (Godiva), 0.75 oz	110	6.5	12
Extra Large (J.Schmidt), 11/2 oz	220	13	24
Turtles (Nestlé), each	85	4.5	10
Twix: Caramel (1), 1 oz	140	7	18
King Size: 1 cookie, 3.35 oz	120	6	16
4 cookies	480	24	64
Fun Size, 0.5 oz	80	4	10
2 oz pkg, 2 bars	280	14	37
Peanut Butter, 0.9 oz	140	8.5	14
Snack, 1 cookie, 0.5 oz	80	5	8
Twizzlers: Candy, aver., 1 pce, 8g	30	0	8
Pull 'n' Peel, Cherry (1), 1 oz	90	1	19
Velamints Sugar Free, 1 pce	10	0	2
Werther's Original, 3 pce, 15g	60	1	13
Whatchamacallit Bar, 1.7 oz	220	10	29
Snack (1), 0.58 oz	80	3.5	10
Whitman's:			
Pecan Roll, 2 oz roll	300	20	26
Sampler, 3 pces, 1.4 oz	200	11	25
Assorted, 1 pce	63	3	9
Dark Chocolate, 1 pce	65	3	8
Snoopy Treats, 2 pces	190	10	24
Yogurt Candy: Plain, 1 oz	120	6	15
Coated Raisins, 1 oz	120	4	21
York Mints: 1.5 oz patty	145	5	34
Snack size, 2	55	1	11
Peppermint Patties, 3	150	5	30
York Peppermint Pattie (9)	90	1.5	19
Zachary Old Fash. Creme Drops, 3	170	3	36
Zagnut: 1.75 oz bar	230	10	31
Snack size (1), 0.5 oz	70	3	9
Zero Bar, 1 pce, 0.6 oz	70	2.5	12

Carob, Cough Drops

Carob Candy

Per Piece/Serving

	C	F	Cb
Carob: Plain/Natural, 1 oz	160	11	9
Carob coated: Raisins, 1 oz	130	8	15
Almonds/Peanuts, 1 oz	150	10	14
Malt Balls, 1 oz	135	8	15
Caramels, 1 oz	110	4	18
Dates, 1 oz	125	5	20
Soybeans	145	9	16
Trail; Party Mix, 1 oz	140	9	15
Carob Chips, unsweetened, 1 oz	140	7	19
Carob Bars, average all brands:			
Plain/Nut, 1 oz	160	11	13
Fruit & Nut, 1 oz	155	10	13
Mint/Orange, 1 oz	160	11	14
Caroby Natural Touch, 3 oz	450	27	36
Carafection: Cashew Coconut Crunch, 1/2 Bar, (42g) 1.5 oz	250	14	5

Cough Drops & Lozenges

Per Piece/Serving

	C	F	Cb
Beech Nut, 1 tablet	10	0	2
Hall's, 1 tablet	15	0	4
Hall's Plus, 1	18	0	5
Helps Cough, all flavors, 1	14	0	3
Listerine Loz. (Amer.Chicle)	9	0	2
Ludens Throat Drops, all flavors, 14	10	0	2
Pine Bros, 1 cough drop	10	0	2
Rite Aid, Menthol Cough, 1 drop	12	0	3
Rolaids/Sodium Free, 1	4	0	1
Sathers Peppermint Lozenges, 1	13	0	3
Squibb Cough/Throat Loz.'s, 1	16	0	4
Sucrets (Beecham) Lozenges, 1	10	0	2
Wintergreen Loz. (Walgreens), 1	13	0	3
Cough Medications - Page 132			

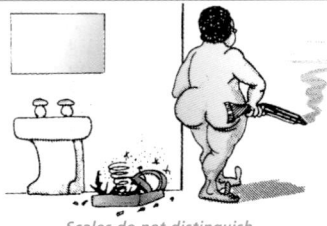

Scales do not distinguish between fat, muscle and fluids.

Unexplained Weight Changes

Body weight fluctuates from day to day due to changes in body fluids. Water makes up 60-70% of total body weight and can be affected by changes in hormone levels, dietary salt and carbohydrates and even exercise.

Weight on the scales doesn't distinguish between weight changes due to water, fat or muscle. This is why we shouldn't allow every fluctuation in weight to rule our lives.

Limit salt and salty foods if you retain excess fluid but do not limit fluid intake. Drink at least 6-8 glasses of water and other fluids daily.

Menopausal Weight Gains

Most women gain an average of 4-5 pounds in the years leading up to the menopause - usually in their middle to late 40's. This can occur even when exercise and eating habits have not changed significantly.

With hormonal changes occurring at that time, body fat also tends to be redistributed from thighs, buttocks and hips to the breast and stomach areas (a greater health risk).

Be sure to eat wisely and continue daily physical activity including strength-training to maintain or build muscles - and to boost metabolism and self-esteem.

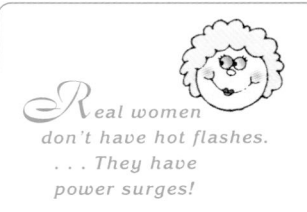

Real women don't have hot flashes. . . . They have power surges!

Home-Popped Popcorn

	C	F	Cb
Popping Corn Kernels:			
2 Tbsp, 1 oz	100	1	22
(makes approx. 3½ cups)			
Air-popped (no oil), plain, 1 oz	100	0	22
1 cup (6g)	20	0	4
Oil-popped, plain, 1 oz	140	8	10
1 cup (11g)	55	3	4
Popcorn Oil, 1 Tbsp	120	14	0

Microwave Popcorn

Average All Brands (Popped)

	C	F	Cb
Butter: Regular, 1 cup	35	2	4
Light, 1 cup	25	1	4
Act II Popcorn:			
Butter, 1 cup, 0.3 oz	35	2	4
4 cups, popped, 1 oz	140	8	16
Light Butter, 1 cup, 0.2 oz	25	1	4
5 cups, popped, 1 oz	125	4	20
Butter Lovers,1 cup, 0.3 oz	45	3	4
3.5 cups, 1 oz	160	10	14
Butter Lovers (Reduced Fat), 1 c.	30	1.5	4.5
4.5 cups, 1 oz	130	6	20
American Fare (K-Mart):			
Butter, 1 cup, 0.3 oz	37	2.5	4
3.5 cups, 1 oz	130	9	14
Light Butter, 1 cup, 0.3 oz	28	1	5
3.5 cups, 1 oz	100	4	17
Healthy Choice: Butter, 6 cups, 1 oz	100	2.5	22
Natural, 6 cups, 1 oz	100	2	22
Newman's Own: Butter, 1 oz	170	11	16
Light Butter Flavor, 3½ cups	110	3	20
Orville Redenbacher:			
Corn on the Cob, 1 cup, popped	35	2.5	3
Movie Theater Butter, 1 cup	30	2	3
4 cups, popped, 1 oz	120	8	12
Light Movie Theater Butter, 1 cup	20	1	2
4 cups, 1 oz	80	4	8
Double Feature Jumbo, 1 cup	30	2	3
Smart Pop!: Lowfat, 1 cup	15	0	3
Butter Light, 1 cup	20	0.5	3

Bagged Popcorn

Average All Brands (Ready-to-Eat)

	C	F	Cb
Regular: Plain, ½ oz pkg	80	5	7
1 oz pkg	160	10	14
4 oz pkg	640	40	56
Box (store/airport), 2 oz	320	20	28
Bag (9" high x 5" wide), 3 oz	480	30	42

Brands ~ Bagged Popcorn

	C	F	Cb
Act II Popcorn:			
Butter Toffee: ¾ cup, 1 oz	110	1	27
w. Peanuts, ¾ cup, 1 oz	120	2.5	24
Caramel w. P'nuts, ¾ cup, 1 oz	120	2.5	24
Supreme w. Pecans, Almonds, ¾ c.	130	5	22
Boston's: Fat Free, ⅔ cup, 1 oz	100	0	23
Lite, 2 cup, 1 oz	140	6	19
Gourmet Super Prem., 2 c., 1 oz	160	11	13
40% Less Fat, 2¾ cup, 1 oz	140	6	17
Cracker Jack: Original, ½ cup, 1 oz	120	2	23
Fat Free varieties, ¾ cup, 1 oz	110	0	26
Crunch 'N Munch: ½ cup, 1 oz	140	5	22
Caramel w. P'nuts, ⅔ cup, 1.2 oz	140	3.5	25
Fiddle Faddle: ¾ cup, 1 oz	140	6	21
Orville Redenbacher:			
Butter Toffee, ⅔ cup, 1.1 oz	140	4.5	24
Skippy P'nut Butter, ¾ cup, 1 oz	130	3	23
Chocolate Lovers Poppycock,			
½ cup, 1 oz	140	5	21
Heath Toffee Candy, ½ c., 1 oz	100	1.5	23
Slimmons (Fat Free): ¾ c., 1 oz	110	0	25
Weight Watchers: Butter, ⅔ oz	90	2.5	14

Movie Theater Popcorn

	C	F	Cb
Small (7 cups): Plain	400	27	30
with Butter	580	47	30
Medium (16 cups): Plain	900	60	70
with Butter	1170	90	70
Large (20 cups): Plain	1150	76	90
with Butter	1500	116	90

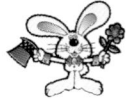
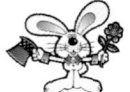
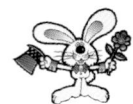

Potato Chips, Pretzels, Tortilla Chips

Potato Chips/Crisps

Average All Brands

		C	**F**	**Cb**
Regular:				
Plain or flavored, 1 chip		9	1	1
17 chips, 1 oz bag		150	10	15
4 oz quantity		600	40	60
Pringles, 14 crisps, 1 oz		160	11	15
5.75 oz can		920	63	86
Ruffles, Buffalo Style, 1 oz		160	10	16
Reduced Fat:				
Pringles, 1 oz		140	7	20
Crunch Tators, 1 oz		140	7	19
Kettle Fry (Eagle), 1 oz		150	8	16
Lowfat/Baked varieties, 1 oz		110	1.5	23
Fat Free:				
Childer's/Louise's, 1 oz		100	0	22
Pringles (Fat Free), 1 oz		70	0	15
Lay's Wow!, 1 oz		75	0	18
Ruffles Wow!, 17 chips, 1 oz		75	0	17
Cheddar Sour Crm, 15, 1 oz		75	0	16

Tortilla Chips

	C	**F**	**Cb**
Tortilla Chips: Average, 1 oz	150	8	22
(1 oz = approx. 11 chips or 12 strips)			
Boston: Baked, 13 chips, 1 oz	110	1.5	23
Doritos: 18 chips, 1 oz	140	6	20
Light, 13 chips, 1 oz	130	5	20
Wow! Nacho Cheesier, 1 oz	90	0.5	16
Keebler Suncheros Light, 1 oz	150	8	18
Kettle: Average, 1 oz	140	6	18
Padrino Reduced Fat, 1 oz	130	4	22
Utz: Lowfat Baked, 8 chips, 1 oz	120	1.5	23

Pretzels

Average All Brands

		C	**F**	**Cb**
Hard Baked Pretzels:				
1 oz		110	2	22
Sticks, thin, 2¹/₄" (9/oz), 1		12	0	3
Twists, thin, ¹/₄" thick, (5/oz), 1		25	0.2	5
Dutch (2³/₄"x 2⁵/₈") ¹/₂ oz, 1		55	1	11
Fat Free: *Snyders* (1), 1 oz		100	0	22
Utz Wheels/Nuggets, 1 oz		100	0	22
Rold Gold: Sticks, 48, 1 oz		100	0	23
Sourdough Nuggets, 12, 1 oz		100	0	23
Thins, 12, 1 oz		110	0	24
Twists, 16, 1 oz		110	1	22
Tiny Twists, 18, 1 oz		100	0	23
Low Fat Pretzels:				
American Fare Mini Twists, 1 oz		120	1	23
Rold Gold: Crispy Thins, 9, 1 oz		110	0.5	22
Choc-coated: *(Nestlé)*, 1 oz		130	6	20
White Fudge covered *(Nestlé)*, 1 oz, 7 pieces		140	6	19
Soft Pretzels (Twists) average:				
Plain: Regular, 2.5 oz		190	0	41
King Size, 5 oz		390	0	83
Big Cheese, 5 oz		380	7	61
Peanut Butter filled *(Tr. Joe's)* 1 oz		160	7	18
Toffee *(Crunch 'n Munch)*, 12		120	1	25
Auntie Anne's: See Fast-Foods Pg. 172				
Snyder's of Hanover: Logs (7) 1 oz		120	1	21
Homestyle (15), 1 oz		120	1	24
Super Pretzel: Jalapeno, 5 oz		360	0	78
Bavarian Twist, 3 oz		210	3	41
Cinnamon Raisin w. Icing, 5 oz		420	4	76
Sweet Dough Twist, 3.7 oz		300	3	60

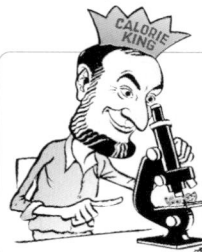

Feedback Welcome!

Please contact the author with comments and suggestions.

Write to: Allan Borushek
POB 1616 Costa Mesa CA 92627
Email: allan@calorieking.com

Snacks	C	F	Cb
Bacon Cheese Crackers, 1 oz	140	6	14
Banana Chips, 1/3 cup, 1 oz	140	7	18
Beef Jerky: Average, 1 oz	70	1	0
Beef Sticks (Frito-Lay's) 0.3 oz	50	4	1
Bugles: Original, 1 1/3 cups, 1 oz	160	9	18
Baked Bugles, 1 1/2 cup, 1.1 oz	130	3.5	23
Cajun Jerky, 1 1/2 oz	150	6	6
Carrot Chips (Hain)	160	9	26
Cheddar Lites (Health Valley) 1 oz	120	3	21
Cheese Crackers, 1 oz	130	6	18
Cheese Filled (Frito-Lay's)	210	11	24
Cheese Curls, 1 1/4 cup, 1 oz	160	9	19
Reduced Fat (Utz), 1 oz	140	6	21
American Fare, 1 1/4 cup, 1 oz	140	5	22
Cheese Puffs: average, 1 oz	150	10	15
Lowfat, 1 oz	140	5	20
Health Valley, 1 1/2 cup	110	3	21
No Fries, 1 oz	110	0	23
Cheese Straws, 4 pieces	110	7	8
Cheese Twists: 23 twists, 1 oz	150	8	19
Cheetos:			
Regular all flavors	160	10	15
Light, cheese flavored	140	6	19
Cheez Balls:			
45 balls, 1 oz	150	10	15
Reduced Fat, 45 balls, 0.73 oz	100	4.5	13
Cheez Bopps (Boston's), (28) 1 oz	130	6	17
Cheez Curls/Doodles, 1 oz	160	10	16
Cheez Mania (Planters), 35, 1 oz	160	3	15
Chex Mix:			
General Mills, 1.1 oz	150	10	15
Bold 'N Zesty (40% less fat), 1/2 c.	140	6	20
Chedder (50% less fat), 1/2 c.	130	5	20
Traditional (60% less fat), 2/3 c.	130	4	21
Chex (Ralston) 2/3 cup, 1 oz	130	5	20
Churros (Mex. Pastry) 10",1.2 oz	140	9	12
Cinna Chips (T.J. Cinn.) 3, 1 oz	110	4	19
Combos (Oven Baked): Per Bag, 1.8 oz			
Cheddar Cheese Crackers	240	11	31
Cheddar/Nacho Cheese Pretzels	240	8	35
Pepperoni Pizza	240	11	30
Corn Chips:			
Average all types, 1 oz	160	10	15
8 oz bag	1280	80	120
Doritos: (12), 1 oz	150	7	20
Nachos; 4-Cheese, 1 oz	140	8	17
3D's Nacho Cheesier, 1 oz (32)	130	5	19

Snacks (Cont)	C	F	Cb
Corn Crunchies/Spirals, 1 oz	160	10	15
Corn Crisps (Pringle), 1 oz	140	7	18
Corn Nuts, 1/3 cup, 1 oz	130	4	20
Corn Puffs (Health Valley) 2 c. 1 oz	120	1.5	25
Dunkaroos, 1 tray, 1 oz	130	4.5	20
FlavorTwists (Fritos), 1 oz	160	10	16
French's Potato Sticks 3/4 c., 1 oz	180	12	16
Fruit a Freeze: Bars, each, 3 oz	170	9	23
Funyun's Onion flavor., 1 oz	140	7	18
Goldfish (Pepperidge Farm) 1 oz	140	7	18
Gold-N-Chees (Lance), 1 3/8 oz	180	7	25
Keebler: Wheatables Snack Mix,			
Toasted Honey, 1/2 cup, 1 oz	130	5	20
Peanut Butter Crunch, 1/2 c., 1 oz	160	7	20
Koolstuf: All flavors, 1 bar, 1.3 oz	130	3	27
Lance Sandwich:			
Bonnie, 1 pkg	160	7	23
Capt. Wafers; Choc-O-Mint, pkg	190	10	23
Sour Dough w. Cheddar, 1 pkg	240	15	23
Other varieties, average, 1 pkg	200	10	22
Munchos, 16 pieces, 1 oz	160	10	16
Nabisco: Oreo, 1.3 oz	160	7	24
Chips Ahoy, 1.3 oz	150	5	25
Sportz, Cheese Nips (38), 1 oz	150	7	19
Sweet Crispers (18), 1 oz	135	3	25
Nibblers (Snyder's): Regular (13)	130	3	23
Sourdough Fat Free (16)	120	0	25
Onion Rings (Lance), 1 pkg	120	6	16
Oriental Mix (rice snacks), 1 oz	155	7.5	15
Original Party Mix (Flavor House):			
1/3 cup	160	10	13
Party Mix (Flavor Tree) 1/4 cup	160	11	14
Pork Skins/Rind:			
Baken-ets, 1 oz	160	10	0
Grande, 2/3 cup	80	5	0
Lance, 1 pkg	65	4	1
Potato Puffs (Health Valley), 1 oz	110	3	21
Potato Sticks (French's), 3/4 c., 1.1oz	180	12	16
Ranch Puffs (No Fries), 1 oz	110	0	23
Rice Chips: Bar-B-Q/Onion, 1/2 oz	70	3	9
Santitas (Frito Lay), 1 oz	140	6	20
Sesame Sticks, 1 oz	155	8	18
Snack Crackers (No Fries), 1 oz	110	0	24
Soy Nuts: Dry Roasted, 1 oz	130	6	9
Choc-coated, 12-15 pces, 1/2 oz	70	4	7
Spicers Wheat Snacks, 1 1/2 oz	150	7.5	18
Sunchips (Frito Lay), 1 oz	140	7	18

Snacks, Granola Bars

Snacks (Cont)

	C	F	Cb
Toast/Cheese Crackers, 1 pkg	205	10	23
Tostitos:			
Regular, average, 1 oz	140	8	18
Fat Free, 1 oz	90	0	20
Trail Mix (Nuts/Seeds/Dried Fruit):			
Regular, 3 Tbsp, 1 oz	130	8	13
Tropical, 3 Tbsp, 1 oz	120	5	19
w. Chocolate Chips, 1 oz	140	9	13
Turkey Jerky Teriyaki *(Oberto)*	80	0.5	0
Vegetable Snacks/Chips, 1 oz	130	4	24
Weight Watchers: Chse Curls, 1/2 oz	70	2.5	10
Apple Chips, 3/4 oz pkg.	70	0	18
Yogurt Raisins, 1 oz	120	4	21

Fruit Snacks

	C	F	Cb
Betty Crocker:			
String Things, 1 pouch, 0.75 oz	80	1	17
Lucky Charms Fruit Shapes, 1 pouch, 0.9 oz (25g)	80	0	20
Squeezit, average, 1 bottle	100	0	25

"They say he's good!"

Granola & Sports Bars

Per Bar

	C	F	Cb
Amway: Positrim Food Bar,			
Cocoa Almond, 1 wrap (2 bars)	190	7	28
Peanut Butter, 1 wrap (2 bars)	210	9	28
Arbonne: Nutrition Bar, 50g	190	4.5	24
Ashfi /Herbal Energy, 51g	190	4	29
Atkins Advantage Bar, 60g	240	10	2
Balance + Bar, 50g (1.76 oz)	200	6	22
Snack, Honey, Peanut, 25g	100	3	11
Barbara's Bakery: Real Fruit	50	0	13
Cereal Bars, fruit filled	110	0	27
Granola Bars	80	2	15
Balance: Oasis, average, 1.7 oz	185	4	26
Coach's Oats: PB & J, 2 oz	240	7	38
Apple Cinnamon, 2 oz	190	2	39
Choc. Chip; Mocha Java, 2 oz	200	4	41
Gold: Caramel Nut Blast, 1.76 oz	210	7	23
Bariatrix: Nutra Bars, 47g	170	5	23
Proti Bars (15g Protein), 41g	130	5	15
Right Choice Bars, 40g	140	3	24
BioX Bio Protein: 81g	300	7	37
Body Smarts: Choc. P'nut Crunch	210	6	34
Yogurt Berry Crunch	200	5	35
Boost: Choc./Strawb. Crunch	190	6	30
Boulder Bar Endurance, 2.5 oz	220	4	13
Burn-IT: 50g bar	180	3	13
Cap'N Crunch, all types, 0.8 oz	90	2	17
Carb Solutions: Protein Bar	230	8	2
Carnation Breakfast Bars, 35g (1.2 oz):			
Granola (Honey/Choc), average	130	2.5	26
Choc Chip/P.nut Butter, chewy	150	5	24
Clif Bar: 2.4 oz, 68g bar	250	6	40
Crunchy, all types, 1 bar	240	5	39
Luna: 48g bar	180	5	24
Apr.; Cranb. Apple Cherry, 1 bar	220	2	44
Choc Almond Fudge, 1 bar	230	4.5	39
Carrot Cake; Choc Chip, 1 bar	240	4	43
Cookies 'n Cream, 1 bar	230	3.5	39
Ginger Snap, 1 bar	230	3.5	42
Choc Brownie, 1 bar	240	4	41
Designer Whey:			
Protein Gourmet, aver, 2.7 oz	260	6	7
Doctor's Diet: Low Carb Bar, 2 oz	234	8	2.5
Choc Mint Cookie; P'nut Butter	234	8	2.5
Banana Nut; Rasp. Choc Truffle; S'Mores	205	4	2.5

...er Bar	C	F	Cb
...r Soy: Protein Bar, Lemon, 1.76 oz	180	2.5	28
Chocolate/Peanut, 1.76 oz	185	4	27
...dgebar, 2 oz, 57g bar	220	2	42
...nergia Bar, 2.25 oz	230	2	41
...nsure Choc Fudge Bar	130	3	20
...ntenmann's: Multi-Grain, 1.3 oz	140	3	25
...xtreme Body, 3 oz bar	340	8	24
...xtreme Ripped Force, 45g	170	3	33
...i-Bar Nectar Granola Bars, 1 oz	100	0	22
Chewy & Nutty Bar, 1.2 oz	140	4.5	23
...-Pro-Tein (R-Kane), 1.2 oz bar	107	1	16
...gurines Diet Bar, aver., 1 bar	110	6	12
...uitein Energy Bar, 1.3 oz	130	3	18
...atorbar Energy Bars, 2.3 oz	260	5	47
...eneral Mills: Milk 'n Cereal			
Chex; Cheerios, 1.4 oz	160	4	26
Cinnamon Toast Crunch, 1.6 oz	180	4	30
...eniSoy: Nature Grains, 2.3 oz	230	3	41
Peanut Butter Fudge	230	5	31
Soy Nutty, 1.76 oz	190	5	26
...lucerna: Nutr'l Bar, 38g	140	4	24
...ain: Mini Munchies Rice	90	1.5	2
...ansen's: Chocolate, 50g	180	3	38
Yogurt varieties, 50g	190	4	38
...ardbody, 2.5 oz, 71g	280	7	41
...ealth Valley: Fruit/Granola Bars	140	0	34
Cereal: Strawberry Cobbler	130	2	27
...ealthy Recipes (Novartis)	150	4	21
...eartBar, Orig., Cranberry, 50g	190	3	27
...MR Benefit Bar, 1.1 oz	160	5	22
...N (Nu Skin): AppSignal, 2 wafers	25	0	5
Glycobar, 42g (1.48 oz)	170	5	28
ProGRAM-16 Bar, 65g (2.28 oz)	250	5	34
...on-Tek: Vanilla Fudge, 2.73 oz	290	5	21
...nny Craig: Meal Bars, 1.97 oz			
Milk Choc; Lemon Meringue	210	5	32
Choc Peanut; Yogurt Peanut	220	5	33
Oatmeal Raisin	210	3	35
...wel Granola Bars: Cereal	140	3	27
Choc Chip/P'nut Butter	130	4.5	20
Lowfat varieties	110	2	22
...t Bar (Nutra Tech) 40g	140	3	24
...shi Golean Bars: Aver. all, 78g	290	5	53
...dos: M&M's	90	2.5	17
Snickers, 23g	100	3.5	14
...Choc Chip/Fudge; P. Butter, 28g	125	5	20

Per Bar	C	F	Cb
Kraft: Philadelphia Cream Cheese,			
average of all bars, 1.5 oz	190	12	18
Lean Body, 76g	300	6	15
Low Carb Diet, 1 pce, 0.5 oz, 14g	62	4	0.5
Metab-o-Lite (w. Ephedra) 1.23 oz	130	4	21
Met-Rx Food Bars, average, 100g	320	3	50
After FX: Choc Chip, 3 oz	300	9	13
Double/Peanut Fudge, 3 oz	250	2	13
Protein Plus, 3 oz	200	0	15
Source One: all types, 1 pkg	190	3	30
MightyBite Choc. Bar, 25g	100	4	11
MLO Bio Protein, 2.85 oz	300	7	15
Mountain Lift Energy Bar	220	4.5	34
Myoplex Plus Deluxe, 90g	340	7	43
Myoplex HP: Mocha, 2.3 oz	250	5	30
Lite, all flavors, 1.97 oz	190	4	27
Natrol Prolab, 1.76 oz bar	190	6	12
Naturade: Total Soy, 2.1 oz	250	8	32
Nature Valley Granola: Oats	180	6	27
Lowfat varieties	110	2	21
Nature's Best: Solid Protein, 2.75 oz			
Honey Almond; Cherry Vanilla;			
Choc Raspberry	290	4	11
Blueberry Cheesecake	280	4	14
Choc. Peanut Butter; S'Mores;			
Chocolate Mint	290	7	12
Cookie Dough Chip; Dble Choc	270	4	10
Nature's Plus:			
Energy Bar, 1.45 oz	140	4.5	24
Chinese Herbal, 1.5 oz	150	4	20
Calcium Almond Blitz, 1.5 oz	150	2.5	29
Spiru-tein, all flavors, 1.4 oz	150	4	20
New Chapter: AB Bar, 1.76 oz	200	4.5	15
The B Bar, 1.76 oz	270	6	17
NiteBite (Time-release Glucose Bar)			
Choc. Fudge; P'nut Butter, 25g	100	3.5	15
NuBar Decadence, 1.3 oz	140	2.5	30
Nutiva (Hemp, Sunflower), 40g	205	14	15
Nutra Blast, average, 47g	160	4	27
Nutri-Grain: Cereal/Twist bars	140	3	27
Low Fat Granola Bars, 21g	80	1.5	16
Fruit-full Squares, 49g bar	190	6	33
Odwalla, 2.2 oz	245	5	45
100% Bar, 50g	190	6	31
Optizone, 50g	190	6	20
Perfect Rx Nutrition Bar, 100g	340	3	50
Planters: Peanut Bar, 1.6 oz	230	11	22

Granola, Sports & Diet Bars (Cont)

Per Bar	C	F	Cb
Pounds Off Bar: All flavors	220	4	35
Power Bar: Harvest, 2.3 oz	240	4	45
Performance, average all, 2.3 oz	230	2.5	45
Protein Plus, 2.75 oz	290	5	38
PR Bar Ironman, 49.6g	200	6	22
Premier Nutr.: Premier Eight	270	6	8
Promax: Dble Fudge Brownie, 75g	270	5	34
Other flavors	280	5	36
Protein Revolution: Lo Carb	230	8	2.5
Prozone Nutrition Bar, 50g	195	6	18
Pure Protein Sports Bar, 78g (2.75 oz)			
Chewy Choc Chip, 1 bar	285	5	16
Peanut Butter, 1 bar	280	7	9
Other varieties, average	270	4	15
Quaker: Chewy Granola Bars			
Butterfinger; Néstlé Crunch; Baby Ruth	120	3.5	21
Other flavors	110	2	22
Restart: Peanut Butter, 1.25 oz	140	4	10
Strawb. Banana; Chocolate	130	2.5	21
Revival Soy Protein: 60g bars,			
Choc. Tempt.; M'mallow Crunch	220	3	30
Peanut Butter/Chocolate Pal	240	6	30
Rice Krispies Bar (Kellogg's), 28g	120	4	20
Coco Pops Bar, 22g	100	3.5	16
Treats Squares, 22g	90	2	18
Slim-Fast Bars:			
Ultra Slim-Fast Snack Bars,			
Crispy Peanut Caramel	120	4	21
Peanut Butter Crunch	130	4	21
Rich Chewy Caramel	120	4	22
Meal On-The-Go Bars (56g),			
average all varieties	220	5	35
Breakfast & Lunch Bars (34g),			
Dutch Chocolate	140	5	20
Peanut Butter	150	6	19
Snacbar (Champion Nutr.), 1 bar	180	3	24
Snackwell's: Cereal Bars	120	0	29
Hearty Fruit & Grain	130	3	26
Chewy Granola, Fudge-Dipped	130	3	26
SoBeBars (Market America):			
Meal Replacement Bars, Choc	296	6	42
Peanut	299	7	44
Tropical	290	4.5	47
Wafers, 2	10	0	3
Source One (Met-Rx), 1 pkg, 62g	190	3	30
Spirutein Energy Bar, 1.4 oz	150	4	20
Energy: Cocoa, 65g (2.3 oz)	210	3	41
Steel Bar, 3 oz, 85g	330	6	52
Steel Pro, 85g	330	6	15
Sweet Rewards: Choc. Chip	110	2	23
Brownie; Fat Free	120	2	30
Sweet Success (Nestlé): Choc Bars	100	3.5	23
Snack Bars, 33g (1.2 oz)	120	4	23
Thermo Speed Bar, 85g	280	5	24
Think!: Interactive Bar, 2 oz, 56g	220	3	43
Protein Bar, 2.3 oz	280	9	18
Thunder Bar, all flavors	220	2	44
Tiger's Milk: 35g Bar	130	2.5	24
Peanut Butter varieties	150	6	19
Protein Rich	145	5	18
Tiger Sport, 65g	230	2	43
Twinlab: Ultra Fuel, 2½ oz	230	0	42
Protein Fuel, 3 oz	340	6	12
Soy Sensations, 1.76 oz	180	5	23
Hi Energy, 2 oz	230	7	25
Ironman Triathlon, 56.8g	230	7	25
Ultimate Lo Carb: 2.1 oz Bar			
Cr. P'nut Butter	270	10	2
Honey Alm; Choc Brownie Nut	240	7	2
Amaretto Irish Cream	240	6	2
Ultimate Protein Bar:			
Choc./Dream; P'nut Butter, 78g	280	6	26
Berries 'N Yogurt, 40g (1.4 oz)	140	3	16
Chocolate Choc Dream, 40g	140	2.5	16
Ultra Slim-Fast: Rich Caramel, 1 oz	110	3.5	24
Peanut Butter Crunch, 1 oz	120	4	26
Universal Muscle, 56.7g	280	5	35
Usana: Nutribar, 41g	150	4	26
Fiberg Bar, 48g	180	2.5	37
Verve (Wholefoods Mkt), 2.4 oz	240	5	4
Viactive (Mead Johnson), 1.6 oz	180	4.5	26
Vita-Trim (Market America):			
Choc./Peanut Bar, 78g	280	6	44
White Lightning, 85g	320	5	2
Whole Foods: Everyday Bars, 1.76 oz			
Choc Fudge/Raspberry	172	4	1
Honey Peanut Yogurt	200	4.5	18
Worldwide Sport Nutrition: Bars, 2.75 oz			
Pure Protein: Lemon Chiffon	290	5	4
Blueberry Cheesecake	270	4	1
Peanut Butter	280	6	
S'Mores	280	4.5	
White Choc. Mousse	290	5	1
You Are What You Eat, 56g	220	5	33
Zone Force/Perfect, aver., 50g	195	6	21

Per 1 oz Unless Indicated	C	F	Cb
Acorns, raw 1 oz	105	7	12
Almonds, Dried/Dry Roasted:			
Whole, 24-28 med., 1 oz	170	15	7
1/2 cup, 2 1/2 oz	420	37	17
Chopped, 1/2 cup, 2 1/4 oz	380	34	16
Sliced, 1/2 cup, 1 2/3 oz	280	25	12
Choc. coated (5-6), 1 oz	160	11	14
Oil Rstd (Blue Diamond), 1 oz	175	17	3.5
Almond Meal (partially defattened)			
1 cup (not packed), 2 1/4 oz	260	11	11
Honey Roasted, 1 oz	170	13	8
Brazil Nuts, 8 medium, 1 oz	185	19	3.5
Cashews, Dry or Oil Roasted:			
14 large/18 med./26 small, 1 oz	165	14	10
1/2 cup, 2.4 oz	400	33	23
Honey Roasted, 1 oz	170	12	10
Chestnuts, aver. all: Dried, 1 oz	105	1	22
Raw/Fresh, 5-6 nuts, 1 oz	60	0	13
Canned, water chestnuts			
sliced/whole/drained, 1 oz	23	0	13
Coconut:			
Flesh (no shell), 1 oz	100	10	4
Raw: 1 pce. (2"x2"x1/2"), 1.6 oz	160	15	7
1/2 medium (4 1/2" diam.)	650	62	30
Dried (Desiccated):			
Unsweetened, 1 oz	187	18	17
Sweetened, shredded, 1 oz	140	9	13
Grated, 1/2 cup, 1.3 oz	185	12	18
Cream (can.), 1/2 c., 5.2 oz	285	26	12
Milk (canned), 1/2 c., 4 oz	225	24	3
Water (center liqr.), 1/2 cup, 4 1/4 oz	23	0	4.5
Filberts or Hazelnuts:			
Shelled, 18-20 nuts	180	18	4.5
Chopped, 1/4 cup	180	18	4.5
Ground, 1/4 cup	120	12	3
Ginko Nuts, can., 14 med., 1 oz	32	0	6
Hickory, 30 small nuts	190	18	5
Macadamia Nuts, shelled:			
Raw, 7 med./14 small, 1 oz	200	21	4
1/2 cup, 2.3 oz	460	48	10
Oil roasted, 1 oz	205	22	3.5
1/2 cup, 2.4 oz	490	52	8
Choc. coated, 2-3 pces, 1 oz	180	13	15
Mixed Nuts: 18-22 nuts, 1 oz	175	13	7
Planters: Dry Roasted/Honey	170	15	7
Oil Roasted, all types	180	16	7
Sweet Roasts, 26 pces, 1 oz	160	12	10
Kettle: Choc Lover's Mix, 1 oz	130	17	16

Per 1 oz Unless Indicated	C	F	Cb
Nut Toppings:			
Chopped, 1 Tbsp, 1/4 oz	40	4	1.5
Peanuts:			
Raw/Dried: In shell, 1 oz	117	10	3
Shelled, 1 oz	160	14	4.5
Boiled: 1/2 cup, 1.1 oz	102	7	7
Roasted, 30 lge./60 sml., 1 oz	165	14	6
1 cup, 5.1 oz	840	71	31
Chopped, 3 Tbsp, 1 oz	165	14	6
Planters: Oil Roasted, 1 oz	170	15	5
Beer Nuts, 1 oz pkg	180	14	7
Choc-coated, 1/2 cup, 2 1/2 oz	380	25	36
Cocktail, oil roasted, 1 oz	170	14	5
Dry Roasted, 1 oz	160	14	6
Honey Roasted, 1 oz	170	13	8
Honey/Dry Roasted, 1 oz	160	13	7
Spanish Oil Roasted, 1 oz	170	14	5
Sweet 'n Crunchy, 1 oz	140	8	16
Pecans: Kernel halves, 1 oz	190	19	5
(20 Jumbo or 31 large halves)			
1 cup halves, 3.8 oz	720	73	20
Chopped, 1/2 cup, 2 oz	380	30	10
Oil Roasted, 1 oz	195	20	4.5
Honey Roasted, 1 oz	200	18	5
Pilinuts, dried, 1/4 cup, 1 oz	205	23	1
Pinenuts, dried, 1 Tbsp, 10g	50	5	1.5
Pistachios:			
Unshelled, 1/2 cup, 2 oz	165	14	7
Shelled, 1/4 c., 45 nuts, 1 oz	165	14	7
Lance, 1 1/8 oz package	180	14	8
Planters: Dry Roasted, 1oz	170	15	6
Fruit 'n Nut Mix, 1 oz	150	9	13
Nut Topping, 1 oz	180	16	6
Tavern Nuts, 1 oz	170	15	6
Trail Mix, 3 Tbsp, 1 oz	140	9	15
Sesame Nut Mix: Planters, 1 oz	160	12	8
Soy Nuts: Dry Roasted, 1 oz	130	6	9
1/2 cup, 3 oz	390	18	28
Dr Soy: Choc coated, 1 oz pkg	130	4.5	18
Honey Roasted, 1 oz pkg	140	6	21
Flavors, average, 1 oz	150	7	8
Walnuts:			
Black, 15-20 halves, 1 oz	175	16	3.5
Chopped, 1/4 cup	190	18	4
Ground, 1/4 cup	120	12	2.5
English/Persian:			
14 halves, 1 oz	185	18	5
Chopped, 1/4 cup	195	19	5

Seeds, Peanut Butter, Supplements

Seeds

	C	F	Cb
Alfalfa Seeds, sprout., 1/2 c., 1/2 oz	5	0	1
Caraway, Fennell, 1 tsp	10	0.5	1
Cottonseed Kernels, rst., 1 Tbsp	50	4	2
Flax Seeds, 3 Tbsp, 1 oz	160	12	7
Lotus Seeds, dried, 1/2 c., 1/2 oz	50	0.5	10
Poppy Seeds, 1 tsp	15	1	1
Pumpkin & Squash Seeds, whole:			
Roasted/Tamari, 1 oz	125	5.5	3
1/2 cup (32g)	140	6	3.5
Dried, 1 oz	155	13	5
Safflower Kernels, dried, 1 oz	150	11	10
Sesame Seeds: Dried, 1 Tbsp, 9g	50	4.5	2
Roasted/Toasted, 1 oz	160	14	7
Sunflower Kernels/Seed:			
Dry Roasted, 1 Tbsp, 8g	45	4	1.5
1/4 cup, 1 oz	160	14	6
Oil Roasted, 1/4 cup, 1 oz	180	17	6
Watermelon, dried, 1/4 cup, 1 oz	160	14	4.5

Quick Guide

Peanut Butter

	C	F	Cb
Average All Brands:			
1 tsp, 6g	35	3	1.5
1 Tbsp, 0.6 oz, (17g)	105	8.5	3.5
2 Tbsp, 1.2 oz, (34g)	210	17	7
1 oz Quantity (28g)	170	14	6
1/2 cup, 5 oz	850	70	30
Jif "Sensations" Berry Blend, 1 T.	100	8.5	5
Chocolate Silk, 1 Tbsp, 0.6 oz	95	7.5	7
Peanut Wonder, 1 Tbsp	50	2	5.5
Smucker's Honey Swtnd., 1 Tbsp	100	8	4
Goober Grape/Strawb., 1 Tbsp	90	5	4
Skippy, honeynut, 1 Tbsp, 16g	95	8	4

Other Nut & Seed Butter

	C	F	Cb
Almond Butter, 1 Tbsp, 1/2 oz	105	9	2.5
Almond Butter Honey Roasted	90	7	5.5
Beanut Butter, 1 Tbsp, 1/2 oz	88	5.5	7
Cashew Butter, 1 Tbsp	92	7	4.5
Cashew Peanut Date Butter	95	7	4
Hazelnut Butter, 1 Tbsp	100	10	2.5
Pecan Butter, 1 Tbsp	110	11	3.5
Pistachio Butter, 1 Tbsp	100	8.5	5
Sesame Butter/Tahini, 1 tsp	30	3	1
1 Tbsp, 1/2 oz	90	8.5	2
Sunflower Seed Butter, 1 Tbsp	95	8	4

Supplements

	C	F	Cb
Aloe Vera Juice, undil., 2 fl.oz	5	0	1
Cod Liver Oil, 1 Tbsp	120	13	0
Evening Primrose Oil, capsules, 1	5	0.5	0
Fiber Supplements: Tabs, 1	1	0	0
Bios Life 2, 1 packet	10	0	2
Metamucil, 1 packet	5	0	1
Regular, 1 rounded Tbsp	34	0	8
Sugar-Free, 1 Tbsp	6	0	1
Fish Oil Capsules, aver., each	10	1	0
Flax Oil Capsules, 2	10	1	0
Garlic Tablets/Capsules, each	3	0	1
Lecithin Granules, 1 Tbsp, 10g	50	5	1
Protein; Powders, aver., 1 oz	100	0.5	0
Tablets, 20 tabs., 1/2 oz	70	0	0
Seaweed: Dried, 1 oz	85	0.5	22
Soaked, drained, 1 oz	15	0.5	3
Spirulina, 1 tablet	2	0	0.5
Vitamins/Minerals: Tabs/Caps, 1	2	0	0
Vitamin E Capsules, each	5	0.5	0
Yeast: Tablets, 2 tabs.	4	0	0.5
Flakes, 1 heaping Tbsp, 1/3 oz	30	0.5	4
Powder, 1 heaping Tbsp, 1/2 oz	50	0.5	6

Cough & Pharmaceutical

	C	F	Cb
Cough/Cold Syrups: 1 tsp	36	0	9
Regular, average, 1 Tbsp	120	0	30
Sugar-free, 1 Tbsp	0	0	0
Cough Drops/Lozenges ~ See Page 125			
Antacids: Average, 1 tablet	4	0	1
Liquid, 1 Tbsp	6	0	1
Sudafed Syrup, 1 tsp	14	0	3
Tylenol Liquid: Child, 1 tsp	17	0	4
Extra Strength, 1 tsp	11	0	3

Nut eaters are healthier and live longer say medical researchers.

Nuts are a nutritious source of protein, vitamins, minerals and fiber

Their fat and fiber content can help to lower blood cholesterol, but watch the quantity if overweight

Veights As Purchased	C	F	Cb
cerola, 1 cup, 20 pcs, 3 1/2 oz	30	0	7.5
pples: whole, average all varieties:			
1 small (4 per lb), 4 oz	70	0	17
1 medium (3 per lb), 5 1/2 oz	90	0	23
1 large (2 per lb), 8 oz	135	0	34
l extra large, 11 oz	185	0	46
without skin, 1/2 medium	35	0	9
Caramel Apple, 1 medium	170	0	42
Nut Coated, 1 medium	230	5	46
pricots: 1 small (12 per lb)	17	0	4
1 medium (8 per lb), 2 oz	25	0	6
1 large (5-6 per lb), 3 oz	35	0	8
temoya, 1/3 cup	95	0	22
vocado (w/out seed/skin):			
Average, 1/2 medium, 3 1/2 oz	160	15	6
1 salad slice, 1/2 oz	25	2	1
Mashed/Puree, 2 Tbsp, 1 oz	50	4.5	2
1/4 cup, 2 oz	90	9	5
Californian, 1/2 medium, 3 oz	150	14	8
Mashed/Puree, 1/2 c., 4 oz	200	18	12
Florida, 1/2 medium, 5 1/2 oz	170	13	14
Mashed/Puree, 1/2 c., 4 oz	125	10	10
1/2 cup cubed, 3 oz	95	8	8

ote: Avocados are nutritious and contain no
olesterol. Fat is mainly monounsaturated and
enefits blood cholesterol. Excellent substitute
r butter or margarine on bread.

anana: 1 small (4 lb), 4 oz	55	0	12
1 medium (3 per lb), 5 oz	80	0	18
1 large (2 1/2 per lb), 7 oz	105	0	24
W/out skin, 1 medium., 3 1/4 oz	80	0	18
1/2 cup, mashed, 4 oz	105	0	24
erries: Average all types,			
lack/Boysenberries/Blueberries)			
1/2 cup, 2.5 oz	40	0	10
1 pint, 14 oz	220	1	56
readfruit, 1/2 cup, 4 oz	115	0	28
antaloupe, 1/2 med. (5" diam.)	100	0	25
1 slice, 2.5 oz (w/out skin)	20	0	6
1 cup pieces/balls, 5.5 oz	55	0	13
arambola (Star Fruit), 1 med	50	0	4
assava, 1/3 cup	120	0	27
herimoya (Custard Apple), 5 oz	130	0	33
herries: Sweet, 8 fruit, 2 oz	40	0	10
1/2 lb (30 cherries)	145	0	38
Sour, 8 fruit, 2 oz	25	0	6
1/2 lb (30 cherries)	100	0	23

Weights As Purchased	C	F	Cb
Coconut: Fresh, 1 piece, 1 oz	100	10	4
Shredded, fresh, 1/2 cup	140	14	6
Sweetened, dried, 1/2 cup	235	16	22
Crabapples, 1/2 cup slices, 2 oz	40	0	9
Cranberries, 1/2 cup, 2 oz	20	0	5
Currants: *Per 1/2 cup*			
European Black, raw, 2 oz	35	0	8
Red & White, raw, 2 oz	30	0	7
Custard Apple, raw, 4 oz	115	1	27
Dates ~ See Dried Fruits			
Durian, flesh, 4 oz	165	6	30
Elderberries, 1/2 cup, 2 1/2 oz	55	0	13
Feijoas, 1 medium, 2 1/2 oz	35	0	7
Figs, green/black: 1 med., 2 oz	40	0	10
1 large, 3 oz	60	0	15
Fruit Salad, fresh, average,			
1/2 cup, 3 1/2 oz	60	0	15
1 cup, 7 oz	120	0	30
Gooseberries, raw, 1/2 c., 2 1/2 oz	30	0	7
Grapefruit: average all types,			
1/2 fruit, 8 1/2 oz (4 1/2 oz flesh)	40	0	10
1 cup sections w. juice, 8 oz	75	0	17
Grapes: Average, 1 cup, 5 1/2 oz	100	0	24
1 small bunch, 4 oz	70	0	15
1 medium bunch, 7oz	125	0	31
1 large bunch, 16 oz	285	0	71
Granadilla, flesh, 3 1/2 oz	95	0	23
Groundcherries, 1/2 cup, 2 1/2 oz	35	0	8
Guava: 1 fruit, 4 oz	80	0	15
1/2 cup, 3 oz	40	0	9

Continued Next Page

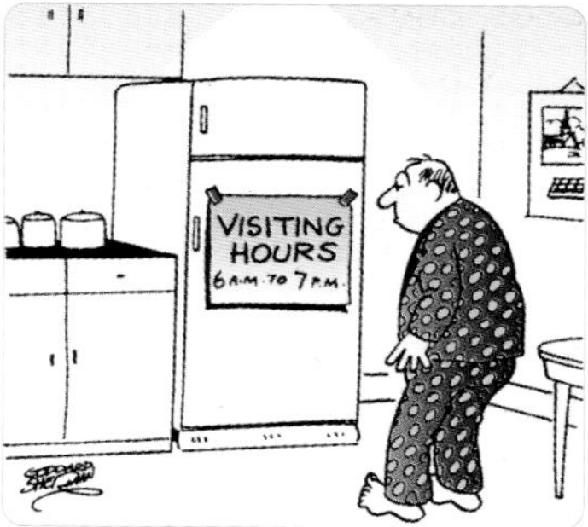

Weights As Purchased	C	F	Cb
Honeydew, 1 wedge (7"x2" wide),			
8 oz (with skin)	45	0	10
1 cup cubes/balls, 6 oz	60	0	14
Honey Murcots, 1 only, 5 oz	45	0	11
Jaboticaba, flesh, 4 oz	75	2	15
Jackfruit, flesh, 1/8 average, 4 oz	105	0	25
Jambos (Brazil Cherry), flesh 4 oz	35	0	8
Java-Plum, 4 plums, 1/2 oz	25	0	6
Jujube, 3 oz	65	0	16
Kiwifruit, 1 medium, 3 oz	45	0	11
1 large, 4 oz	60	0	15
Kumquats, 5 medium, 3 1/2 oz	60	0	15
Kiwano, 1/2 medium, 5 oz	35	0	8
Langsat, Duku, 2 oz	25	0	5
Lemon: 1 medium, 4 oz	20	0	5
1 wedge, 1 oz	5	0	1.5
Peel, 1 Tbsp	4	0	0.5
Limes, 1 only, 2 oz	20	0	7
Loganberries, froz., 1/2 c., 2 1/2 oz	40	0	9
Longans, 5 fruit, 1/2 oz	10	0	2.5
Loquats, 4 fruit, 2 1/4 oz	20	0	6
Lychees, 4 fruit, 2 1/4 oz	25	0	6
Mamey Apple, 1 whole, 3 lb	430	4	100
1/4 fruit (1 cup flesh), 7 oz	100	1	24
Mandarin: 1 small, 3 oz	25	0	6
1 medium, 4 oz	35	0	8
1 large, 6 oz	55	0	13
Mango: flesh, 1/2 cup sl., 3 oz	48	0	11
1 whole, medium, 11 oz	140	0	34
Melons: Average all types			
1 cup, cubes/balls, 6 oz	60	0	14
Monstera Deliciosa (Taxonia),			
Edible part, 4 oz	50	0	11
Mulberries, 20 fruit, 1 oz	15	0	3
Nashi Fruit (Asian Pear),			
1 medium, 4 1/2 oz	50	0	11
Nectarines, 1 medium, 4 oz	50	0	12
1 large, 5 1/2 oz	70	0	17
Oheloberries, 1/2 cup, 2 1/2 oz	20	0	5
Olives (Pickled): Green, 10 lrg, 1 1/2 oz	45	5	0.5
Ripe, Grk. Style, 10 med., 1 oz	70	7	2
Ripe (Black), Californian:			
1 small/medium	4	0.5	0.3
1 large/extra large	6	0.5	0.5
1 jumbo	7	0.5	0.5
1 colossal	9	1	0.5
1 super colossal	13	1	1

Weights As Purchased	C	F	Cb
Oranges, average all varieties:			
1 small, 5 oz (with skin)	50	0	12
1 medium (3" diam.), 7 oz	70	0	17
1 large, 10 oz	100	0	24
Flesh only, 1 cup, 6 oz	80	0	19
Californian Valencia,			
1 medium (2 3/4" diam.), 6 oz	60	0	15
Californ. Navels (3" diam.), 7 oz	60	0	15
Sunkist Navel, 14 oz	130	0	32
Florida Orange, 1 medium, 7 oz	70	0	17
Peel, 1 Tbsp	0	0	0
Papaya, 1/2 cup, cubed, 2 1/2 oz	30	0	7
1 medium, 16 oz	120	0	28
Passionfruit, 1 medium, 1 1/4 oz	20	0	4.5
PawPaw (see Papaya)			
Peaches: 1 med. (4 per lb), 4 oz	35	0	8
1 large, 6 oz	55	0	13
Pears: Bartlett, 1 small, 4 oz	60	0	15
1 medium, 6 oz	90	0	22
1 large, 8 oz	120	0	30
Bosc, 6 oz	90	0	22
D'Anjou, 1 medium, 8 oz	120	0	30
Red Pear, 5 oz	80	0	20
Seckel (Wash'ton), 2 1/4 oz	35	0	9
Asian (Nashi), 1 large, 7 oz	80	0	20
Pepino, 1/2 medium, 4 oz	20	0	4
Persimmons: Native, 1 oz	30	0	7
Japan. (2 1/2"d. x 2 1/2"h), 7 oz	120	0	30
Seedless (Maui), 1 md., 5 oz	100	0	25
Pineapple (flesh only), 1 slice			
(3/4" thick, 3 1/2" diam.), 3 oz	40	0	10
1 cup, diced, 5 1/2 oz	80	0	20
1 medium, 1 1/2 lb	525	0	130
Pitanga, 3 fruit, 1 oz	6	0	1
Plaintains, 1/2 cup slices, 2 1/2 oz	90	0	22
Plums, average all types:			
Mini/Damson, (1" diam.), 1/2 oz	8	0	2
Small (1 3/4" diam.), 2 oz	30	0	7
Medium (2 1/4" diam.), 3 oz	45	0	10
Large (2 1/2" diam.), 4 oz	65	0	15
Pomegranates, 1/2 fruit, 5 oz	55	0	13
Pummelo, flesh, 1/2 cup, 4 oz	35	0	8
Prickly Pears, 1 fruit, 5 oz	50	0	11
Quinces, 1 medium, 3 1/2 oz	55	0	14
Rambutan (Rambotang),			
Red/Yellow, 1 med., 2 oz	15	0	4
Raspberries, 1/2 cup, 2 oz	30	0	6

Weights As Purchased	C	F	Cb
Rhubarb, raw, 1/2 cup, 2 oz	15	0	3
Sapodilla (Chico), 1 md., 7 1/2 oz	140	2	34
Sapotes, 1/2 medium, 5.5 oz	150	0.5	38
Soursop, 1 cup pulp, 8 oz	150	0	38
Strawberries:			
1 cup, 5 1/2 oz	45	0	10
6 medium/3 large, 2 oz	15	0	3
1 pint, 12 oz	95	0	22
Chocolate Dipped, 2 medium	45	2.5	6
Sugar Apples, 1/2 cup pulp, 4 oz	120	0	30
Tamarillo, 1 medium, 3 oz	20	0	4
Tamarind: 1 fruit, 1/4 oz	5	0	0
Tangelo: 1 small, 4 oz	30	0	1.5
1 medium, 5 oz	40	0	2
1 large, 7 oz	55	0	2.5
Tangerine, 1 medium, 4 oz	50	0	12
Tangor, 1 medium, 4 oz	35	0	7
Tomato:			
Cherry, 1 med., 3/4 oz	5	0	1
1 small, 3 oz	25	0	6
1 medium, 5 oz	35	0	7
1 large, 7 oz	45	0	9
1 medium slice	5	0	1
Canned Tomatoes/Products ~ Page 78-81			
Tree Tomato (Tamarillo), 3 oz	20	0	5
Ugli Fruit, Tangelo type, 5 oz	40	0	2
Watermelon (flesh only): 1 sl, 8 oz	70	0	15
1 cup cubed, 5 1/2 oz	50	0	12
Wax Jambu (Rose Apple), 2 oz	10	0	2

Dried Fruit

	C	F	Cb
Apples, 5 rings, 1 oz	75	0	18
Apricots, 8 halves, 1 oz	65	0	15
Banana Chips, 1/2 cup, 1 1/2 oz	160	5	18
Banana Flakes, 4 Tbsp, 1 oz	80	0	20
Cranberries, sweetened, dried, 1/3 cup, 1.5 oz	130	0	33
Currants, 1/4 cup, 1 1/4 oz	100	0	24
Dates: 5 medium dates, 1 1/2 oz	120	0	28
Large Calif., 3 dates, 2 oz	160	0	37
1/2 cup, chopped, 3 oz	240	0	57
Figs, 3 medium figs, 2 oz	145	0	34
Longans; Lychees, 1 oz	80	0	19
Mango Slices, 4 strips, 1 oz	70	0	16
Mixed Fruit, 1 oz	70	0	17
Papaya Spears, 1 oz	75	0	17
Peaches, 2 halves, 1 oz	60	0	14
Pears, 3 halves, 2 oz	75	0	17
Pineapple, 1 oz	80	0	18
Prunes: with pits, 1 oz	60	0	14
1 Medium (60/lb)	16	0	4
1 Large (50/lb)	22	0	5
1 Extra Large (40/lb)	27	0	6
Without pits, 4 med., 1 oz	70	0	17
Cooked: w. sugar, 1/2 c, 5 oz	200	0	45
w/out sugar, 1/2 c, 4 1/2 oz	125	0	28
Raisins: 2 Tbsp, 1 oz package	85	0	19
1/2 cup, 2 1/2 oz	215	0	50
Sunsweet: Fruitlings, 1/3 c., 1.5 oz	130	0	31

Candied Glacé Fruit

	C	F	Cb
Apricot, 1 medium, 1 oz	100	0	25
Cherry, 3 large, 1/2 oz	50	0	12
Citron/Fruit Peel, 1 oz	90	0	21
Fig, 1 piece, 1 oz	90	0	21
Ginger, 1 oz	95	0	23
Pineapple, 1 slice, 1 1/4 oz	120	0	30

Fruit Leather/Rolls

	C	F	Cb
Average All Brands: 1 oz	100	0	24
Fruit By The Foot, 1 roll, 3/4 oz	80	0	17
Fruit Gushers, 1 pouch, 1 oz	90	1	20
Fruit Roll-Ups, 1 roll, 1/2 oz	50	0	12
Stretch Island Leathers, 2 pces, 1 oz	90	0	21
Sunkist Fruit Roll, 1 roll	75	0	18
Other Fruit Confectionery/Snacks/Bars			
~ See Snacks/Granola Bars Page 127-130			

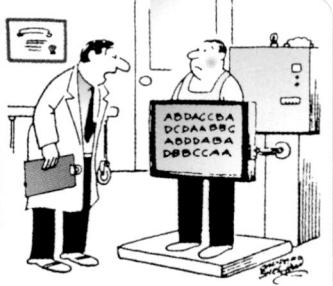

"You have a Vitamin E deficiency."

135

Canned Fruit & Snacks

Canned Fruit

Solids & Liquids:
Per 1/2 Cup (Approx. 4 1/2 oz)

	C	F	Cb
Apples: sweetened	70	0	17
Apricots: In water/diet	35	0	9
In juice/light	60	0	15
In syrup	105	0	27
Blackberries/Blueberries			
In heavy syrup	115	0	30
Cherries, pitted, in water	55	0	14
In light syrup	85	0	21
In heavy syrup	110	0	28
In extra heavy syrup	130	0	33
Fruit Cocktail: In water/diet	40	0	11
In juice/light	55	0	15
In light syrup	80	0	21
In heavy syrup	95	0	25
Fruit Salad: In water/diet	35	0	9
In juice/Light	60	0	16
In heavy syrup	95	0	25
Gooseberries: Light syrup	90	0	23
Grapefruit: Juice pack	45	0	15
In light syrup	75	0	20
Mixed Fruit: In water/diet	40	0	10
In fruit juices	60	0	15
In light syrup	60	0	15
In heavy syrup	100	0	25
Mandarin Oranges: In water	40	0	11
In light syrup	80	0	21
Peaches (halves or slices):			
In water/diet	30	0	8
In juice/light	50	0	14
In light syrup	70	0	20
drained, 1/2 peach	40	0	11
In heavy syrup	100	0	26
Pears: In water/diet	35	0	10
In juice/light	60	0	16
In heavy syrup	100	0	26
Pineapple:			
(Chunks/Crushed/Spears/Wedges/Slices)			
In own juice	70	0	18
In heavy syrup	90	0	23
Slices, drained, 2 slices			
In own juice	30	0	8
In heavy syrup	45	0	11

Canned Fruit (Cont)

Per 1/2 Cup

	C	F	Cb
Plums: In water	50	0	14
In juice	75	0	20
In light syrup, 3 plums	85	0	21
In heavy syrup, 1/2 cup,	160	0	41
3 plums	120	0	31
Prunes: In heavy syrup	120	0	32
4 prunes	70	0	18
Raspberries, in heavy syrup	120	0	30
Strawberries: In water	25	0	7
In heavy syrup	120	0	31
Tropical Fruit Salad:			
In light syrup	80	0	18
In heavy syrup	95	0	21

Fruit Snack Cups

Del Monte Fruit Cups: Per 4 oz

	C	F	Cb
Diced Peaches/Pears/Mixed,			
In heavy syrup	80	0	20
In extra light syrup	50	0	13
In fruit juices	50	0	13

Miscellaneous

	C	F	Cb
Cherries: Maraschino, 5, 1 oz	50	0	12
Sour Pitted, drained, 5, 1 oz	40	0	11
Lychees: Canned, 1/2 cup, 4.5 oz	106	0	26
Prunes: in Liqueur, 1/2 cup, 125g	280	0	70

Rev. Dr Robert Schuller

Inch by inch
Life's a cinch

You'll never win
If you don't begin!

Vegetables - Fresh or Frozen

Edible Portion
(Raw Weight Unless Indicated)

	C	F	Cb
Alfalfa Sprouts, 1/2 cup, 1/2 oz	5	0	1
Artichokes, Globe/French:			
1 medium, 4 1/2 oz	65	0	15
Artichoke Heart, 1/2 cup, 3 oz	40	0	10
Asparagus, raw/froz.: 4 med. spears	15	0	3
Cuts & tips, 1/2 cup, 3 oz	25	0	5
Bamboo Shoots, ckd, 1/2 c, 4 oz	15	0	3
Beans: Green/Snap, 1/2 c, 2 oz	20	0	4
Broadbeans, ckd, 1/2 cup, 3 oz	90	0	16
Butterbeans, 1/2 cup, 3 oz	90	0	20
Lima, baby, 1/2 cup, 3 oz	90	0	17
Dry Beans, average all types:			
(Kidney, Brown, Haricot, Lima,			
Mung, Navy, Pinto, Red, White)			
Raw, 2 Tbsp, 1 oz	95	0.5	18
1 cup, 7 oz	665	3	126
Cooked, 1 oz	35	0	7
1/2 cup, 3 oz	105	0	21
Soybeans: Mature, dry, 1 oz	110	5	7
Dry, 1/2 cup, 3 1/2 oz	385	18	22
Cooked, 1/2 cup, 3 oz	105	5	6
Bean Sprouts, aver., 1/2 c., 3 oz	25	0	3
Beets, cooked, 1/2 c, slices, 3 oz	25	0	6
1 beet, 2" diam., 2 oz	17	0	4
Beet Greens, ckd, 1/2 c., 2 1/2 oz	20	0	4
Bell Pepper: See Peppers			
Black Eyed Peas, ckd, 1/2 c., 2 oz	160	0	32
Bok Choy (Chinese Chard), 3 oz	12	0	2
Broccoli: Raw, 1/2 cup, 1 1/2 oz	12	0	3
1 spear (5 oz edible)	40	0	8
Cooked, 1/2 cup, 3 oz	25	0	5
Brussel Sprouts, ckd, 1/2 c, 3 oz	35	0	7
Cabbage, average all varieties:			
Raw, shred., 1/2 cup, 1 1/4 oz	8	0	1
Cooked, 1/2 cup, 2 1/2 oz	15	0	2
Carrot: Ckd, 1/2 cup sl., 2 1/4 oz	35	0	8
Raw, 1 medium (7 1/2"), 3 oz	33	0	8
Raw, 1 lb, (5-6 med)	175	0	40
4 sticks (4"), 1 1/2 oz	15	0	3
Shredded, 1/2 cup, 2 oz	25	0	6
Cauliflower, cooked:			
3 floret, 1/2 c. 1" pcs, 3 oz	15	0	3
1/2 medium (15 oz raw)	100	0	20
Celeriac, raw, 1/2 cup, 2 3/4 oz	30	0	7
Celery, 1 stalk, 7 1/2", 1 1/2 oz	5	0	1
Diced, 1/2 cup, 2 1/4 oz	10	0	3

Edible Portion
(Raw Weight Unless Indicated)

	C	F	Cb
Chard (Swiss), 1/2 cup, ckd, 3 oz	20	0	4
Chick Peas (Garbanzo Beans):			
Dry, 1 cup, 6 oz	550	10	92
Cooked, 1 cup, 6 oz	270	4	45
Chicory/Witloof ~ See Endive			
Chicory, Greens, 1/2 cup, 3 oz	20	0	4
Chives, chopped, 1 Tbsp	1	0	0
Collards, 1/2 cup, 3 oz	15	0	4
Corn, yellow/white:			
Raw, kernels, 1/2 cup, 2 3/4 oz	65	1	14
Ear (5"x 1 3/4"), 5 1/2 oz	80	1	17
Trimmed to 3 1/2" long	60	1	14
Cooked, kernels, 1/2 cup	35	<1	7
(Also see Frozen & Canned Corn Page 140)			
Cress, Garden, 1/2 cup, 1 oz	10	0	2
Cucumber, 1 whole, 11 oz	40	0	12
1/2 cup slices, 2 oz	5	0	1
Dandelion Greens, 1/2 cup, 1 oz	15	0	3
Eggplant: 1 whole, 4 1/2 oz	40	0	10
1/2 cup, 1" pieces, 1 1/2 oz	10	0	2
1 slice, fried, 1 oz	40	4	10
Endive, Belgian/French:			
1 med. head (6"), 2 1/2 oz	12	0	3
Fennel, 1/2 cup, 2 oz	10	0	2
Garlic, 1 clove	4	0	1
Ginger: 1/4 cup slices, 1 oz	20	0	4
Crystallized (sugared), 1 oz	95	0	20
Horseradish, 1 pod, 3/4 oz	4	0	1
Jerusalem Artichoke, 1/2 cup	60	0	14
Jicama, raw, 1/2 cup	25	0	5
Kale, 1/2 cup, 2 oz	20	0	4
Kohlrabi, 1/2 cup, cooked, 3 oz	25	0	6
Leek, cooked, 1 whole, 4 oz	40	0	9
Lentils, green/brown: Dry, 1 oz	95	0	17
Dry, 1 cup, 6 1/2 oz	620	0	108
Cooked, 1/2 cup, 3 1/2 oz	115	0	20
Lettuce: 1 c., chop./shred., 2 1/2 oz	10	0	2
Butterhead 2 leaves, 1/2 oz	2	0	0.5
Cos/Romaine, 1/2., shred., 2 1/2 oz	4	0	1
Iceberg, 1 leaf, 3/4 oz	3	0	1
1 medium head, 15-16 oz	60	0	15
Lotus Root, 10 slices, ckd, 3 oz	60	0	15
Mung Bean Sprouts, 1/2 cup	15	0	3
Mushroom: Raw, 1/2 cup, 1 oz	10	0	2
Cooked, 1/2 cup, 2 1/2 oz	20	0	3
Mustard Greens, 1/2 cup, 1 oz	7	0	1

Edible Portion (Raw Weight Unless Indicated)	C	F	Cb
Okra, ckd., 1/2 cup, slices, 2 3/4 oz	25	0	6
Onions: Raw, 1 medium, 4 oz	40	0	9
1/2 cup, chopped, 3 oz	30	0	7
Dehydrated flakes, 1/4 c, 1/2 oz	45	0	11
Rings, breaded/fried, 2 rings	80	5	9
Ore-Ida, 4 pces	220	11	27
Scallions, 1/2 cup, 2 oz	15	0	4
Spring, 1/4 cup, chopped, 1 oz	6	0	1
Parsley, chopped, 1/2 cup, 1 oz	10	0	2
Parsnips, 1 medium, 4 oz	80	0	20
Cooked, 1/2 cup slices, 2 3/4 oz	65	0	16
Peas: Green, 1/4 cup, 1 1/2 oz	35	0	6
raw, with pods, 1/2 lb	70	0	13
Snow Peas (8-9 pods), 1 oz	10	0	2
Split, dry, hulled, 1 oz	50	0	14
cooked, 1 cup, 7 oz	230	1	41
Peppers: Bell, 1 medium, 5 oz	25	0	6
1/2 cup, chopped, raw, 1 3/4 oz	12	0	3
1 ring (3" diam. x 1/4" thick)	2	0	0
Sweet, 1 medium, 5 oz	35	0	10
Chili: Green/Red, 1 1/2 oz	18	0	4
Habanero, 1 only, 8g	11	0	2
Pigeon Peas, cooked, 1/2 cup	85	1	16
Pimientos, 3 medium, 3 1/2 oz	25	0	5
Poi, 1/2 cup, 4 1/4 oz	135	0	33
Potatoes: Raw (with skin)			
1 Baby, Gourmet, 2 oz	45	0	11
1 small, 3 oz	65	0	15
1 medium, 5 oz	110	0	26
1 peeled, 4 oz	90	0	21
1 large, 8 oz	180	0	41
1 Extra large. (Russet), 12 oz	270	0	62
Mashed w. milk and fat, 1/2 c.	110	4	14
Baked (no fat); large, 10oz raw:			
Plain, with skin, 7 oz	220	0	51
without skin, 5 1/2 oz	145	0	34
With Toppings:			
+ 2 tsp fat	290	8	51
+ Sour Cr./Chives, 2 Tbsp	270	6	53
+ Plain Yoghurt, 2 Tbsp	240	1	55
+ Grated Cheese, 1 oz	330	9	56
+ Cottage Cheese, 2 oz	280	2	56
Roasted (w. fat), 1 small	155	8	36
Garlic Potatoes, 4 oz	120	2	22
Hash Browns: w. Butt. Sce, 2 1/2 oz	125	6	10
Homemade, 1/2 cup, 2 1/2 oz	165	10	10

Edible Portion (Raw Weight Unless Indicated)	C	F	Cb
Potatoes (Cont):			
French Fries: small serve, 2 1/2 oz	220	12	14
medium serve, 4 oz	350	20	22
Froz., uncooked, 18 fries, 4 oz	185	7	22
Oven-heated, 18 fries, 4 oz	185	7	22
Take-Out: 1 cup, 5 oz	440	25	28
McDonald's: Small, 2 1/2 oz	210	10	26
Large, 5.2 oz	450	22	57
Supersize, 6.2 oz	540	26	68
Fried: 18 fries, 3 oz	275	15	16
Au Gratin, 1/2 cup, 4.3 oz	160	9	22
Pancakes, 1 only, 5 oz	90	5	9
Kugel, 5 oz	300	20	26
Puffs, fried, 4 puffs, 1 oz	65	3	37
Scalloped, 1/2 cup, 4 1/4 oz	105	4	13
Stuffed Baked Potatoes:			
See *1-Potato-2* ~ Fast-Food Section			
Ore-Ida Frozen Potatoes (As Purchased):			
Steak Fries, 8 fries, 3 oz	110	3.5	17
Frozen Crispers, 3 oz	220	13	24
Country Fries, 15 fries, 3 oz	120	3.5	19
Crispy Crunchies, 13 fries, 3 oz	160	8	20
Fast Fries, 22 fries, 3 oz	150	6	20
Pixie Crinkles, 22 pces, 3 oz	130	1.5	21
Golden Curls, 17 pces, 3 oz	160	7	22
Golden Fries, 16 pces, 3 oz	120	4	20
Golden Patties, 1, 2.5 oz	140	7	16
Hash Browns: Average, 3 oz	80	0	17
Oven Chips, 7, 3 oz	180	8	25
Potatoes O'Brien, 3/4 c., 2 oz	60	0	14
Season'd Crinkle Cuts, 15, 3 oz	120	3	23
Shoestrings, 3 oz	150	5	22
Sweet Potatoes: 1 patty, 60g	70	0	17
Center Cut: Prime, 2 pce	70	0	16
Petite, 3 oz, 117g	80	0	18
Mashed/Casserole, 1/2 cup	80	0	20
Tater Tots, 9 pces, 3 oz	150	8	20
Taters, 8 pces, 3 oz	150	7	20
Twice Baked, all types, 1, 5 oz	190	7	16
Waffle Fries, 9, 3 oz	150	7	21
Zesties, 12 pces, 3 oz	160	9	21
Potato Salad, 1/2 cup, 4 1/2 oz	180	10	14
Pumpkin, mashed, 1/2 c., 4 oz	25	0	6
Purslane, cooked, 1/2 c., 2 oz	10	0	2
Radish: aver., 10 only, 1 1/2 oz	10	0	2
Oriental, 1/2 c. slices, 1 1/2 oz	10	0	2

Edible Portion
Raw Weight Unless Indicated

	C	F	Cb
Rutabagas, ckd., 1/2 c. cubes, 3 oz	30	0	7
Salsify, ckd, 1/2 c. slices, 2 1/2 oz	45	0	11
Sauerkraut, 1/2 cup, 4 oz	25	0	5
Seaweed, aver. all: Dried, 1 oz	50	0	13
Soaked, drained, 1 oz	15	0	4
Nori/Laver, dried, 6 sheets, 1/2 oz	35	0	5
Shallots, chopped, 1 Tbsp	7	0	1
Soybeans ~ See Beans Page 70-72, 137			
Soy Products/Tofu/Tempeh ~See Pages 69)			
Sorrel, raw, 1/2 cup, 4 oz	23	0.7	4
Spinach, cooked, 1/2 cup, 3 oz	20	0	4
Creamed, 1/2 cup, 4 1/2 oz	140	12	10
Squash: Summer, average			
raw, 1/2 cup slices, 2 1/4 oz	13	0	3
cooked, 1/2 cup slices, 3 oz	18	0	4
Winter, cooked:			
Acorn, 1/2 cup cubes, 3 1/2 oz	55	0	15
1/2 medium (10 oz raw wt.)	85	0	22
Butternut, 1/2 c. cubes, 3 1/2 oz	40	0	11
1/4 medium (9 oz raw wt.)	95	0	26
Hubbard, 1/2 c. cubes, 3 1/2 oz	50	0	11
Spaghetti, 1/2 cup, 2 3/4 oz	23	0	5
Succotash, ckd, 1/2 cup, 3 1/3 oz	110	1	23
Sweetcorn ~ See Corn.			
Sweet Potatoes: Cooked with Skin			
No fat, 1 only, 4 oz	120	0	28
No skin, mash, 1/2 c., 5 1/2 oz	170	0	40
Swedes, 1/2 cup, 3 oz	45	0	10
Taro, cooked, 1/2 cup, 2 oz	95	0	23
Tomatoes: See Fruit ~ Page 135			
1 small, 3 oz	20	0	5
1 medium, 5 oz	35	0	8
1 large, 7 oz	45	0	10
Cooked, 1/2 cup, 4 1/4 oz	30	0	7
Fried, 1 small, 3 oz	60	4	5
Tomatillo, 1 oz	7	0	1
Turnips: White, ckd, 1/2 cup, 3 oz	15	0	4
Greens, ckd, 1/2 cup, 2 1/2 oz	15	0	3
Water Chestnuts, 4 nuts	40	0	10
1/2 cup slices, 2 1/4 oz	65	0	15
Watercress, 10 sprigs, 1 oz	4	0	1
Yam, cooked, 1/2 cup, 2 1/2 oz	80	0	20
Baked Yam, medium, 8 oz	260	0	62
Yardlong Bean, 1 pod, 1/2 oz	7	0	1
Yucca Root, 1/2 cup, 2.5 oz	60	0	14
Zucchini: 1 medium, 10 oz	45	0	10
1/2 cup slices, cooked, 3 oz	13	0	3

Frozen Vegetables (Mixed)

Birdseye	C	F	Cb
Brocc./Carrots/W. Chestnuts, 1 cup	35	0	6
Broccoli/Corn/Red Peppers, 3/4 cup	50	0.5	11
Broccoli/Cauli./Carrots, 1 cup	30	0	4
Brussels Sprouts/Cauli./Carrots	35	0	5
Carrots/Corn/Green Beans, 2/3 cup	60	0.5	11
Cauliflower/Carrots/Pea Pods, 1 cup	30	0	5
Chopped Spinach, 1/3 cup	20	0	2
Baby: Corn Blend, 2/3 cup	60	0.5	11
Bean & Carrot Blend, 1 cup	30	0	5
Broccoli Blend, 1 cup	70	1.5	8
Broccoli Florets, 1 cup	25	0	4
Gold & White Corn, 2/3 cup	80	1	15
Pea Blend, 3/4 cup	40	0	7
Sweet Pea, 2/3 cup	70	0.5	12
Pasta Secrets: Primavera, 1 cup	230	10	26
Zesty Garlic, 1 cup, cooked	240	10	31
Stir Fry: *Prepared (Includes Pasta)*			
Asparagus, 2 cup	90	0.5	16
Green Bean, 1 3/4 cup	100	0.5	19
Voila: Garlic Chicken, ckd, 1 cup	260	11	27
Pesto Chicken, ckd, 1 cup	250	9	25
Green Giant			
Vegetables: Asparagus Cuts, 2/3 c.	25	0	4
Corn: Nibblers, 1 ear	70	0.5	14
Extra Sweet Niblets, 2/3 cup	70	1	13
Sthwestern & Rst Peppers, 3/4 c.	90	1	18
Green Bean Casserole, 2/3 cup	100	5	11
Honey Glazed Carrots, 1 cup	90	3.5	13
Le Sueur Baby Sw. Peas, 2/3 cup	60	0.5	11
Spinach, 1/2 cup	25	0	3
Veges In Cheese & Cream Sauce: *Prepared*			
Alfredo Vegetables, 3/4 cup	80	3	9
Broccoli & Cheese, 2/3 cup	70	2.5	9
Brocc., Cauliflower, Carrots, 2/3 c.	70	2.5	10
Cauliflower in Cheese Sce, 1/2 cup	60	2.5	8
Creamed Spinach, 1/2 cup	80	3	9
Cream Style Corn, 1/2 cup	110	1	23
Green Bean Casserole, 2/3 cup	90	5	9
Rice & Vegetables: *Prepared*			
Cheesy Rice & Brocc., 1 pkt, 10 oz	300	5	56
Oriental Rice, 1 pkt, 10 oz	340	12	52
Rice Medley, 1 pkt, 10 oz	280	4	52
Rice Pilaf, 1 pkt, 10 oz	230	3.5	44
White & Wild Rice, 1 pkt, 10 oz	280	6	51

Continued Over Page

Vegetables - Canned/Bottled

Frozen Vegetables (Cont)

Green Giant (Cont)

	C	F	Cb
Pasta Accents: Per 1 Cup, Cooked			
Alfredo Broccoli	105	4	14
Cr. Cheddar w. Broc./Carrots	125	4	18
Garden Herb	115	3.5	16
Garlic Seas. w. Broc./Corn/Carrots	130	5	18
Primavera	140	4.5	19
Three Cheese	150	4.5	21
White Cheddar	135	4	18

La Choy

	C	F	Cb
Mixed Fancy Vegetables, 1/2 cup	12	0	3

Veg-All

	C	F	Cb
Succotash, 1/2 cup	80	1	17

Westpac

	C	F	Cb
Just Add: As Prepared, Per 10 oz			
Beef: Oriental Garlic & Ging. 1 1/4 c.	280	7	25
Chicken, 1 1/4 cup	290	2	34
Hamburger: Vegetable Stroganoff	320	12	32

Canned/Bottled

Solids & Liquid

	C	F	Cb
Artichoke Hearts: Plain, 1 oz (1)	30	0	8
Marinated, 1 oz	60	5	2
Asparagus (Tips/Cuts/Spears),			
1/2 cup, 4 1/2 oz	20	0	3
Bamboo Shoots, 1 cup, 4 1/2 oz	25	0	4
Bean Salad, 1/2 cup, 3 oz	90	0	23
Bean Sprouts, 2/3 cup	10	0	2
Beans:			
Green, 1/2 cup, 4 1/4 oz	20	0	4
Baked Beans, 1/2 cup, 4 1/2 oz	120	<1	18
Butter Beans, 1/2 cup, 4 1/2 oz	90	0	20
Italian, cut, 1/2 cup, 4 1/2 oz	30	0	7
Kidney Beans, 1/2 cup, 4 1/2 oz	105	<1	20
Lima Beans, 1/2 cup, 4 1/2 oz	80	0	15
Pinto Beans, 1/2 cup, 4 1/2 oz	100	<1	20
Wax Beans, cut, 1/2 cup, 4 1/2 oz	20	0	4
(Also see Canned Products ~ Pages 70-72)			
Beets:			
Sliced/Whole, 1/2 c., 4 1/2 oz	35	0	7
Crinkle/Pickled (Del Monte) 1/2 c.	80	0	20
Carrots:			
Sliced, 1/2 cup	35	0	8
Honey Glazed (Green Giant) 1/2 c.	45	3.5	13

Canned/Bottled (Cont)

	C	F	Cb
Corn: Whole kernel, sweet:			
1/2 cup, 4 1/2 oz	80	0.5	20
Drained Solids, 1/2 cup, 3oz	65	0.5	15
Creamed style, 1/2 cup, 4 1/2 oz	100	0.5	24
Eggplant, 2 Tbsp, 1 oz	25	2	5
Garbanzo/Chick Peas, 3 oz	100	2	20
Green Chilies: diced, 2 Tbsp, 1 oz	5	0	1
Hearts of Palm, (1), 1.2 oz	9	0	2
Mushrooms: 1/2 cup, 2 1/2 oz	20	0	4
in Butter Sauce, 2 oz	30	1	3
Olive Salad (Progresso), drain, 2 T.	25	2.5	1
Onions: Pickled, 1 med., 3/4 oz	10	0	2
Cocktail, 1 onion	2	0	0.5
Peas, 1/2 cup, 3 oz	60	0	11
Peppers: Hot Chilli, 1 only, 1 oz	8	0	2
Sweet, undrained, 2 1/2 oz	15	0	3
Jalapeno, w. liq., 1/2 c. chopped	17	0	3
Cherry (Progresso), dr., 2 T., 1 oz	25	2	2
Fried, drain, 2 Tbsp, 1 oz	60	5	3
Pepper Salad (Progresso), dr., 2 T.	15	1	1
Potatoes, 1/2 cup, 3 oz	55	0	12
Salsa: Average all types, 2 Tbsp	15	0	3.5
Sauerkraut, undrained, 1/2 c., 4 oz	25	0	6
Spinach, 1/2 cup, 3 1/2 oz	25	0	3.5
Straw Mushrooms, 1/2 cup, 4.3 oz	20	0	3
Succotash: Per 1/2 cup, 4 1/2 oz			
w. Cream Style Corn	100	1	23
w. whole kernels, undrained	80	1	17
Sweetcorn: See Corn.			
Sweet Potato, 1/2 cup, 3 1/2 oz	105	0	24
Candied (Green Giant) 3/4 cup	240	7	41
Tomatoes, Sundr.: Natural, 5-6 pce	22	0	5
In Oil, drained, 6 pces, 1/2 oz	60	4	4
Tomato Products ~ See Page 80-83			
Vegetables, mixed, 1/2 cup, 4 oz	45	0	8
Yams in Light Syrup, 1/2 cup, 4 oz	105	0	25
Zucchini in Tom. Sce., 1/2 c., 4 oz	30	0	8

Take-Out Vegetable Dishes

	C	F	Cb
Appetizers: Caponata, 1/4 cup	30	1	5
Curried Vegetables, 8 oz serving	400	33	22
Pakoras, 1, 2 oz	110	5	13
Ratatouille, 1 cup, 9 oz serving	200	16	10
Samosa, 2, 4 oz	500	45	25
Succotash, 1 cup	110	1	23
Spring Roll, 2, 3 oz	200	9	28

Salads - Fresh, Deli, Restaurant)

Average All Outlets
Per Serving

	C	F	Cb
Antipasto Salad, 1 cup	140	10	2
Bean Salad, 1/2 cup	110	4	17
Bulgur Salad, 1/2 cup	70	2	12
Caesar Salad, Classic, 1 cup	200	14	15
Side Salad, no dressing	25	0	6
Carrot Raisin: No dress., 1/2 cup	20	0	5
with dressing, 1/2 cup	65	5	5
Chef Salad: Regular, no dressing	620	37	8
w. 2oz 1000 Island	860	61	8
Chicken Salad Platter, 6 oz	200	8	12
Coleslaw: Traditional, 1/2 cup	150	8	18
w. low cal dressing	60	1	12
Corn, Mexican, 1/2 cup	240	12	33
Cucumber, non-oil dress, 1/2 cup	60	0	14
w. Oil dressing, 1/2 cup	140	12	14
Eggplant Salad, 1/2 cup	75	5	7
Fettucini w. veges, 1/2 cup	110	5	15
Garden Salad, no dressing	35	0	8
Greek Salad, 1 cup	120	10	7
Greek Vegetables, 1/2 cup	140	12	7
Lettuce, hearts, 1/4 head	20	0	4
Lobster Salad Platter, 6 oz	200	8	12
Macaroni Salad, 1/2 cup	140	8	16
Nicoise, 1 cup	450	32	16
Pasta Salad, 1/2 cup	160	8	16
Pineapple Coconut Slaw, 1/2 cup	150	10	14
Potato Salad: Dijon	140	7	17
w. Mayonnaise, 1/2 cup	170	10	17
Lowfat, 1/2 cup	110	1.5	21
Rice Salad, 1/2 cup	150	10	13
Saffron Rice, 1/2 cup	130	3	24
Spinach Salad	180	13	13
Tomato & Mozzarella, 1/2 cup	180	14	10
Tabouli, 1/2 cup	150	6	22
Three Bean Salad, 1/2 cup	80	5	9
Tortelini w. Basil Pesto, 1/2 cup	170	10	19
Waldorf w. mayo, 1/2 cup	160	12	12

Signature Salads: Per 6 oz Serving
(Supplied to Deli's and Institutions)

	C	F	Cb
Antipasto Salad, 6 oz	510	50	4
Artichoke Salad, marinated	400	41	8
California Medley	120	7	15
Cheese Agnolotti	250	8	23
Chicken Salad	420	33	11
Crabmeat Flavored	450	38	20
Egg Salad	300	23	14

Signature Salads (Cont):

	C	F	Cb
Fresh Button Mushroom	190	16	6
Garden Olive, 6 oz	630	67	3
Ham Salad	400	32	14
Prima Pasta Salad	360	30	18
Seafood Pasta Del Mar	170	10	21
Seafood with Crab & Shrimp	420	34	20
Shrimp Salad	360	32	8
Tuna Salad	450	36	14

Fast-Food Restaurant Chains ~ See Page 167

Fresh Salad Packs

Pre-Packaged (Supermarkets)

	C	F	Cb
Dole: Complete: Caesar, 3 1/2 oz	170	13	8
Oriental, 3 1/2 oz	120	6	13
Romano, 3 1/2 oz	150	12	9
Spinach Bacon, 3 1/2 oz	170	10	18
Sunflower Ranch, 3 1/2 oz	160	16	5
Lunch For One: Ranch, 1 kit	350	29	20
Special Blends (no added dressing):			
Aver. all varieties, 2 cups, 3 oz	15	0	3
Regular Salad Packs (no added dressing):			
Classic Coleslaw, 3 oz	25	0	5
Classic Iceberg, 3 oz	15	0	4
Zesty Italian, 7 oz	110	0	4
Fresh Express: Per 1 1/2 cups			
Salad Kits: Caesar Salad	170	14	9
Fat Free Caesar Salad	70	0	1
Taco Fiesta	110	8	7
Garden Salad; Italian Salad Mix	20	0	3
European/Riviera Salad Mix	15	0	3
Hearts of Romaine Salad Mix	20	0.5	3
Garnden w. Romaine Salad	20	0	3
Ready Pac: Aver. all types	15	0	2
Weight Watchers			
Caesar/Garden/European, 3.5 oz	60	0	12
Caesar Salad w. cookies, 4 oz	160	3	30
Garden Salad w. cookies, 4 oz	120	1.5	24
European Salad w. cookies, 4 oz	160	3	11

Salad Toppings

	C	F	Cb
Bacon Bits, aver., 1 Tbsp	30	1.5	2
Chow Mein Noodles, dry, 1/2 c.	120	5	13
Croutons, 2 Tbsp, 10g	35	1	6
Olives, 5 medium	25	2	0
Potato Chips, 1 oz	150	10	15
Sunflower Seeds, 1 Tbsp, 8 g	45	4	1.5
Tortilla Chips, 1 oz	150	8	16

Fruit & Vegetable Drinks & Juices

Quick Guide | C | F | Cb

Orange Juice
Average ~ Fresh or Sweetened:

	C	F	Cb
1/2 Cup, 4 fl.oz	55	0	13
Small Glass, 6 fl.oz	82	0	20
Regular Glass, 8 fl.oz	110	0	26
8 3/4 fl.oz Box	120	0	28
10 fl.oz Bottle	140	0	32
11 1/2 fl.oz Can	160	0	36
16 fl.oz Bottle	220	0	52
20 fl.oz Bottle	280	0	72
64 fl.oz Bottle	880	0	208

Juices ~ Generic

Average All Brands
Per 8 fl.oz Unless Indicated

	C	F	Cb
Aloe Vera Juice, unsweet., 2 oz	5	0	1
Apple Juice: 8 fl.oz	115	0	30
10 fl.oz Bottle	145	0	36
16 fl.oz	230	0	60
Blueberry Juice, 8 fl.oz	90	0	25
Carrot Juice: Fresh, 6 fl.oz	60	0	14
Sweetened, 6 fl.oz	75	0	17
Cranberry Juice, Cocktail/Blend	120	0	34
Grape Juice, 8 fl.oz	160	0	40
Grapefruit Juice, 8 fl.oz	100	0	23
Lemon Juice: 1 Tbsp	4	0	1.5
1 cup, 8 fl.oz	60	0	21
Concentrate, 1 tsp	0	0	0
Lime Juice, 1 Tbsp	4	0	1.5
Noni Juice, 1/2 cup, 4 fl.oz	50	0	12
Orange Juice, 8 fl.oz	110	0	26
Passion Fruit Juice (Fresh):			
Purple, 1 cup, 8 fl.oz	125	0	34
Yellow, 1 cup, 8 fl.oz	150	0	36
Papaya/Peach Nectar, 8 fl.oz	140	0	35
Pear Nectar, 8 fl.oz	150	0	40
Pineapple Juice, 8 fl.oz	110	0	27
Prune Juice, 8 fl.oz	180	0	43
Strawb./Raspberry Juice, 8 fl.oz	100	0	23
Tangerine Juice, 8 fl.oz	100	0	25
Tomato Juice, 8 fl.oz	50	0	12
Vegetable Juice, 8 fl.oz	50	0	12
Fruit Blends, average, 8 fl.oz	120	0	31
Fruit Nectars, average, 8 fl.oz	140	0	35

Juice Brands | C | F | Cb
Per 8 fl.oz Unless Indicated

	C	F	Cb
Apple & Eve			
Naturally Cranberry	120	0	30
Cranberry/Raspberry Apple	120	0	30
Arizona			
Crazy Carrot; Lemonade/Pink	110	0	27
Grape/Kiwi/Strawberry	120	0	29
Mucho Mango	100	0	25
Bright & Early			
Orange Juice (Chilled/Frozen)	120	0	30
Grape Juice (Frozen)	140	0	33
Campbell's			
Tomato Juice, 8 fl.oz	50	0	10
10.5 fl.oz	60	0	12
V-8 Healthy Request, 8 fl.oz	50	0	12
V-8 Splash Tropical Blend, 8 fl.oz	120	0	30
Capri Sun			
Average all flavors, 6.75 oz	100	0	28
Chiquita			
Frozen Concentrates, prepared:			
Average all varieties, 8 fl.oz	130	0	32
Del Monte			
Pineapple Juice: Fresh, 8 fl.oz	110	0	27
From Concentrate, 8 fl.oz	130	0	32
Prune Juice, 8 fl.oz	170	0	42
Tomato Juice:			
Fresh, 8 fl.oz	40	0	10
From Concentrate, 8 fl.oz	50	0	12
Snap-E-Tom Cocktail, 6 fl.oz	40	0	10
Fruit Smoothie Blenders: *Per 6.5 fl.oz*			
Mango-Pineapple-Banana;			
Strawberry-Peach-Banana	180	0	45
Peach-R'berry/P'apple-Or.-Ban.	210	0	53
Dole			
100% Fruit Juice Blends:			
Average all varieties, 8 fl.oz	120	0	29
Fruit Drink Blends:			
Average, 8 fl.oz	130	0	31
Spicy Vegetable Blend, 12 fl.oz	80	0	16
Dominick's			
Orange Juice (100% Pure), 8 fl.oz	110	0	27
Tropical Fruit Blend	130	0	32

Fruit & Vegetable Drinks & Juices (Cont)

Per 8 fl.oz Unless Indicated	C	F	Cb
Eden: Organic Apple, 8 fl.oz	80	0	23
Five Alive: Citrus beverage, 8 fl.oz	120	0	30
Fresh Samantha			
Banana Strawberry	150	1	12
Carrot/Orange; The Big Bang	100	0	8
Grapefruit	90	0	7
Mango Mama/Tangerine	120	0	10
Raspberry Dream	120	1	10
Protein Blast	160	1	10
Desperately Seeking C	110	0	5
Fruitopia			
Apple Raspberry, 8 fl.oz	75	0	19
20 fl.oz Bottle	190	0	48
Other flavors, average, 8 fl.oz	115	0	29
20 fl.oz Bottle	290	0	72
Goya Nectar			
Apricot Nectar, 1 can	130	0	31
Pear Nectar, 1 can	240	0	59
Hansen's: Natural Juice Cocktail			
Regular, all flavors, 8 fl.oz	110	0	28
Low Calorie Peach Mango	10	0	4
Hawaiian Punch			
Fruit Juicy, Red, 6 fl.oz	90	0	22
Box, 8.45 fl.oz	120	0	30
Hi-C			
Orange Juice			
Chilled/Premium Choice, 8 fl.oz	110	0	30
10 fl.oz bottle	140	0	36
Calcium Rich, 8 fl.oz	120	0	33
Other Juices Drinks: Aver., 8 fl.oz	130	0	32
8.45 fl.oz box, average	135	0	33
11.5 fl.oz can	180	0	45
Hood: Grapefruit Juice (Select)	100	0	23
Natural Blenders, average	130	0	32
Orange Juice: Select	120	0	30
Calcium Rich	120	0	30
Jui2ce: All flavors, 8 fl.oz bottle	95	0	23
Juicy Juice			
Apple Grape, 8.45 fl.oz box	120	0	10
Berry, 8.45 fl.oz box	130	0	30
Punch, 8.45 fl.oz box	140	0	32
Tropical, 8.45 fl.oz box	150	0	26

Per 8 fl.oz Unless Indicated	C	F	Cb
Kern's Nectars			
Pineapple Coconut Nectar, 6 fl.oz	140	0	26
11.5 fl.oz box	210	0	48
Other nectars, average, 6 fl.oz	110	0	27
Kool Aid			
Koolers, average, 8.45 fl.oz	140	0	37
Fruit Drinks, average, 8 fl.oz	100	0	25
Sugar Free, 8 fl.oz	5	0	0
Knott's: Sparkling Ciders, 325 ml	110	0	25
Knudsen			
Fruit Juices: Apple	110	0	28
Apple Blends, all varieties	120	0	30
Black Cherry; Prune	180	0	43
Grape; Pomegranate	150	0	37
Grapefruit	100	0	23
Just Cranberry; Tomato	60	0	14
Orange	100	0	23
Pear	120	0	30
Nectars: Coconut	140	5	26
Other Nectars, average	130	0	36
Blends: Average all flavors	120	0	30
Citrus Juices:			
Rio Red Grapefruit	140	0	35
Lemonade (Natural)	120	0	30
Simply Nutritious: Per 8 fl.oz			
Ginseng Boost	110	0	27
Lemon Ginger Echinacea	120	0	30
Mega C	130	0	31
Mega Green; Gingko Alert	120	0	30
Morning Blend; VitaJuice	120	0	30
Floats: Orange	140	0	33
Spritzers:			
Average all flavors, 12 oz	170	0	43
Lights, all flavors, 12 oz	110	0	28
TeaZers: All flavors, 12 oz	110	0	28
Very Veggie: 8 fl.oz	50	0	10
Krasdale			
Cranberry Apple	170	0	42
Cranberry Juice Cocktail	130	0	32
Cranberry Raspberry	150	0	37
Libby's			
Orange Juice, 8 fl.oz	105	0	25
Juicy Juice, average, 8 fl.oz	140	0	34
Nectars, 1 can, 11.5 fl.oz	220	0	52

Fruit & Vegetable Drinks & Juices (Cont)

Per 8 fl.oz Unless Indicated	C	F	Cb
Mauna La'i Hawaiian: 8 fl.oz	130	0	32
Mistic (Mega 24 fl.oz)			
Average All flavors, 8 fl.oz	120	0	30
24 fl.oz	360	0	90
Minute Maid			
100% Juices: *Per 8 fl.oz*			
Apple/ Orange Juice	115	0	27
Fruit Drinks/Punch: *Per 8 fl.oz*			
Average all flavors	115	0	30
Chilled Singles: *Per 16 fl.oz Bottle*			
Berry/Tropical Punch	240	0	60
Lemonade/ Orange Juice	220	0	55
Juices to Go: *Per 10 fl.oz Bottle*			
Average all flavors	160	0	40
Boxed Juices: *Per 8.45 fl.oz*			
Cherry Grape; Tropical Punch	130	0	32
Orange/Apple Juice; Berry; Fruit	120	0	31
Calcium Juices: *Per 8 fl.oz*	120	0	29
Mott's			
Apple Raspb., Fruit Punch, 10 fl.oz	145	0	36
Apple Cranb., Grape Apple, 10 fl.oz	180	0	42
Clamato Tomato Cocktail, 8 fl.oz	60	0	11
Fruitsations: all flavors, 4 oz	85	0	22
Grapefruit (from conc.), prep.	120	0	28
Juice Paks: All flavors, 8.45 fl.oz	120	0	30
Mini Motts, 4.23 oz	60	0	14
Orange Juice (from conc.)	130	0.5	30
Naked Juice			
Apple Juice, 8 fl.oz	120	0	29
Banana Blueberry; Boysenberry	140	2	34
Banana Date	240	4	46
Berry Blast; Wise Guy	130	0	30
Carrot Beet/Celery/Spinach	100	0	21
Chocolate Dream	190	2	38
Grapefruit Juice	110	0	23
Green Machine	140	0.5	35
Mighty Mango; Orange Jce Nirvana	110	0	24
Papaya Strawberry	100	0	24
Protein Drink (6g protein)	170	1.5	33
Protein Zone (17g protein)	220	4	32
Strawberry Banana/Lemonade	140	0	33
Turbo C	110	0	27
Vanilla Creme	150	1	28
Watermelon	80	1	18
Zippitea	80	0	32

Per 8 fl.oz Unless Indicated	C	F	Cb
Nantucket Nectars			
100% Juices: Apple Raspberry	140	0	34
Grape Juice	160	0	39
Grapefruit Juice	100	0	24
Orange Passionfruit	120	0	29
Pineapple Orange Banana	140	0	35
Premium Orange Juice	120	0	29
Pressed Apple Juice	100	0	25
Ruby Red Grapefruit	100	0	25
The Original Peach	120	0	30
Juice Cocktails: Cranberry	140	0	34
California Melonberry	110	0	28
Cranberry Apple	140	0	34
Diet Green Tea	5	0	1
Diet Iced Tea	5	0	1
Fruit Punch	130	0	32
Grapeade	130	0	33
Guava	130	0	33
Kiwi Berry	120	0	30
Orange Mango	130	0	32
Papaya	120	0	30
Pineapple Orange Guava	120	0	30
Watermelon Strawberry	120	0	30
Lemonades: Authentic/Pink	120	0	30
Super Nectars: Chai Green Tea	90	0	23
Gingko Mango	150	0	38
Green Angel	140	0	39
Protein Smoothie	120	1	38
Red Guarana Tea	110	0	26
Strawberry Smoothie	120	0	30
Vital C	130	0	32
Vitamin Smoothie	110	0	27
Newman's Own			
Lemonade, 10 fl.oz	140	0	34
Ocean Spray			
Apple Juice (from conc.)	110	0	28
Bl. Cherry; Crazy Kiwi; Mega Melon	130	0	33
Cranberrry: Cranberry Grape	170	0	41
Cranberry Juice Cocktail	140	0	34
Light Style (Low Calorie)	40	0	10
Other Cranberry flavors, aver.	150	0	35
Caribbean Colada; Cran-Mango	130	0	32
Cranicot; Cranapple; Cranblueberry	160	0	41
Crantastic Fruit Punch	150	0	37
Fruit/Holiday Punch; Tangerine	130	0	32

Per 8 fl.oz Unless Indicated

	C	F	Cb
Ocean Spray (Cont)			
Grapefruit: 100% Juice	100	0	24
Other flavors, average	125	0	31
Lemonade flavors, average	130	0	32
Orange Juice (from concentrate)	120	0	31
Kiwi Strawb.; Summer Cooler	120	0	31
Ruby Red & Strawberry	140	0	34
Ruby Red & Mango/Tangerine	130	0	33
Odwalla: *Per 8 fl.oz Unless Indicated*			
Boyzenberry Mango	140	0	34
C Monster, 16 fl. oz	300	0	72
Fruitshake Blackberry	160	0	40
Grapefruit Juice	90	0	34
Guanaba Dabba Doo!	130	0	30
Lotta Colada	160	0	33
Mango Tango	150	0	37
Mo Beta, 16 fl. oz	280	0	70
Orange Juice	120	0	34
Raspberry Smoothie	140	0	35
Strawberry Banana/Go Man Go	100	0	25
Super Protein, 16 fl.oz	400	0	40
Vegetable Cocktail	70	0	18
Orange Julius: *Per 16 fl.oz*			
Orange	265	0	65
Pina Colada	300	0	75
Strawberry	340	0	85
Raspberry Cream Supreme	510	20	82
Tropical Cream Supreme	510	25	71
Realemon - Realime *(Borden)*			
Lemon/Lime Juice (from concentrate)			
1 teaspoon	0	0	0
2 Tbsp, 1 fl.oz	6	0	2
1/2 cup, 4 fl.oz	24	0	8
Santa Cruz			
Natural 100%: Aver. all varieties	120	0	30
Sparkling varieties, 8 fl.oz	150	0	33
S&W: Apple Juice, 8 fl.oz	120	0	30
Orange Juice, 6 fl.oz can	90	0	22
Grapefruit Juice, unswt'd, 8 fl.oz	105	0	25
Tomato Juice, 8 fl.oz	30	0	7
Squeezit			
Average all flavors, 6.75 fl.oz	90	0	23

Per 8 fl.oz Unless Indicated

	C	F	Cb
Snapple			
Cranberry Royal, 10 fl.oz	150	0	38
Fruit Drink Blends, 8 fl.oz	120	0	30
Grapeade; Orangeade 8 fl.oz	120	0	30
Orange Juice, 10 fl.oz	130	0	30
Whipped Snapple (Fruit Smoother):			
Aver. all flavors, 297ml bottle	160	0	40
Sunny D			
Enriched Citrus Beverage (5% Jce)	130	0	31
Sunny Delight			
Florida Citrus, 6 fl.oz	90	0	22
Calcium Rich, 6 fl.oz	150	0	37
Sunny Delight Lite, 6 fl.oz	20	0	5
Tropical Fruit Punch, 6 fl.oz	90	0	22
Sunsweet			
Prune Juice/w. Pulp, 8 fl.oz	180	0	43
Tang			
Fruit Box (8.45 fl.oz): Aver. all flav.	140	0	34
Pouches, average all flavors (1)	100	0	26
Mix: *Made up, 6 fl.oz*			
Regular (2 Tbsp dry)	90	0	22
Sugar Free	7	0	0
Tree of Life: Black Cherry	180	0	43
Concord Grape	160	0	40
Cranberry Nectar	150	0	38
Other varieties, average	130	0	33
Tree Top: *Per 6 fl.oz*			
Apple Juice; Apple Citrus/Pear	120	0	30
Apple Cranberry/Grape	130	0	32
Fruit Juice Punch, 10 fl.oz	150	0	37
Grape/Grape Fruit Juice; Sparkling	120	0	30
Orange Juice	120	0	28
Tropicana			
Blends: Berry; P'apple, 8 fl.oz	130	0	32
Pure Premium:			
Orange Juice + Fiber	120	0	30
Ruby Red	120	0	28
Season's Best: Orange Juice	110	0	27
7 fl.oz bottle	90	0	23
10 fl.oz bottle	130	0	33
11.5 fl.oz can	140	0	36
Grapefruit Juice, 8 fl.oz	160	0	40
Tropics: Average all flav., 8 fl.oz	110	0	26

Fruit Juices (Cont) • Smoothies

Per 8 fl.oz Unless Indicated

Tropicana

Twister: Average, 8 fl.oz	120	0	32
10 fl.oz bottle	150	0	40
11.5 fl.oz can	160	0	40
Light: average, 8 fl.oz	35	0	10
10 fl.oz bottle	50	0	11

V-8 Splash

Regular, 1 cup, 8 fl.oz	110	0	28
Diet V-8 Splash, 1 cup	10	0	3

Veryfine

Apple Cranberry	130	0	33
Fruit Punch	140	0	36
Grape Juice (100%)	150	0	37
Grape Drink	110	0	28
Grapefruit Juice (100%)	90	0	20
Pink	120	0	30
Guava Straw.; Lemon Lime	120	0	30
Orange Juice (100%)	120	0	24
Orange Drink	140	0	35
Papaya Punch	120	0	30
Pineapple Orange	130	0	32

Welch's

Regular Juices:			
Average all blends, 8 fl.oz	160	0	40
Tomato, 8 fl.oz	50	0	10
8.45 fl.oz Box, average	150	0	37
Mini Drinks, 5.5 fl.oz	100	0	25
Healthy Tropical Sensation,			
8 fl.oz	120	0	30
Frozen Juice Concentrates: *Per 8 fl.oz*			
(Reconstituted)			
Grape	160	0	41
White Grape Juice Blends	150	0	36
Cranberry/Raspberry	150	0	37
Lite Cranberry/Grape/Raspberry	50	0	13
Other flavors, average	130	0	33

Quick Guide   C F C

Fruit Smoothies

Average All Brands

Fruit Only: 8 fl.oz cup	105	0	25
12 fl.oz	160	0	38
16 fl.oz	210	0	50
24 fl.oz	320	0.5	76
Fruit + Nonfat Milk/Soy:			
12 fl.oz	190	0.5	40
16 fl.oz	250	0.5	53
24 fl.oz	380	1	80
Fruit + Nonfat Frozen Yogurt/Sherbet:			
12 fl.oz	210	0.5	47
16 fl.oz	280	0.5	62
24 fl.oz	420	1	94

Brands - Fruit Smoothies

Hansens: Per 11 fl.oz can

Fruit flavors, regular	170	0	43
Lite: Cranberry; Raspberry	50	0	13
Energy: Island Blast	170	0	42
Super Energy: Tropical Blast	170	0	40
Super Power: Berry Splash	170	0	41
Super Protein: Banana Citrus	290	1	59
Super Vita: Orange Carrot	170	0	40

Jamba Juice (California): See Page 206

Jera's Juice (Boston): Per 24 fl.oz

Mango Passion	300	0.5	71
Raspberry Madness	425	1	100
Spring Fever	400	1.5	91
Soy Smoothie	360	4.5	79

Whippy Snapple: Per 10 fl.oz

Citrus	150	0	39
Pineapple Orange	100	0	41

Fruit Whips: Per 8 oz bottle

Berry/lemon/Orange/Tropical			
All flavors, 236ml (8 oz)	125	0	29

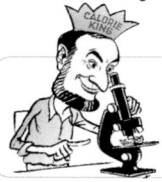

ℱor full nutritional data and product updates
check the database of the author's website
www.CalorieKing.com

Nutritional Shakes & Drinks

Nutritional Shakes/Drinks

	C	F	Cb
Amway Positrim Drink Mix			
Regular Mix, 1 pkt, 43g	160	4	27
Fat Free Mix, 1 pkt, 65g	230	0	50
Arbonne Int'l Meal Shake	190	4.5	24
Balanced: Diet, 11 fl.oz can	180	1	34
Choc Royale; Fr. Vanilla 11 fl.oz	180	2	35
Strawb.; Vanilla 11 fl.oz can	230	3	36
Kids Chocolate, 8 fl.oz can	160	3	30
Bariatrix Shakes, 1 serving	100	2	6
Proti-Max Meal, 67g	250	3	20
Boost: Ready-To-Drink, 8 oz	240	4	41
Boost High Protein, 8 oz	240	6	33
Boost Plus, 8 fl.oz	360	14	45
Bulk Force, 1 pint bottle	750	0	163
Carnation Instant Breakfast:			
Powder: 1 reg. envelope, 37g	130	1	28
No Sugar Added, 1 envel., 21g	70	1	12
Ready-To-Drink, aver., 10 oz	220	3	37
Champion Nutrition:			
Heavyweight Gainer 900, 4 scoops, 154g	630	10	101
Lean Gainer, 3 scoops, 76g	280	4	11
Super H. Wt Gainer, 4 scp, 154g	900	29	108
Choice dm (Mead Johnson), 8 fl.oz	250	12	25
Ensure: Regular, 8 oz can	225	6	31
Ensure Bal'd Bkfst, choc pouch	140	0.5	31
Ensure Fiber, 8 fl.oz can	250	6	42
Ensure Light, 8 fl.oz can	200	3	33
Ensure Plus, 8 fl.oz can	360	13	47
Glucerna, 8 fl.oz can	220	11	22
Powder, made up, $^1/_2$ cup	250	9	34
Gatorade Nutrition Shake:			
Choc./Vanilla, 325ml can	370	6	62
Genisoy: Shake, 1 scoop, 35g	120	0	17
Protein Powder, 1 scoop, 29g	100	0	0
Health Source Soy, 2 scoops, 1 oz	100	1	4
Herbalife (Thermogetics F.1), 1 oz	100	1	14
HMR 500 Shakes, 1 pkt	100	0	16
HMR 120, 1 serving	120	1.5	16
IDN (Nu Skin):			
Aloe Fountain, 2 fl.oz	20	0	5
Amino Build, 3 scoops, 1$^1/_2$ oz	160	1	12
Appeal: French Delight, 2 oz pkt	210	2	33
Swiss Truffle, 2 oz pkt	220	2.5	33
Appeal Lite HT	120	1.5	26
Sports Drinks: See Next Page			

	C	F	Cb
Kashi GoLEAN Shakes:			
Chocolate, 325ml can	230	3	32
Vanilla, 325ml can	220	2.5	36
Powdered, 1 pkt, 71g	250	1.5	30
Mass Recovery, 1 pint bottle	380	0	60
Metabolife Meal Shakes, 11 oz can	220	3	40
Metabolol: Endurance, 2 scps, 52g	200	5	24
Metabolol II, 2 scoops, 66g	260	3	40
Met-Rx: Nutrition Drink Mix, 72g	260	2	22
RTD 40 Shake, 15 fl.oz	250	3	15
Metaform: Lean Mass, 2 scoops	140	0	11
Protein Powder, 76g pkt	270	2	21
Proton, 45g pkt (1.6 oz)	170	1	15
Nutrament (Mead Johnson): 12 fl.oz	360	10	52
Optifast 800: Powder, 1 serving	160	3	20
Ready-to-Drink, Chocolate	160	3	20
Power Dream (Imagine Foods):			
Java Jolt, 11 fl.oz	240	4.5	42
Mango Passion, 11 fl.oz	320	4.5	65
Chai, 11 fl.oz	200	3	35
ProBalance, 8.45 fl.oz	300	10	39
Pro-Cal 100 (R-Kane), 1 pkt	105	2	7
Pure Pro, 22 fl.oz bottle	170	0	1
Resource (Novartis): Plus, 8 fl.oz	360	11	52
Standard, 8 fl.oz pak	250	6	40
Diabetic, 8 fl.oz pak	250	11	23
Fruit Beverage, 8 fl.oz pak	180	0	36
Yogurt Flav'd Beverage, 8 fl.oz	250	4	45
Rite Aid Nutritional Suppl. 8 oz	250	6	40
Sav-on Nut'l: 8 fl.oz can	360	13	47
Light, 8 fl.oz can	200	3	33
Slim-Fast:			
Ready-To-Drink (cans):			
Shakes, all flavors, 325ml	220	3	40
Juices, all flavors, 340ml	220	1	46
Slim-Fast Powder Mix:			
All flavors, 1 scoop, 1 oz	100	1	20
w. 8 oz fat free milk	190	1	32
Ultra Slim-Fast Mixes:			
Regular flavors, average 1 scoop, $^1/_3$ cup, 33g	120	1	24
w. 8 oz fat free milk	200	1.5	36
Choc Delite w. Soy Protein, 2 scoops, $^1/_2$ cup, 48g	170	2	25
w. Fruit Juice Mix, 1 scoop, $^1/_4$ cup, 31g	100	1	17
w. 8 oz fruit juice	220	1	42

Nutritional Shakes & Drinks (Cont)

Nutritional Shakes (Cont)

	C	F	Cb
SoBeShakes *(Market America):*			
Chocolate, Vanilla, 1 pkt	210	2	26
Peach Mango, 1 pkt	210	2	26
Sustacal: Liquid, 8 fl.oz can	240	6	33
Basic, 8 fl.oz can	250	9	34
Sustacal Plus, 8 fl.oz	360	14	45
Powder, 2 oz + water	200	1	36
Sweet Success *(Nestlé):*			
Healthy Shake, 10 fl.oz can	200	3	37
Fruit Flavors, 10 fl.oz	200	0.5	39
Powder, 2 scoops, 32g (1.1 oz)	100	1	25
Total Balance, 9.5 oz can	230	7	25
Twin Lab RxFuel, 1 pkt	250	0	62
Ultra Slim-Fast ~ see Slim-Fast			
Usana: Nutrimeal, 2 scoops, 43g	150	4	20
Fibergy, 2 scoops, 33g	90	1	23
SoyaMax, 2 scoops, 1 oz	105	1	1
Vita-Trim Shake *(Mkt America):*			
Chocolate/Vanilla, 57g pkt	210	2	26

	C	F	Cb
Walgreens Nutritional Supplements:			
Advanced Formula, 8 oz can	250	6	40
Plus, 8 oz can	355	13	47
Light, 8 oz can	200	3	33
Weider *(Powders):*			
Creatine ATP, 2 scoops, 2 oz	230	0	37
Complete Rx, 70g pkt (2.5 oz)	240	2.5	27
Lean Pro, 2 scoops, 50g (1.76oz)	180	1.5	22
Ultra Whey Pro, 1 scp, 30g (1oz)	110	1	2
Women's Natural Replace., 33g	120	1	13
Dynamic: Body Shaper, 35g	140	0.5	22
Muscle Builder, 2 scoops, 45g	190	0	27
Weight Gainer, 4 scoops, 85g	330	0.5	62
Victory Pure Protein: 2 scoops,			
Egg/Beef/Vege. average	140	0	14
Victory Mass 1000, 7 oz	740	2.5	148
Mega Mass 4000, 3 scoops	1640	4	319
Super Mega Mass 2000, 2 sc.	520	1.5	102

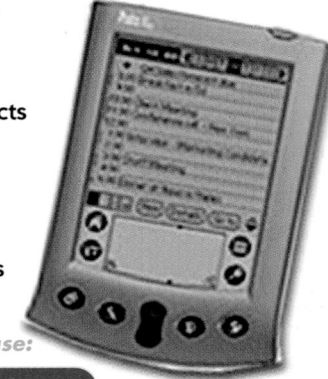

Sports, Energy & Herbal Drinks

luid Replacement, Carbohydrate Rich er 8 fl.oz Unless Indicated	C	F	Cb
08 Energy Drink, 12 fl.oz	120	0	33
0-K (Suntory)	60	0	15
llSport, all flavors, 8 fl.oz	70	0	18
merican: Maximum Fat, all flav.			
1/2 bottle, 8 fl.oz	5	0	<1
mino Force, 22 fl.oz	390	0	75
rizona: Rx Energy	120	0	30
Rx Stress/Memory/Health, aver.	70	0	18
Rx Power	100	0	25
Total Sport; Ginseng, 8 fl.oz	60	0	15
awls Guarana, 8 fl.oz	130	0	32
laa Energy Drink, 12 fl.oz	50	0	13
lue Thunder, 22 fl.oz	400	0	68
ody Fuel (w. NutraSweet), 8 fl.oz	4	0	1
ody Works (Shasta), 12 fl.oz	90	0	22
arboplex (Nutra Life), 31g	120	0	30
arb Mate, bottle, 16 fl.oz	28	0	7
eraSport, 34g pkt (makes 16 fl.oz)	150	0	32
ytomax, 8 fl.oz	65	0	13
xceed (Weider): Powder, 2 Tbsp	70	0	17
Liquid, 12 fl.oz box	105	0	26
-Up, 8.4 fl.oz can	220	0.5	55
atorade: Frost, 8 fl.oz	50	0	14
Energy Drink, 12 fl.oz	310	0	78
ThirstQuencher, 8 fl.oz	50	0	14
o-Go: Sports, 8.4 fl.oz	90	0	24
Relax, 8.4 fl.oz	80	0	26
Immune, 8.4 fl.oz	90	0	24
Hansen's: Anti-Ox, 243ml can	110	0	31
Energy: Original, 246ml can	120	0	32
Endurance Formula, 246ml can	110	0	27
Power Formula, 246ml can	140	0	36
Energade: Stamina, 243ml can	110	0	31
Citrus/Orange, 243ml can	60	0	16
Slim Down, 246ml can	0	0	0
b. well; d. stress, 243ml can	110	0	31
Hydra Fuel (Tury Labs)	65	0	16
Hype Energy, all flavors, 12 fl.oz	90	0	22
IDN (Nu Skin): Splash C w. Aloe, 1 sc.	80	0	20
Creatine Blast, 1 scoop, 1 1/2 oz	130	0	32
Sportalyte, 1/2 pkt (makes 8 fl.oz)	70	0	17
Jones Whoop Ass Energy, 250ml	110	0	28
Knudsen: Isotonic Sports, 8 fl.oz	60	0	15
ReCharge, all flavors	80	0	18
Simply Nutritious, 1/2 bot., 16 fl.oz	60	0	14
Lipovitan: EB[3], 8.2 fl.oz	110	0	29

Per 8 fl.oz Unless Indicated	C	F	Cb
Max, made-up, 8 fl.oz	96	0	24
Met-Rx: Defense, 8.3 fl.oz can	120	0	32
Energy, 8.3 fl.oz can	120	0	32
Met-Rx ORS, Endura (Metagenics)	60	0	15
Nitro Speed, all flavors, 18 fl.oz	110	0	7
Pedialyte (Abbott)	25	0	6
Powerade: All flavors,			
Regular, 8 fl.oz	70	0	19
20 fl.oz bottle	175	0	48
Light, 8 fl.oz	25	0	7
20 fl.oz bottle	65	0	17
PowerBar Energy Gel:			
Chocolate, 41g pack	120	1.5	28
Other flavors	110	0	28
Pro-formance, all flavors	100	0	25
Recharge (Knudsen), all flavors	80	0	18
Red Bull Energy Drink, 8.3 fl.oz	113	0	28
Red Devil Energy Drink, 12 fl.oz	120	0	31
Red Tiger Energy Drink, 8.2 fl.oz	115	0	28
Relode Gel, 0.75 oz pkt	80	0	20
Revenge Pro (Champ. Nutr.),			
1 oz scoop	100	0	20
Sport, 25g scoop	90	0	23
Ripped Force, 16 oz	90	0	22
Snapple Sport, all flavors	80	0	20
SoBe: Energy/Power, 8 fl. oz	120	0	30
Juice Elixers, 8 fl.oz	100	0	25
Liz Blizz; Lizard Lightning	130	0	33
Adrenaline Rush, 8.3 oz can	140	0	36
SoBe Lean: All flavors, 8 fl.oz	5	0	1
Synergy: Per 1/2 bottle, 8 fl.oz			
Cosmic Cranberry	30	0	7
Mystic Mango	50	0	12
Other flavors	35	0	8
The Juice, 11 fl.oz	260	0	65
Thermo Force, 16 oz	260	0	65
Tiger's Milk (mix):			
Energy Booster, 3 heap Tbsp.	120	0	30
Twin Lab Ultra Fuel, 16 oz	400	0	100
Ultima Replenisher, 12g pkt	40	0	10
Upper Deck: All flavors	80	0	19
Venom Energy Drink (Elements),			
8.2 fl.oz	130	0	29
Worldwide: Carbo Rush, 20 fl.oz	280	0	60
Fat Shredder, 20 fl.oz bottle	0	0	0
Pure Protein, 22 fl.oz bottle	170	0	0
XS Energy: Citrus Blast, 8.4 fl.oz	8	0	0

Soft Drinks • Soda

Quick Guide
Cola Soda Drinks

Average All Brands
Coca-Cola and Pepsi

	C	F	Cb
8 fl.oz Cup	100	0	25
12 fl.oz Can	150	0	37
16 fl.oz Bottle	200	0	50
20 fl.oz Bottle	250	0	63
24 fl.oz (*Pepsi*)	300	0	75
1 Liter Bottle	400	0	100
2 Liter Bottle	800	0	200

Other Soda Drinks

	C	F	Cb
Club Soda, 12 fl.oz	0	0	0
Club Soda Cream, 12 fl.oz	170	0	42
Diet Soft Drinks: Aver., 12 fl.oz	0	0	0
Ginger Ale, 12 fl.oz	120	0	30
Lemon Lime, 12 fl.oz	220	0	55
Orange, 12 fl.oz	180	0	45
Root Beer, 12 fl.oz	165	0	41
Tonic Water, 12 fl.oz	135	0	34
Mineral Water: Plain, 12 fl.oz	0	0	0
Sweetened/flavored, 12 fl.oz	150	0	37
w. Fruit Juice, 12 fl.oz	120	0	30
Seltzers: Plain/Diet, 12 fl.oz	0	0	0
Sweetened/flavored, 12 fl.oz	150	0	37
w. Fruit Juice, 12 fl.oz	120	0	30

Movie Theater & Take-Out

Average All Flavors (Figures allow for 25% Ice)

	C	F	Cb
Small, 12 fl.oz	110	0	27
Regular, 16 fl.oz	150	0	37
Medium, 22 fl.oz	210	0	5
Large, 32 fl.oz	300	0	75
Cinnabon: Icescapes, 16 fl.oz			
Orange Cream	360	16	50
Root Beer	470	22	63
Mochalatta	390	12	62

Soda Brands

Per 12 fl.oz Unless Indicated

	C	F	Cb
A&W: Cream Soda	165	0	41
Diet Cream Soda/Root Beer	1	0	0
Root Beer	180	0	45
Albertson's: Cola	160	0	43
Lemon Lime	140	0	38
Other flavors, average	170	0	47

Soda Brands (Cont)

Per 12 fl.oz Unless Indicated

	C	F	Cb
Arizona: Lemonade(s), 8 fl.oz	110	0	28
Kiwi Strawb./Grape, 8 fl.oz	120	0	30
Pina Colada, 8 fl.oz	140	1	34
Diet Peach/Raspberry	0	0	0
Barq's: Root Beer	165	0	41
Barrelhead: Rootbeer	165	0	41
Big Red: 12 fl.oz	150	0	38
Bodyworks (Shasta), all flav.	90	0	23
Canada Dry: Birch Beer; Cactus	165	0	41
Club Soda	0	0	0
Collins Mixer	120	0	30
Ginger Ale, all flavors	135	0	37
Diet, all flavors; Seltzer	0	0	0
Half & Half; Hi-Spot; Wild Cherry	165	0	41
Lemon Sour	150	0	37
Sour Mixer	135	0	34
Tahitian Treat	225	0	56
Tonic Water/Twist Lime	150	0	37
Diet	0	0	0
Clearly Canadian, 11 fl.oz, aver.	120	0	30
Coca-Cola: Classic	140	0	35
Coke II	160	0	40
Diet Coke; Diet Cherry Coke	1	0	0
Cherry Coke	150	0	42
Cragmont: Cola	165	0	41
Cherry	180	0	45
Diet, all flavors	0	0	0
Crush, all flavors	210	0	52
Crystal Light, all flavors	8	0	2
Diet Rite, all flavors	1	0	0
Doc Shasta	160	0	40
Dr Diablo, Cola	140	0	35
Dr Nehi	150	0	41
Dr Pepper: Regular	150	0	40
Diet (Reg.; Caffeine Free)	3	0	0.5
Fanta: Orange; Grape	180	0	45
Ginger Ale	130	0	33
Root Beer	165	0	41
Fresca	4	0	1
Frutopia ~ See Page 143			
Hansen's: Average all flavors	130	0	37
Orange Creme Soda, 8 fl.oz	110	0	31
Natural Lemonade(s), 16 fl.oz	200	0	52
Health Valley: Wild Berry	140	0	35
Ginger Ale; Sarsp. Root Beer	150	0	41
Rootbeer Old Fashioned	120	0	30

Per 12 fl.oz Unless Indicated	C	F	Cb
Hires: Cream; Root Beer	180	0	45
Jolt Cola	150	0	41
Kick (Royal Crown)	180	0	45
Knudsen: Spritzers, average	170	0	43
Lights, all flavors	110	0	28
Lucozade, 7 fl.oz	136	0	34
Mello Yello: Regular	180	0	45
Diet	5	0	0
Minute Maid: Diet Orange	3	0	0.5
Berry; Black Cherry; Orange	165	0	41
Fruit Punch; Grape; Strawberry	180	0	45
Lemonade	160	0	40
Peach; P'apple; R'berry; Grapefr.	165	0	41
Mountain Dew, 24 fl.oz Bottle	170	0	46
Mr Pibb: Regular	150	0	37
Diet	2	0	1
Mug: Root Beer	160	0	43
Natural Brew: Apple, Cream	170	0	43
Cafe Mocha, Cherry Amaretto	160	0	40
Ginseng Cola, Ginger Ale	170	0	43
Nehi (Royal Crown): Cream	180	0	45
Ginger Ale, Quinine Water	135	0	45
Other flavors, average	195	0	45
Orangina, 10 fl.oz Bottle	120	0	45
Orbitz, 300ml Bottle, average	130	0	30
Pepsi: Regular; Caffeine Free	150	0	41
Diet Pepsi	0	0	0
One	1	0	0
Sierra Mist Lemon Lime	150	0	39
Wild Cherry	160	0	43
Perrier: Regular or flavors	0	0	0
Ramblin' Root Beer	180	0	45
RC Cola: Regular	160	0	40
Diet Cola	1	0	0
Cherry	165	0	41
Royal Mistic: Punch, 16 fl.oz	230	0	57
'N Juice, average	155	0	38
Sparkling, average, 11.1 fl.oz	115	0	28
Santa Cruz: Sparkling, all types	150	0	37
Orange	195	0	48
Schweppes: Bitter Lemon	165	0	41
Ginger Ale, regular; Raspberry	120	0	30
Ginger Beer; Lemon Lime	150	0	37
Grapefruit; Lemon Sour	165	0	41
Seltzer	0	0	0
Tonic: Regular	120	0	30
Diet	0	0	0

Per 12 fl.oz Unless Indicated	C	F	Cb
Sensa (Guarana flavored)	135	0	34
7UP: Regular	140	0	38
Cherry, Gold	155	0	38
Shasta: Black Cherry	170	0	46
Cherry Cola; Doc Shasta	160	0	40
Club Soda; Diet, all flavors	0	0	0
Cola, regular	170	0	46
Caffeine Free	160	0	40
Fruit Punch, Pineapple	200	0	50
Ginger Ale	130	0	33
Shasta Plus: all flavors	170	0	46
Slice: Lemon Lime	150	0	38
Diet Lemon Lime	0	0	0
Dr. Slice	140	0	40
Fruit; Grape; Pineapple; Red	190	0	51
CherryLime; Slice Cola	160	0	43
Snapple: Average all flavors	180	0	45
SoBe Drinks ~ See Page 149			
Spree (Shasta): all flavors	170	0	43
Sprite: Regular	150	0	37
Diet	4	0	1
Squirt: Regular Soda Citrus	150	0	40
Ruby Red Soda	170	0	46
Sunkist: Average all flavors	210	0	52
Diet Citrus	0	0	0
Diet Orange	7	0	1.5
Surge Citrus	170	0	46
TAB	1	0	0
Think!: Root Beer, 8.4 fl.oz	118	0	27
Sparkling Citrus, 8.4 fl.oz	130	0	31
Cola, 8.4 fl.oz	112	0	29
Upper 10 (RC): Regular	150	0	37
Diet	4	0	1
Vernor's: Ginger Ale	150	0	37
Welch's: Sparkling, average	180	0	45
Wink	195	0	48

Kool-Aid, Tang

	C	F	Cb
Bright & Early, 6 fl.oz	90	0	23
Kool-Aid, unsweetened, 6 fl.oz	2	0	0.5
Sugar, sweetened, 6 fl.oz	80	0	20
Sugar Free (NutraSweet), 6 fl.oz	5	0	1
Tang, all flavors, 6 fl.oz	90	0	23
Sugar-Free, 6 fl.oz	5	0	1

Coffee

Instant Coffee

	C	F	Cb
Powder/Granules: Regular or Decaffeinated,			
1 level tsp	2	0	0.5
1 rounded tsp	4	0	1
Ground, 1 Tbsp	5	0	1
Brewed/Percolated, 1 cup, 8 fl.oz	5	0	1
Coffee With Milk/Cream/Creamers:			
1 Cup Coffee (8 fl.oz):			
w. Whole Milk: Dash, 1 Tbsp	10	0.5	1
2 Tbsp, 1 fl.oz	20	1	1.5
w. 2% Milk, 2 Tbsp	15	0.5	1.5
w. 1% Milk, 2 Tbsp	12	0.3	1.5
w. Fat Free Milk, 2 Tbsp	10	0	1.5
w. Half & Half: 2 Tbsp	45	4	1
w. Cream (light coffee): 2 Tbsp	65	6	1
w. *Coffee Mate:* Liquid, reg., 1T.	40	2	5
Liquid Fat Free, 1 Tbsp	15	0	2
Powder, 1 heaping tsp	20	1	2
Sugar ~ Add Extra: 1 heaping tsp	25	0	6
Single portion, 1 pkt	25	0	6

Flavored Coffee Mixes

	C	F	Cb
Caffé D'Vita: 1 tsp	20	1	4
Coffee Essence, 1 tsp	16	0	4
General Foods, Cafe Intl: Regular	60	3	10
Sugar-free, average	30	2	3
Maxwell House: Mocha, 1 envelope	100	2.5	17
Mocha, sugar-free, 1 envelope	60	3	7
Van., Irish Cream, 1 envelope	90	1	20
Nescafé: Frothé, all flavors, average	90	1.5	19
Chicory: Instant Coffee, 1 tsp	6	0	1
Coffee Essence, 1 tsp	16	0	4

Coffee Substitute Mixes

	C	F	Cb
Roasted Cereal Beverages:			
Cafix Instant Beverage, 1 tsp	6	0	1
Kaffree Roma (Natural Touch) , 1 tsp	6	0	1
Postum, Instant Hot Beverage, 1 tsp	12	0	3
Revival Soy "Coffee", 1 Tbsp	5	0	1
Teeccino Caffe, 1 tsp	10	0	2

Bottled Coffee

	C	F	Cb
Main St: Fr. Vanilla, 12 fl.oz	190	3	31
Nescafé: Caffe Latte, 9.5 fl.oz	140	3.5	23
Mocha, 9.5 fl.oz	140	3	26
Starbucks: All types,. 9.5 fl.oz	190	3	40

Coffee Shops/Restaurants

Per 8 fl.oz Cup (Unless Indicated)	C	F	C
Coffee (Regular/Percolated/Filtered)	5	0	1
Americano Drip Coffee, 1 cup	5	0	1
Cafe Au Lait: 1 cup, 8 fl.oz	65	2.5	6
Nonfat Milk,1 cup	45	0	7
Caffe Latté:			
8 fl.oz cup: w. Whole Milk	100	5	8
w. 2% Milk	80	2.5	8
w. Nonfat Milk	60	0	8
12fl. oz: w. Whole Milk	180	10	14
w. Nonfat Milk	110	0.5	15
Cafe Mocha (Mochaccino): 1 c.	120	3	15
12 fl.oz	180	4.5	15
16 fl.oz	240	6	15
Cappuccino:			
8 fl.oz cup: w. Whole Milk	70	3.5	6
w. 2% Milk	60	2	6
w. Nonfat Milk	40	0	6
12 fl.oz: w. Whole Milk	110	6	9
w. 2% Milk	80	3	9
w. Nonfat Milk	60	0	9
Mocha, with Cream			
8 fl.oz: w. Whole Milk	180	12	16
w. Nonfat Milk	150	8	16
Tall, 12 fl.oz: Whole Milk	290	18	25
w. Nonfat Milk	230	11	26
Iced Mocha (no cream)			
Tall, 12 fl.oz: w. Whole Milk	190	9	24
w. Nonfat Milk	140	2	24
Espresso: Regular	4	0	1
Doppio (Double)	8	0	2
Espresso Con Panna			
(w. dollop whipped cream)	30	3	1
Espresso Macchiato	15	0.5	2
Frappuccino: Tall, 12 fl.oz	200	3	39
Grande, 16 fl.oz	270	4	52
Frappuccino Mocha:			
Large/Tall, 12 fl.oz	230	3	44
Grande, 16 fl.oz	310	4.5	59
Iced Latte: Similar to Caffe Latte			
Intellicino: 12 fl.oz	150	7	15
Lowfat (2% milk)	120	3.5	5

Irish & Liqueur Coffees

	C	F	C
Irish Coffee (no sugar)	175	10	0
Liqueur Coffee, aver. all types	200	10	16

Cocoa & Hot Chocolate

	C	F	Cb
Cocoa:			
8 fl.oz cup: w. Whole Milk	210	14	19
w. Nonfat Milk	80	8	2
Tall (12 fl.oz): w. Whole Milk	300	20	26
w. Nonfat Milk	120	11	5
Hot Chocolate:			
8 fl.oz cup: w. Whole Milk	200	10	25
w. Nonfat Milk	140	2	25
Tall (12 fl.oz): w. Whole Milk	300	15	38
w. Nonfat Milk	210	3	38
Cinnabon: Mocholatta Chill, 16 oz	410	18	54

Coffee Extras

	C	F	Cb
Chocolate (Cocoa) Topping, 1/2 tsp	10	0	2
Flavored Syrups, 2 Tbsp	80	0	20
Sugar-free, 2 Tbsp	0	0	0
Hershey's Chocolate Syrup, 2 Tbsp	100	0	24
Half & Half Cream, 2 Tbsp	40	3	3
Light Whipped Cream, 2 Tbsp	30	2	2
Marshmallows, miniature, 2	20	0	5

Starbucks

Hot Beverages: *Grande (16 fl.oz)*

	C	F	Cb
Caffe Americano	15	0	3
Caffe Latte: w. Whole Milk	270	14	22
w. Lowfat Milk (2%)	220	7	22
w. Nonfat Milk	160	1	23
w. Soy Milk	150	8	10
Breve	570	42	16
Caffe Misto/Au Lait: Whole Milk	150	8	12
Caffe Mocha: w. Whole Milk	370	21	40
w. Lowfat Milk (2%)	340	16	40
w. Nonfat Milk	290	11	40
w. Soy Milk	320	14	44
Breve	580	40	36
Cappuccino: w. Whole Milk	180	9	15
w. Lowfat Milk (2%)	140	5	15
w. Nonfat Milk	110	0	15
w. Soy Milk	100	5	7
Caramel Apple Cider	370	8	74
Caramel Macciato: Whole Milk	250	9	36
w. Lowfat Milk (2%)	225	5	36
w. Nonfat Milk	190	1	36
w. Soy Milk	210	3	44
Chai Tea Latte: 16 fl.oz	320	13	36
w. Nonfat Milk	210	0.5	37
Egg Nog Latte: w. Whole Milk	500	27	49

Starbucks (Cont)   C F Cb

Hot Beverages (Cont): *Grande (16 fl.oz)*

	C	F	Cb
Drip Coffee	10	0	2
Espresso: Solo	5	0	1
Doppio	10	0	2
Espresso Con Panna: Solo	110	9	3
Doppio	115	9	4
Espresso Macchiato: Solo	15	0.5	2
Doppio	20	0.5	3
Hot Chocolate w. Whole Milk	450	24	49
Mocha Valencia w. Whole Milk	480	25	60
Steamed: Whole Milk, 16 fl.oz	300	16	23
Lowfat Milk (2%)	240	9	23
Nonfat Milk	170	1	24
Soy Milk	160	9	9
Breve	560	48	16
Steamed Cider	230	0	57
Tazo Chai	320	9	52
White Chocolate: w. Whole Milk	480	20	60
w. Lowfat Milk (2%)	450	18	61
w. Nonfat Milk	400	11	61
w. Soy Milk	430	13	65
Breve	690	40	56

Blended Drinks: *Grande (16 fl.oz)*

	C	F	Cb
Frappuccino®: Caramel	350	9	61
Chocolate Brownie	490	14	88
Coffee	270	3.5	55
Eggnog	330	9	57
Expresso	230	3	46
Mocha	290	4	61
Tazo Berry®, Grande (16 fl.oz)	210	0	53
Tazo Berry® & Cream	600	23	63

Cold Beverages: *Grande (16 fl.oz)*

	C	F	Cb
Iced Caffe Americano	15	0	3
Iced Caffe Latte: w. Whole Milk	160	8	13
w. Lowfat Milk (2%)	130	4.5	14
w. Nonfat Milk	100	0	14
w. Soy Milk	90	4.5	88
Iced Mocha: w. Whole Milk	310	16	35
White Choc. Mocha, Whole Milk	320	8	52
Iced Tazo Chai w. Whole Milk	320	5	66

Beverage Additions: *Per Serving*

	C	F	Cb
Caramel Sauce	10	0	2
Fontana® Syrup, all flav., 4 pumps	80	0	21
Mocha Syrup	100	2	24
Power Packet	110	0	23
Sweetened Whipped Crm Topping	100	10	2

Tea & Iced Teas

Teas

	C	F	Cb
Regular: Bag, Loose or Instant			
Brewed, 1 cup, 8 fl.oz	1	0	0
(Add extra for sugar/milk)			
Herbal: Average all varieties, 1 cup	1	0	0
Bigelow: Apple Orchard, 1 cup	5	0	1
Other Varieties	2	0	0.5
Celestial Seasonings:			
Bengal Spice; Spearmint	5	0	0.5
Lemon Zinger	4	0	1
Roastaroma	10	0	2
Other varieties	2	0	0.5
Chai Tea Latté (Starbucks): See Previous Page			

Quick Guide

Iced Tea

Average All Brands

	C	F	Cb
Pre-Sweetened: 8 fl.oz	100	0	25
12 fl.oz	150	0	38
16 fl.oz	200	0	50
Unsweetened: 8 fl.oz	2	0	0

Iced Tea Mixes

Per Serving

	C	F	Cb
4C Instant	90	0	22
Bigelow, Nice Over Ice	1	0	0.5
Celestial Seasonings, Iced Delight	4	0	1
Crystal Light, Sugar Free	3	0	0
Kool-Aid Fruit T's	70	0	17
Lipton: Instant	0	0	0
Instant Lemon/Raspberry	3	0	1
Lemon	55	0	14
Peach/Raspb, Sugar Free	5	0	1
Nestea: 100% Instant	2	0	0
Decaffeinated	6	0	1
Ice Teasers, all flavors	6	0	1
Peach, Raspberry	90	0	22

> *A woman is like a teabag. You never know her strength until she's in hot water.*
>
> ~ Nancy Reagan

Bottled & Canned Teas

Per 8 fl.oz Unless Indicated

	C	F	Cb
Arizona: Green Tea w. Ginseng & Honey			
20 fl.oz Bottle: 1 cup, 8 fl.oz	70	0	18
Diet Green/Lemon	0	0	0
15.5 fl.oz Can: Average, 1 Can	190	0	50
w. Ginseng Extract	60	0	15
Herb Tea w. Honey, 8 fl.oz	70	0	17
Lemon/Raspberry, 8 fl.oz	90	0	22
Brisk: 1 liter Bottle, aver., 1 cup	90	0	24
12 fl.oz Can: Lemon, 1 Can	120	0	33
Raspberry, 1 Can	130	0	35
24 fl.oz Bottle: Lemon, 1 cup	80	0	22
Hansen's: Natural Iced Tea, 8 fl.oz	70	0	20
Low Calorie Blueberry/Raspberry	10	0	3
Knudsen: Coolers, all flavors	90	0	23
Lipton (16 fl.oz Bottle): Per 8 fl.oz			
No Lemon	70	0	18
Lemon	90	0	21
Peach; Raspberry	110	0	26
Mistic: Tropical Cooler, 8 fl.oz	45	0	12
Nantucket: Blueberry Tea, 8 fl.oz	80	0	20
Original Lemon Tea	90	0	23
Diet Lemon Tea	10	0	2
Half & Half	90	0	23
Nestea Iced Tea: Diet Lemon	3	0	0.5
Cool from Nestea, 1 cup, 8 fl.oz	80	0	20
Diet Cool from Nestea	2	0	0.5
Lemon/Peach/Raspberry	80	0	20
Sweetened Ice Tea	65	0	17
Oregon Chai: Herbal Bliss, 1/2 cup	70	0	18
Nirvana/Kashmir Green, 1/2 cup	80	0	20
Royal Mistic: Regular, 12 fl.oz	145	0	36
Diet, 12 fl.oz	8	0	2
Schweppes, 8 fl.oz	90	0	20
Shasta, 8 fl.oz	80	0	20
Snapple: Regular, sweetened	70	0	17
Diet/Unsweetened	0	0	0
Lemon; Peach, Raspberry	100	0	25
Sobe: Green/Lemon Tea, 8 fl.oz	90	0	24
Ssips (Johanna Farms), 8.45 fl.oz	100	0	25
Tropicana: Lemonfruit	100	0	25
Diet Lemon Fruit	15	0	4
Peach/Rasp./Tangerine, 8 fl.oz	120	0	28
11.5 fl.oz Can	160	0	40
Twister: Apple Berry, 8 fl.oz	100	0	28
Turkey Hill: Regular	90	0	22
Raspberry Cooler	110	0	28

♦ Health Hazards: Excess alcohol contributes to obesity, high blood pressure, stroke, heart and liver disease, some cancers, and even impotence.
Concentration and short-term memory are reduced as well as sporting performance.
Other alcohol hazards include stomach upsets, menstrual problems, anxiety, headaches, insomnia, work absenteeism and family arguments.

♦ Alcohol contributes to obesity through its high calories and by lessening the body's ability to burn fat. Fat storage is promoted, particularly in the belly - a danger zone. Alcohol can also stimulate appetite.
♦ Alcohol is potentially more harmful while dieting. Blood sugar levels may drop with resultant tiredness and further impairment of concentration, reflexes and driving skills - and maybe the dieter's resolve!

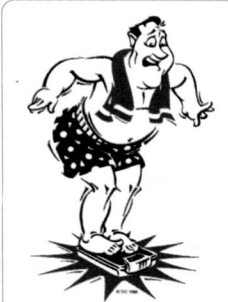

Excess alcohol contributes to obesity and high blood pressure

SAFE ALCOHOL LIMITS

Women: No more than **1 drink** per day.
Men: No more than **2 drinks** per day.
(At least 2 days a week should be alcohol-free.)

1 Drink = 12 fl.oz regular beer, or 5 fl.oz wine,
or 1½ fl.oz spirits (80 proof).
Each drink contains approximately 14g alcohol.

For some people, **safe drinking** will mean no alcohol drinks at all. (Even one drink may impair driving skills, particularly if tired; and 3-4 drinks daily has been linked to brain shrinkage in some social drinkers.)

♦ It is advisable not to drink at all if you are:
  • pregnant or trying to conceive
  • taking drug medication (unless approved by your doctor or pharmacist)
  • have a condition such as liver or heart disease
  • planning to drive or use machinery
  • studying or needing to concentrate
  • a child or adolescent

♦ Women and adolescents are more prone to alcohol's ill-effects due to their lower body weight, smaller livers and lesser capacity to metabolise alcohol.
Note: You cannot save daily drinks for one occasion.
  Binge drinking is particularly harmful ~
  4 drinks 'in a row' for males or 3 drinks for females.

HOW TO CALCULATE ALCOHOL CONTENT

Percent alcohol on label refers to alcohol volume (ml alcohol/100ml).

100ml = 3½ fl. oz

To convert to grams (weight) of alcohol, multiply the percent volume by 0.8 - since 1 ml of alcohol weighs only 0.8 grams (actually 0.789g).

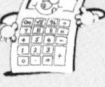

EXAMPLE
12 fl.oz Can Beer
(5% alcohol)

5% alc.volume = 5% of 12 fl.oz
            = 0.6 fl.oz
            = 18ml alcohol
            (1 fl.oz=30ml)

Weight (18ml x 0.8)
            =14.4g alcohol

Beers ✦ Ales ✦ Malt Liquors

Quick Guide   C   Alc   Cb

Beer: Alc ~ Alcohol (Grams)

Beer Contains Zero Fat

Malt Liquor/Ale (5.6% Alc. Vol.)

	C	Alc	Cb
12 fl.oz Can/Bottle/Glass	180	16	17
22 fl.oz Can/Bottle/Glass	330	29	32

Regular Beer (5% Alc. Vol.)

	C	Alc	Cb
7 fl.oz Glass	80	8.5	4
12 fl.oz Bottle/Can/Glass	140	14	10
16 fl.oz. Bottle/Can	185	19	11
22 fl.oz Bottle	260	26	20
32 fl.oz Bottle	370	37	28
40 fl.oz. Bottle	470	47	35

Light Beer (4.2% Alc. Vol.)

	C	Alc	Cb
7 fl.oz Glass	65	7	4
12 fl.oz Bottle/Can/Glass	110	12	6
16 fl.oz. Bottle/Can	145	16	8
22 fl.oz Bottle	200	22	11

Low Alcohol Beer (2.3% Alc. Vol)

	C	Alc	Cb
(Example: *Blatz LA*),12 fl.oz	75	7	6

Non-Alcoholic/Near Beer

(Less than 0.5% alcohol by volume)

	C	Alc	Cb
Average All Brands, 12 fl.oz	70	1	16

Beer Brands   C   Alc   Cb

Per 12 fl.oz Serving
Percentage alcohol listed below
is by volume - not by weight.

	C	Alc	Cb
Amber Ice (5.3% alcohol)	130	15	6
Anchor Steam (4.6%)	155	13	16
Anheuser Light (3.2% alcohol)	75	9	7
Artic Ice (5.3%)	150	15	8
Artic Ice Light 3.2 (3.9%)	100	11	6
Augsburger Bock (4.9%)	170	14	17
Augsburger Golden/Dark (4.9%)	170	14	17
Augsburger Red (4.9%)	160	14	14
Ballard Bitter (4.7%)	180	14	19
Beck's (5%)	150	14	12
Big Sky (4.8%)	150	14	12
Big Sky Light (4.5%)	105	13	5
Black & Tan (4.5%)	185	13	22
Black Label (5.6%)	155	16	11
Black Label Light (3.7%)	100	11	6
Blackhook Porter (4.9%)	160	14	14
Blatz (4.3%)	135	12	10
Blatz LA (2.3%)	75	7	6

Brands (Cont)   C   Alc   Cb

Beer Contains Zero Fat

	C	Alc	Cb
Blatz Light (3.7%), 12 fl.oz	100	11	3
Blue Moon Ale: Belgian (4.8%)	160	14	13
Honey Blond Ale (5.5%)	200	16	20
Nut Brown Ale (5.1%)	180	15	16
Raspberry Cream Ale (4.9%)	190	14	20
Bud Dry (4.9%)	130	14	8
Bud Light (4.2%)	110	12	7
Bud Ice (5.5%)	150	16	9
Bud Ice Light (4.1%)	95	12	4
Budweiser (4.9%)	150	14	11
Busch (4.9%)	145	14	11
Busch Light (4.2%)	110	12	7
Carling (4.4%)	140	13	10
Carlsberg (5%)	135	13	10
Castlemaine XXXX (4.7%)	140	13	9
Colt 45 Malt (5.6%)	155	16	12
Coors (4.9%)	150	14	12
Coors Dry (4.9%)	120	14	6
Coors Light 3.2 (4%)	100	11	4
Corona Extra (4.6%)	130	13	9
Dos Equis Lager (5%)	130	14	9
Elk Mountain Amber Ale (5.5%)	190	16	18
Elk Mountain Red (4.9%)	160	14	13
Extra Gold (4.9%)	150	14	10
Extra Gold 3.2 (4%)	120	11	10
Faust (5%)	170	14	17
First Reserve (4.9%)	170	14	16
Fosters Lager (4.9%)	135	14	9
George Killian's: Irish Brown(5.2%)	185	15	15
Irish Red (5%)	160	14	13
Wilde Honey Ale (5.3%)	170	15	14
Goebel (4.1%)	130	12	12
Goebel Light (3.9%)	110	11	8
Grolsch Premium (5%)	140	14	10
Guinness Draught (4.3%)	155	12	18
Heileman's: Old Style (4.9%)	147	14	12
Old Style Light (4.1%)	110	12	6
Heineken (5.4%)	170	15	15
Heineken Dark (5.2%)	175	15	16
Herman Joseph's			
Special Premium (4.9%)	150	14	12
Highland Ale: Black (5.6%)	180	16	16
Amber (5.6%)	160	16	14
Hurricane (5.5%)	150	16	10
Icehouse, Miller (5.0%)	135	14	9
Icehouse, Miller (5.5%)	150	16	

Beers ✦ Ales ✦ Malt Liquors

Brands (Cont)

Beer Contains Zero Fat
Per 12 fl.oz Serving

	C	Alc	Cb
Keystone Regular/Dry (4.9% alc.)	125	14	6
Ice (5.3%)	145	15	8
Light, 3.2 (4%)	100	14	4
Amber Light (3.8%)	110	11	8
King Cobra (5.9%)	180	17	15
Kirin Lager (Japan) (4.8%)	135	13	9
Labatt's Blue (5%)	145	14	9
Lowenbrau Dark/Special (4.9%)	160	14	15
Magnum Malt Liquor (5.9%)	155	17	23
Meister Brau (4.5%)	130	13	11
Meister Brau Light (4.5%)	105	13	5
Memphis Brown (4.6%)	120	13	6
Michelob: Regular (5%)	160	14	12
Light (4.3%)	135	12	12
Dry (4.9%)	130	14	8
Amber Bock (5%)	160	14	15
Centennial (5.5%)	175	16	15
Classic Dark (5%)	160	14	15
Golden Draft (4.8%)	150	14	13
Golden Draft Light (4.2%)	110	12	7
Hefeweizen (5%)	165	14	14
Malt (5.8%)	160	17	9
Miller, Regular (5%)	150	14	12
Miller Genuine Draft (5%)	145	14	11
Light (4.5%)	100	13	4
Miller High Life (5%)	145	14	9
Miller High Life Ice (5.5%)	142	16	7
Miller High Life Light (4.5%)	100	13	4
Miller Lite (4.5%)	95	13	4
Miller Lite Ice (5.5%)	125	16	4
Miller Lite Ice (5%)	115	14	3
Milwaukee's Best (4.5%)	130	13	11
Milwaukee's Best Ice (5.5%)	135	16	5
Milwaukee's Best Light (4.5%)	100	13	8
Minnesota's Best (4.9%)	140	14	10
Moosehead (5%)	125	14	14
Natural Ice, Budweiser (5.9%)	160	14	10
Natural Light, Budweiser (4.2%)	110	12	7
Natural Pilsner, Budweiser (4.9%)	150	14	12
Newcastle Brown Ale (4.5%)	140	12	13
Northstone Amber Ale (4.9%)	150	14	8
Old Milwaukee (4.5%)	145	13	13
Light (4.3%)	122	12	10
Ice (5.5%)	155	16	10
Red (4.5%)	135	13	11

	C	Alc	Cb
Pabst (5%), 12 fl. oz	155	14	14
Pete's Wicked Ale (5%)	180	14	20
Piels (4.7%)	135	13	10
Piels Light (4.5%)	127	13	9
Primo (4.3%), 12 fl.oz	140	12	13
Ranier (4.6%)	142	13	12
Red Bull Malt (7%)	192	20	12
Red Dog (5%)	150	14	12
Red Hook ESB (5.4%)	175	16	16
Red Hook Rye (5%)	155	14	14
Red Light (4.1%)	105	12	5
Red River Valley (4.9%)	165	14	15
Red Wolf (5.5%)	155	16	12
Samuel Adams (4.6%)	170	13	17
Samuel Adams Lager (4.7%)	180	13	19
Sapporo Draft (Japan) (4.5%)	140	12	12
Schaefer (4.3%)	140	12	12
Schaefer Light (3.9%)	110	11	8
Schlitz Ice (4.6%)	145	13	13
Schlitz Ice Light (4.3%)	120	12	8
Schlitz Malt (5.9%)	180	17	14
Schmidt (4.6%)	142	13	12
Sheaf Stout, 5.7%	180	16	17
Sierra Nevada: Pale Ale (5.6%)	175	16	16
Big Foot Ale (10.1%)	210	29	2
Pale Bock (6.6%)	190	19	20
Porter (6%)	185	17	18
Silver Thunder (5.9%)	165	17	11
Stella Artois, 5%, 330ml	135	14	9
Southpaw Light (5%)	125	14	6
Stroh's (4.4%)	145	13	13
Stroh's Light (4.3%)	115	13	7
Stroh's Signature (4.9%)	160	14	15
Wheat Hook (4.8%)	150	14	12
Winterfest (5.7%)	185	16	18
Zeigenbock (5%)	155	14	13
Zima Clear Malt (4.6%)	150	14	13

Homebrewed Beer: Similar to regular beers, according to alcohol content.

Non-Alcoholic Brews

	C	Alc	Cb
Less Than 0.5% Alcohol			
Average All Brands			
(Busch, Kaliber, O'Douls, Old Milwaukee NA, Stroh's NA, Sharp's, Haakebeck, Texas Select)			
12 fl.oz Can/Bottle	70	1	15

Alc ~ Alcohol (Grams)

Cider ◆ Wine ◆ Liquor

Alcoholic Lemon Brews

	C	Alc	Cb
Average All Brands			
(Average of 5% Alcohol)			
Hooper's Hooch/Lusty, 12 fl.oz	150	14	12
Hard/Spiked Lemonade,12 oz	250	14	37

Cider

Alc ~ Alcohol (Grams)

	C	Alc	Cb
Alcoholic Cider: Average,			
5.5% alcohol, Dry, 12 fl.oz	130	16	12
Sweet, 12 fl.oz	160	16	12
Hardcore Crisp Hard Cider (6% alc)			
12 fl.oz	190	17	19
Hornsby's Draft Cider (6% alc)			
12 fl.oz bottle	170	17	15
Woodchuck Draft Cider (5% alc)			
Amber, 8 fl.oz	135	14	14
Dark & Dry, 8 fl.oz	120	14	11
Granny Smith, 8 fl.oz	110	14	7

Quick Guide

Table Wine

	C	Alc	Cb
Average All Varieties (11.5% Alcohol)			
4 fl.oz (1/2 large wine glass)	85	11	2
6 fl.oz (3/4 large wine glass)	125	16	3
1/2 Carafe/Bottle, 375ml	265	34	6
1 Bottle, 750ml	530	68	13

Table Wines

	C	Alc	Cb
Red: Claret/Burgundy/Chianti, 4 fl.oz	80	11	0
Sparkling Reds, 4 fl.oz	90	11	3
Rose: Medium, 4 fl.oz	80	11	0
White: Dry (Chablis/Hock/Riesling) 4 fl.oz	75	11	0
Zinfandel Sweet			
(Moselle/Sauterne), 4 fl.oz	85	11	2
Sparkling, 4 fl.oz	95	11	4
Champagne: *Per 4 fl.oz Serving*			
Average 1 glass, 4 fl.oz	85	11	2
w. Orange Jce (3:1 orange)	75	8	4
w. Orange Jce (1:1 orange)	65	5	7
Cold Duck, 4 fl. oz	108	11	8
Sake: Rice Wine (16% alc.), 4 oz	125	15	5
Mulled Wine: (Gluhwein), 4 oz	180	14	20
Non-Alcoholic Wine, aver., 4 oz	50	0	12
Reduced Alcohol Wine (6%):			
Average all types, 4 fl.oz	50	0	12

Dessert Wines

	C	Alc	Cb
Madeira (18% alc), 2 oz	85	9	5
Marsala (18%), 2 oz	110	9	11
Port, Muscatel, (18%), 2 oz	85	9	5
Sherry (18%), 2 oz			
Dry, 1 Sherry glass	65	9	0.5
Sweet/Cream, average	85	9	5
Vermouth: Dry (18%), 2 oz	65	9	0.5
Sweet (15%), 2 oz	85	7	8

Cooking Wine

	C	Alc	Cb
Average All Brands			
Red/White, 2 Tbsp, 1 oz	20	3	1
Marsala. 2 Tbsp, 1 oz	35	4	2
Sherry, 2 Tbsp, 1 oz	40	4	2

Cooking with Wine

For alcohol to evaporate, sufficient heat and cooking time (at least 30 minutes) is required.

Red and white table wines would then contain negligible residual calories.

Sweetened wines (marsala/sherry) would contain 10 calories per 1 fl.oz used.

Flambé Desserts: Only surface alcohol is burnt off.

Spirits/Liquors

All Contain Zero Fat

Includes Bourbon, Brandy, Gin, Rum, Scotch, Tequila, Vodka, Whiskey.

Note: All spirits with same proof (alcohol) have similar calories and zero fat.

Average All Brands	C	Alc	Cb
80 Proof (40% Alcohol by Volume):			
1 fl.oz	65	9.5	0
11/2 fl.oz Jigger	100	14.5	0
1/2 Bottle, 375 ml	810	120	0
1 Bottle, 750 ml	1620	240	0
86 Proof (43% Alcohol):			
1 fl.oz	70	10	0
11/2 fl.oz Jigger	105	15	0
1/2 Bottle, 375 ml	870	125	0
1 Bottle, 750 ml	1750	250	0
100 Proof (50% Alcohol):			
1 fl.oz	82	12	0
11/2 fl.oz Jigger	125	18	0
1/2 Bottle, 375 ml	1025	150	0
1 Bottle	2050	300	0

Coolers & Premix Cocktails

Zero Fat Unless Indicated
Calorie & Carbohydate estimates
given where no data available.

	C	Alc	Cb
Bacardi Fruit Mixers (Frozen Conc.)			
Made up (2 oz mix + 1 oz Rum + Ice)			
Margarita	160	10	22
Pina Colada	230	10	40
Other varieties, average	200	10	32
(If 2 oz Rum used, add extra 70 cals/10g alcohol)			
Bartles & Jaymes:			
Wine Cooler/Cocktails (5%): Per 12 fl.oz			
Berry; Kiwi Strawberry	230	14	35
Fuzzy Navel, Margarita	260	14	44
Original	200	14	30
Strawberry Daiquiri; Tropical	230	14	39
Malt Based Coolers (3.9% alc.): Per 12 fl.oz			
Berry; Black Cherry; Peach	210	11	33
Margarita; Pina Colada	270	11	48
Fuzzy Navel; Tropical	230	11	38
Strawberry Daiquiri	220	11	36
Boone's Farm Wine Coolers:			
Snow Crk Berry; Sun Peach (5%)	150	10	20
Sangria; Strawberry Hill (7.5%)	190	14	23
Breezer By Bacardi (3.2% alc): Per 12 fl.oz			
Passionfr.; Calypso Berry	220	9	39
Pina Colada (contains 6g fat)	250	9	33
Strawberry Daiquiri	250	9	47
Tahitian Tangerine	200	9	34
Heublein Premium Classics:			
Long Is. Ice Tea (15% alc), 2 oz	130	7	20
Manhattan (22.5%), 2 oz + ice	160	11	20
Mai Tai (22%), 2 oz + ice	160	11	20
Pina Colada, 4 oz (10g fat) + ice	280	4	40
Jack Daniels Country Cocktails (5.9%)			
Average all flavors, 200ml	170	9.5	25
Jose Cuervo Cocktails (5.9%):			
Margarita/Lime/Strawb., 200ml	180	9.5	27
Seagram's Coolers (3.2%), 12 fl.oz			
Wild/Berry flavors, average	230	12	36
Smirnoff Ice (5%), 12 fl.oz	245	14	36
TGI Friday's Frozen Cocktails (12.5%):			
Per Serving (3 fl.oz Premix & Ice):			
Margarita; Strawberry Daiquiri	145	9	20
Note: All drinks below contain 6g fat/serving.			
B52; Strawberry Shortcake	230	9	29
Mint Choc. Chip; P.Colada	250	9	32
Mudslide; Orange Dream	240	9	31

Premix Cocktails (Cont)

The Club
(Premix Cocktails): Per 4oz

	C	Alc	Cb
Long Island Ice Tea; Manhattan	220	16	30
Margar.; Scr'driver; Vod. Martini	210	7	40
Mudslide (9g fat)	270	12	41
P. Colada; Or. Craze; Whisk. Sour	260	10	40

Shooters — Alc ~ Alcohol (Grams)

Kamakazi	150	20	2
Mud Slide	160	13	17
Fuzzy Navel	120	13	7
Pineapple Bomber	130	11	13
Turbo	110	14	3
Shots: Average all types, 1$\frac{1}{2}$ fl.oz	110	14	3

Flavorings/Syrups

Non-Alcoholic, Fat Free

	C	Alc	Cb
Angostura Bitters, $\frac{1}{4}$ tsp	3	0	0
Grenadine/Cassis, 2 Tbsp, 1 oz	70	0	17
Lime Juice, 2 Tbsp, 1 oz	10	0	2
Sugar Syrup, 2 Tbsp, 1 oz	70	0	17
Sour Mix, 2 Tbsp, 1 oz	10	0	2
Tonic Water, 8 fl.oz	90	0	22

Cocktail Mix 'N Drinks

No Alcohol Added

	C	Alc	Cb
Bloody Mary Mix (Mr & Mrs T),			
8 fl.oz	40	0	9
Pina Colada Mix: Daily's, 3 fl.oz	160	0	37
Mr & Mrs T, 4.5 fl.oz	180	0	43
Margarita Mix (J.Cuervo), 4 fl.oz	100	0	24

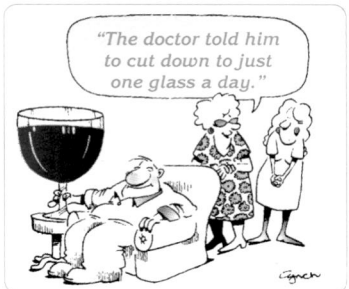

"The doctor told him to cut down to just one glass a day."

Cocktails + Liqueurs

Cocktails

Alc ~ Alcohol (Grams)

Zero Fat Unless Indicated
(Made to Standard Recipes)

	C	**Alc**	**Cb**
Bloody Mary	120	14	5
Blushin' Russian (9g fat)	365	14	47
Bourbon & Soda	110	15	1
Brandy Alexander (16g fat)	300	16	11
Cerebral Hemorrhage (5g fat)	290	17	32
Chupa Naranjas (w. 1½ oz Tequila)	150	16	8
Collins (w. 2 oz gin)	180	20	11
Daiquiri	110	14	3
Gin & Tonic	170	16	14
Harvey Wallbanger (2 oz Vodka)	250	30	11
Highball (1½ oz Whiskey)	110	14	3
Irish Coffee (contains 9g fat)	210	14	8
L.A. Sunrise	280	26	21
Leprechaun's Libation	285	31	17
Long Island Iced Tea (w. 8 oz Cola)	230	19	25
w. Diet Cola	130	19	0
Mai Tai (w. 2 oz Rum)	260	27	17
Manhattan	130	17	3
Margarita	170	21	4
Martini	160	22	1
Mind Eraser	160	17	10
Mint Julep	165	20	8
Mosito (w. 2 oz Rum)	170	19	10
Pina Colada (contains 12g fat)	260	14	12
Screwdriver	180	14	20
Spritzer (3 oz Wine)	70	8	3
Tequila Sunrise	190	20	14
Tom Collins	120	16	2
Whiskey Sour	125	15	5

Liqueurs/Cordials *Per 1 fl.oz*

	C	**Alc**	**Cb**
Baileys Irish Cream (34 Proof; 5g fat)	95	4	5
Lite (30 Proof; 2g fat)	75	4	7
Cherry Brandy (48 Proof)	80	6	9
Coffee Liqueur (53 Proof)	90	6.5	11
Amaretto (56 Proof)	110	6	17
Benedictine (80 Proof)	90	10	5
Cointreau (80 Proof)	100	10	7
Creme de Cacao (54 Proof)	100	6	15
Creme de Menthe (60 Proof)	120	7	14
Drambuie (80 Proof)	105	10	9
Grand Marnier (80 Proof)	100	10	7
Kahlua (53 Proof)	90	6.5	11
Kirsch (68 Proof)	80	8	6
Midori (42 Proof), average all types	80	5	11

Ten Hints to Avoid Harmful Drinking

1. **Add up the alcohol** you typically drink each day and on social occasions. How does this compare with 'low risk' amounts?

2. **Compare the alcohol content** of different drinks and select the lowest. Request half ounces of alcohol in cocktails and mixed drinks. Dilute them and keep topping off with non-alcoholic drinks.

3. **Try low alcohol** or non-alcohol alternatives such as fruit juices and mineral water. Take your own to parties.

4. **Before drinking alcohol,** quench your thirst with water and non-alcoholic drinks - particularly after vigorous exercise or sport.

5. **Slow the rate of drinking.** Chugging or drinking fast is the major cause of illness and death from alcohol poisoning.

6. **Avoid drinking in 'rounds'.**

7. **Have a non-alcoholic 'spacer'** between drinks (e.g. mineral water, orange juice).

8. **Don't drink on an empty stomach.** Food slows the rate of alcohol absorption.

9. **Keep track of the number of drinks** and know when to stop. Stick to a set limit.

10. **Do not drive, swim, or operate machinery** while under the influence.

Note: Alcohol can be very dangerous when taken with prescription or street drugs or when you are very tired.

Liqueurs/Cordials (Cont)

Per 1 fl.oz

	C	**Alc**	**Cb**
Ouzo (80 Proof)	90	10	7
Sambuca (84 Proof)	100	10	5
Schnapps (80 Proof)	100	10	7
Southern Comfort (78 Proof)	75	9	3
Tia Maria (64 Proof)	90	8	9
Triple Sec (60 Proof)	80	7	4
Coffee Liqueurs: *Average All Types*			
(Includes Benedictine, Cointreau, Kahlua):			
1 serving	200	10	10

Note: Figures for these dishes are only a guide. Large variations occur with serving size, recipe ingredients and cooking methods.

Chinese & Asian Dishes

Appetizers	C	F	Cb
Curried Meat Triangles, 1 pce	150	5	12
Dim Sum (Dumplings), 1 ball	65	2	5
Egg Rolls, mini, 3 rolls	100	3	11
Spring Roll, Small, 1 1/2 oz	100	7	10
Medium, 3 oz	200	12	20
Large, 5 oz	350	15	33
Wonton, 1 only	55	3	4
Soup: Clear, 1 bowl	30	1	4
with Noodles	100	3	12
Chicken & Corn	150	8	8
Fortune Cookie: each	25	<1	5

Entrees & Main Dishes	C	F	Cb
Per Whole Dish (2-3 Serves)			
Beef Satay, 17 oz	760	50	15
Beef with Broccoli, 16 oz	650	30	31
Beef in Black Bean Sce, 17 oz	530	33	17
Chicken & Almonds, 18 oz	685	50	18
Chop Suey: Chicken, 20 oz	560	37	17
Pork, 20 oz	680	50	17
Chow Mein: Beef/Chick., 24 oz	940	60	50
Crispy Fried Chicken, 8 oz	485	33	12
Lemon Chicken, 10 oz	580	32	25
Omelet: Chick/Shrimp, 16 oz	990	82	10
Sweet & Sour: Fish, 20 oz	1160	58	106
Pork, 18 oz	950	50	92
Duck, 18 oz	1120	71	85
Vegetable Combination, 6 oz	250	17	19
Extra Listings: See Frozen Entrees/Meals.			
Rice: Plain, 1 cup, 5 oz	170	0	36
Fried: 1 cup, 5 oz	320	13	42
Large dish, 16 oz	1010	40	134
Noodles: Chinese Egg, boiled,1 cup	200	3	42

Confucious say:
"Man who eat with one chopstick never have problem with obesity!"

Cajun & Creole

	C	F	Cb
Per Serving			
Alligator, 1 oz ckd	40	0.5	0
Baked Herb Chicken	850	53	2
Bouillabaisse	400	15	10
Cajun Fried Turkey	630	25	0
Cocktail Sauce, 1 Tbsp	15	0	3
Couche-couche, 1/2 cup	80	0	17
Crawfish Bisque	500	10	10
Crawfish, cooked, 2 oz	45	0.5	0
Creole Jambalaya	550	30	15
Dove, cooked, 1 oz	60	3.5	0
Frog's Legs, steamed (2)	45	0	0
Guinea Fowl, flesh, 1 oz, ckd	40	1	0
Hogshead Cheese, 1/4 cup	80	5.5	0
Jambalaya, Shrimp & Crabmeat	520	14	12
Red Beans & Rice	400	17	52
Roasted Quail, w. Bacon on Toast	550	25	15
Remoulade Sauce, 1 Tbsp	55	5.5	1
Shrimp Creole	450	20	10
Stuffed Smothered Steak, w. 1 cup rice	890	50	50
Squab, flesh, 1 oz cooked	60	3.5	0
Turtle, cooked, 1 1/2 oz	60	1.5	0

French Foods

	C	F	Cb
Blanquette d'Agneau (Lamb Stew w. Veg)	800	30	17
Brioche, 1 cake	280	14	34
Bouillabaise (Fish Stew)	400	15	10
Coq au Vin (Chicken in Wine)	800	30	16
Coquilles St. Jacques, fried, 6 lge	300	14	2
Creme Caramel (Caram. Custard)	260	10	38
Crepe Suzette, 1x 6"crepe/sauce	220	10	13
Duck a l'Orange	780	35	47
Escargots (Snails), in garl. butter, (6)	200	10	4
Frogs Legs, fried, 4 med. pairs	400	20	10
Lamb Noisettes, fried, 2 chops	500	40	1
Mousse au Chocolat	380	15	33
Potage Creme Crecy (Carrot Soup)	360	18	14
Salade Nicoise (Tuna/Oliv./Veg.)	450	13	14
Veal Cordon Bleu (Veal/Ham/Ch)	650	25	18
Vichyssoise (Pot./Leek Soup), 1 c.	200	9	15

German

	C	F	Cb
Bavarian Bread Dumpling, 3 small	330	10	28
Beef Goulash with Veges	520	20	46
Black Forest Cake, 1 slice	380	16	30
Bratwurst, grilled, 1 medium, 6 oz	450	37	2
Chicken: Fried, Viennese-style	530	20	28
Livers w. Apple/On., 6 oz	460	28	10
Herring, Pickled: Rollmops, 4 oz	260	16	3
with Sour Cream, 4 oz	310	20	3
Hot Sausage Curry	300	7	6
Kugelhupf Cake, 1 lge slice, 4 oz	400	23	40
Sauerbraten Pork (Pot Roast)	650	35	15
Torte: Linzer (Alm./Raspb. Jam)	430	18	58
Sacher (Choc./Apricot Jam)	260	12	23
Weiner Schnitzel, 1 med.	750	35	38

Greek

	C	F	Cb
Baklava Pastry, 1 only, 3³/4 oz	400	21	45
Calamari, deep fried, 1 cup	300	13	17
Galactobureko, 1 only (Filo, Custard, Pastry in Syrup)	360	11	48
Kataifi, (Filo, Nut, Pastry in Syrup)	350	11	56
Moussaka, 1 serve, 8 oz	350	22	22
Souvlakia (Lamb), each, 2 oz	120	6	1
Stuffed Tomatoes, 2 only	250	12	17
Taramasalata, 1 Tbsp, ¹/2 oz	40	3	2
Tyropita (Filo/Egg/Cheese Pastry)	350	26	31
Tzatziki (Cucumber/Yog. Dip), 1 T.	20	1	1
Vine Leaves, stuffed, 3 rolls, 6 oz	200	5	13

Indian & Pakistan

Per Serving
(Meat dishes allow 4 oz meat/serving)

	C	F	Cb
Aloo Samosa, each (Savory Pastries w. Potato fill.)	150	12	12
Alu Gosht Kari (Meat/Pot. Curry)	600	40	23
Ande ki Kari (Egg, Tom Sce), each	250	23	7
Bhona Gosht (Mint Broil Lamb)	560	28	5
Chicken Pilaf (Murgh Biriyani)	700	53	50
Chapati/Roti, 7" diam. piece (Baked Whole Wheat Bread)	60	<1	11
Dal (Lentil Puree), 1 cup, no oil	230	1	37
1 Tbsp Tadka (oil topping)	120	13	0
Dhakla, 1 oz	105	5	13
Dhansak, ¹/2 cup	105	3.5	11
Fish Jhol (Fish in Gravy)	230	10	5

Indian & Pakistan (Cont)

	C	F	Cb
Gosht Kari (Meat Curry/Tom./Pot.)	460	25	17
Imli Chatni (Chutney), 1 Tbsp	30	0	7
Lamb Pilaf	520	35	40
Machchi Molee (Fish, C'nut Milk)	690	45	15
Masala Gosht (Beef/Tom./Gravy)	400	25	18
Mulligatawney Soup, average	300	15	8
Murgh Tikka, 1 cup	300	4	7
Naan, 1 cup	75	2	11
Pappadom, 1 large/2 small	50	3	5
Pesrattu, 9" crepe	130	5	15
Pork Vendaloo Curry	620	47	3
Rajmah (Kidney Bean Curry)	400	17	56
Rogan Josh (Lamb/Yoghurt Sce.)	500	30	5
Saag Gosht (Beef/Spinach Sce.)	430	26	10
Shahi Korma (Braised Lamb)	430	28	3
Tandoori Chicken: Breast	260	13	5
Leg/Thigh portion	300	17	5

Italian Dishes

	C	F	Cb
Cannelloni, 1 tube, 6 oz	280	15	18
Chicken Cacciatore	370	22	4
Gnocchi, Spinach	300	18	17
Lasagne with meat, 10 oz	400	17	36
Manicotti, cheese/tomato	230	14	18
Minestrone Soup, 1 cup	260	6	28
Osso Buco (Veal/Tom./Mushr.)	550	28	5
Ravioli, 8 oz	300	12	30
Risotto (Chicken)	420	12	70
Spaghetti: Plain, 1 cup, 5 oz	185	1	44
Restaurant: 2 cups, plain	370	2	88
+ Bolognese (Meat Sce)	650	16	90
+ Marinara (Seafoods)	700	20	90
+ Napoletana (Tom. Sce)	540	13	105
Saltimbocca (Veal/Ham/Cheese)	430	28	5
Tortellini, 20 pieces	530	20	74
Veal Marsala	400	20	11
Veal Parmigiana	350	20	5
Pizza: Per ¹/2 Pizza (12")			
Vegetarian/Cheese:			
Thin Crust	650	26	63
Thick Crust	850	35	108
Sausage/Pepperoni: Thin Crust	700	32	68
Thick Crust	900	62	135
(Also see Pizza Hut, Domino's, Shakey's, Godfather's Pizza ~ **Fast Foods Section.)**			

Japanese

Sushi

	C	F	Cb
Lunch Menu (Assorted Sushi)			
Regular, 1 serving	330	3	56
Deluxe, 1 serving	430	4	72
Sushi Rice, ckd, 1 Tbsp	25	<1	5
1 cup, 5¼ oz	380	3	82
Nigiri-Zushi: (Fish wrapped Sushi)			
Per 1 oz piece:			
Ebi-zushi (Jumbo Shrimp)	20	<1	3
Kani-zushi (Surimi Crab)	30	<1	5
Maguro-zushi (Tuna)	25	<1	4
Sake-zushi (Salmon)	35	1	4
Suzume-zushi (Baby Snapper)	30	<1	4
Tai-zushi (Red Snapper)	30	<1	4
Nori-Maki-Zushi: *Per Piece*			
(Seaweed-wrapped Sushi Rolls)			
Anago-maki (Conger Eel)	20	1	2
California-maki (Crab/Caviar/Avocado)			
	70	1	10
Futo-maki (Egg Omelet, Shellfish, Veg.),			
1 piece	70	1	10
Kobana-maki (Egg Om., Cucum.)	35	<1	6
Kappa-maki (Cucumber)	15	0	3
Tekka-maki (Tuna)	20	<1	4
Uni-maki (Sea Urchin)	20	<1	4
Inari-Zushi (Bean Curd Pouches w. Sushi)			
1 pouch, 3 oz	130	2	23
Tamago-Yaki (Omelet-wrapped Sushi)			
1 piece	45	1	5
Sashimi (Slice Raw Seafood/Beef)			
Ika (Squid), 4 oz	105	2	0
Hamachi (Yellowtail), 4 oz	165	6	0
Naguro (Yellowfin Tuna), 4 oz	120	1	0
Niku (Beef), 5 oz	200	10	0
Saba (Mackerel), 4 oz	160	7	0
Suzuki (Sea Bass), 4 oz	110	<1	0
Tako (Octopus), 4 oz	95	1	0
Dipping Sauces: Aver., 2 Tbsp	30	0	7
Ginger Vinegar Dress., 2 Tbsp	20	0	5
Miso Soup w. tofu pces, 1 cup	85	3	11
Sukiyaki (Beef/Tofu/Veg.), 8 oz	400	24	32
Tempura (Batter-fried Shrimp & Veges.)			
3 large shrimp & veges	320	18	25
1 shrimp only	60	4	3
Teppan Yaki (Steak, Seafood & Veges.)			
10 oz serving	470	30	15
Teriyaki Beef, 4 oz serving	350	25	4
Sake Wine (16% alc.), 3 fl.oz	115	0	7

Kosher/Deli Foods

	C	F	Cb
Bagel/Bialy,			
½ small, 1 oz	80	1	16
Beiglach (Cheese Knish)	350	17	35
Blintzes, average, 1 only	120	1	25
w. Sour Crm. & Preserves	370	10	30
Borscht, (no cream), 1 cup	85	3	14
Diet/Reduced Cal., 1 cup	30	1	7
Cabbage Roll (meat/rice), 5 oz	170	6	21
Chicken Broth, 1 cup	80	8	0
with vegetables	100	8	5
with noodles	150	9	16
Lowfat, plain, 1 cup	25	1	0
Cholent, 1 med serve, 1 cup	350	16	48
Chopped Liver: 1 serve, 3 oz	110	6	5
with Egg Salad, ¼ cup	100	7	3
Farfel, dry, ½ cup	90	<1	21
Hallah (Yeast Bread), 1 sl., 1 oz	85	2	14
Gefilte Fish Balls:			
Regular, medium, 2 oz	55	2	4
with jelled broth	80	2	6
Cocktail size, 1 oz	30	1	2
Sweet, medium, 2 oz	65	2	4
with jelled broth	95	2	9
Herring: Smoked, 2 oz	120	8	0
in Sour Cream, 2 oz	150	10	0
Kasha, cooked, ½ cup	100	<1	20
Kipfel (Vanilla/Almd. Cookie), 1 pce.	60	2	7
Knaidlach, 1 ball	40	2	5
Knish: Kasha/Potato, 1 only	130	4	22
Cheese, 1 only	350	17	35
Kreplach, beef, 1 piece	40	1	6
Kugel, potato/noodle, 1 serve	150	7	20
Latkes (Potato Pancake), 2 oz	200	11	22
3 Latkes w. Sour Cr./Apple Sce	750	25	95
Lochshen: Plain, 1 cup	130	2	26
Pudding, 1 cup	380	13	48
Lox (Smoked Salmon), 2 oz	65	2	0
Mandelbrot (Almond Bread), 1 slice,			
¼" thick	45	2	5
Matzo: 1 board, 1 oz	110	<1	21
(Also see Matzoh ~ Page 98)			
Matzo Balls, 2 small, 1 large	90	3	12
Soup, with 1 large ball	180	7	24
New York Cheesecake, 4 oz	350	24	26
Pierogi, potato/cheese, 1 pce	90	4	11
Reuben Sandwich	920	60	28
Schmaltz (Rend'd chick. fat), 1 T.	90	10	0

Lebanese/Middle East

	C	F	Cb
Baba Ghannouj, 2 Tbsp, 1 oz (Eggplant/Seasame Dip)	70	6	2
Baklava, 1 pastry, 1 3/4 oz (Pastry, Nuts, Syrup)	245	18	18
Cabbage Rolls, 1 roll, 3 oz (Cabbage Leaf, Meat, Rice)	100	3	12
Cous Cous, 1 serve (Semolina, Milk, Fruit, Nuts)	400	21	43
Felafel (Chick Pea Fritter): Fried, 1 medium, 1 oz	60	4	4
Hummus, 1/4 cup, 2.2 oz	105	3	5
Fried Kibbi, 1 piece, 3 oz (Wheat, Meat, Pinenuts)	180	8	15
Kafta, 1 skewer, 1 1/2 oz (Ground Lamb Saus. on Skewer)	85	5	2
Kibbeh Naye, 1 cup, 9 oz (Raw Lamb, Bulgur & Spices)	450	18	28
Lebanese Omelet, 1 serving, 4 oz (Egg, Spinach, Pinenuts, Onion)	200	12	13
Pilaf, 1 cup (Rice, Onion, Rais., Apr. Spice)	400	11	60
Shawourma, 1 serve, 4 oz (Spit Roast Beef)	280	15	2
Shish Kabob, 1 stick, 2 1/2 oz	130	7	2
Spinach Pie, 1 piece, 3 1/2 oz	290	21	20
Sweet Almond Sanbusak, 1 pce (Pastry, Almonds, Spices)	200	15	11
Tabouli, 1 serve, 4 oz	170	14	7
Tahini Sauce, aver., 1 Tbsp	90	8	2

Mexican

	C	F	Cb
Black Bean Soup, 1 bowl	200	3	34
Bueso Fresco, 1/4 cup	80	4.5	2
Burritos (Taco Bell): Bean	380	12	54
Big Beef Supreme	520	23	51
Chili, plain, 1/4 cup	90	6	8
Chili con Carne, w. Beans, 1 cup	310	17	15
w/out Beans, 1 cup	370	28	10
Corn Chips, 1/2 cup, 1 oz	160	10	17
Empanadas, average, 1 small	230	10	28
Enchilada, average	330	10	49
Fajitas: Chicken (Soft)	200	7	20
Guacamole, 2 Tbsp, 1 oz	120	12	4
Horchata 1 cup, 8 fl. oz	120	0.5	27
Margarita (w. 1 1/2 oz Tequila)	160	0	6
Menudo, 1/2 cup	55	1.5	10

Mexican (Cont)

	C	F	Cb
Nachos: Taco Bell, Big Beef	430	24	43
Bellgrande (Taco Bell)	740	39	83
Del Taco: Regular	390	23	39
Macho Nachos	1090	61	110
Quesadilla: Cheese (Taco Bell)	370	20	32
Refried Beans, 3/4 cup, 6 oz	160	3	26
Sopaipillas (flky. pstry.puffs), 1 pc	100	7	10
w. honey & cream	200	14	18
Taco (Taco Bell): Regular	170	10	11
Chicken	180	5	23
Taco Supreme	230	13	13
Big Border Taco	280	16	17
Taco Salad w. Salsa	840	52	85
Taco Sauce, average, 1/4 cup	15	0	3
Taco Shell, regular	50	2	8
Tamales, Van Camp's (can), 1/2 c	150	8	14
Tostada (Taco Bell)	300	14	31
Tortilla, corn, 6" diam.	70	1	14
Tortilla Chips, 1 oz	150	8	18

Extra Listings of Mexican Dishes:
- Frozen Entrees/Meals ~ See Page 57-62
- Fast Foods Section (Taco Bell, Del Taco).
- Canned Bean/Chili Products ~ See Page 66-68

Polish

	C	F	Cb
Cabbage Rolls w. Sour Cr., 2 sm.	220	10	30
Chicken Casserole w. Mush., 1 c.	520	27	5
Kielbasa (Sausages, Onions, fried, 2 large.)	350	28	2
Meatballs w. Sour Cream, 3 x 1 1/2" balls	300	16	11
Pierogi, Fruit/Veg, 3" ball	80	2	15
Pork Goulash (Pork/Veg. Stew)	550	21	38
Pot Roast with Vegetables	630	21	28

OLD McDONALDS FARM
128 FOR PEOPLE WHO WHO BETTER

Brooklyn

Restaurant & Ethnic Foods (Cont)

Soul Foods

	C	F	Cb
Breakfast Sausage, fried, 2 patties	250	17	0
Cornbread, homemade, 3 oz	200	7.5	28
Fatback, raw, 1/4 oz	60	6.5	0
Ham Hock, 1 oz	90	6.5	2
Hog Maw, 1 oz	45	2.5	0
Hominy, 3/4 cup	85	1	17
Hush Puppies, 5 pces, 3 oz	260	12	35
Neck Bones, Pork, 1 oz	65	4	0
Opossum, 1 oz	65	3	0
Oxtail, 1 oz	70	3.5	0
Pig Ear, 1/4 ear	50	3	0
Pig Foot, 1/2 foot	70	4.5	0
Pig Tail, 1/3 tail	115	10	0
Poke Salad, ckd, 1/2 cup	15	0.5	3
Pork Brains, 1 oz	40	2.5	0
Pork Cracklings, 1/2 oz	80	6	0
Pork Chitterlings, simmered, 3 oz	260	25	0
Pork Skin, 1 cup	70	4.5	0
Sousemeat, 1 oz	60	4.5	0
Succotash, 1/2 cup	80	1	17
Sweet Potato Pie, 1/8 of 9" pie	250	12	34
Tongue Pork, 1/3 tongue	75	5.5	0
Tripe, 2 oz	55	2	0
Vienna Sausage, 2 small, 1 oz	90	8	1

Thai Foods

	C	F	Cb
Appetizers: Satay Pork, 1 oz	100	4	2
Spring Roll, 1 1/4 oz	110	6	13
Soups: Tom Yam (Hot & Sour):			
Spicy Shrimp/Seafood, 1 cup	100	4	6
1 bowl	160	7	10
Vegetarian, 1 cup	50	0	11
Curries: Chicken w. Ginger, 1 cup	390	34	4
Thick Red Curry w. Beef, 1 cup	600	50	7
Thai Chicken Curry, 1 cup	340	23	4
Massaman Curry, 1 cup	680	57	8
Green Curry w. Pork, 1 cup	480	44	5
Pad Thai, Large serving, 18 oz	990	38	125
Steamed Fresh Fish w. Spicy Thai Sce	450	8	46
Spicy Chicken (w. veges), stir-fry	450	22	14
Spicy Garlic Tofu w. veges, stir-fry	340	18	18
Sticky Thai Rice, 1 cup, 6 oz	170	0.5	36
Stir-fried Rice Noodles, 1 c., 5 1/2 oz	270	9	40
Stir-fried Vegetables, 1 cup	100	3	18
Salads: Thai Chicken, 1 serving	330	9	17
Thai Beef Salad, 1 serving	260	9	15
Sauces: Peanut Satay, 1/2 cup, 4 oz	160	10	13

Spanish

	C	F	Cb
Arroz Abanda (Fish with Rice)	340	8	31
Arroz Con Pollo (Rice/Chick. Sal)	500	23	50
Clams Marinera, 8 clams	330	16	22
Cochifrito (Lamb w. Lemon/Garlic)	650	25	5
Cochinillo Asado, 2 sl. (Rst Suckling Pig)	300	15	3
Cocido Madrileno			
(Madrid-Style Boiled Dinner)	450	27	18
Flan de Leche (Caramel Custard)	325	9	52
Fritadera de Ternera (Sauteed Veal)	450	27	2
Gazpacho, 1 bowl	60	0	15
Paella a la Valenciana			
(Chicken & Shellfish Rice)	900	42	70
Pollo a la Espanola (Chicken)	475	30	4
Ternera al Jerez (Veal w. Sherry)	660	29	6
Zarzuela (Fish & Shellfish Medley)	530	27	40

Vietnamese

	C	F	Cb
Bo Xao Dau Phong: *Per Whole Dish*			
(Ginger Beef w.Onion, Fish Sce.)	750	30	10
Bo Nuong (Beef Satay), 2 sticks	265	9	4
Ca Chien Gung			
(Whole Snapper w. Ginger)	600	16	6
Canh Chay (Veg./Tofu Soup)	80	3	13
Cuu Xao Lan (Curried Lamb,			
Veges in Coconut)	900	40	80
Ga Chien (Crsp. Chick + Plum Sce)	900	40	105
Ga Nuong (Chicken Satay + Sce.)	240	10	4
Ga Xao Rau(Marinated Chicken			
Braised w. Veg.)	800	26	100
Rau Cai Xao Chay			
(Stir Fried Vege., Soy Sauce)	400	15	65
Thit Heo Goi Baup Cai, each			
(Spicy Cabbage Rolls w. Pork)	200	7	11

Gourmet & Miscellaneous

	C	F	Cb
Ants Eggs/Larvae, 1 Tbsp	20	0	0
Ants, Choc. coated, 3 Tbsp	140	7	2
Bee Maggots, canned, 3 Tbsp	65	2	0
Caviar, black/red, 1 Tbsp	40	3	0
Caterpillars, canned, 2 oz	60	2	0
Frogs Legs, fried, 1 pair (large)	125	7	0
Haggis, boiled, 4 oz	350	24	22
Locusts, raw, 1 oz	35	1	0
Silkworms, raw, 1 oz	60	2	0
Snails (Escargots) ~ See French Foods			
Snake, roasted, 4 oz	160	6	0

Deli, Sandwiches, Wraps • Vending

Sandwiches

	C	F	Cb
No Spreads Unless Indicated			
(Includes 2 Slices Bread ~ 3 oz)			
BLT (5 strips Bacon, 2 Tbsp Mayo)	600	40	46
Breaded Chicken & Salad	540	28	46
Chicken (5 oz) Salad w. Mayo.	580	30	49
Chopped Liver, Egg, Mayo.	630	25	44
Corned Beef (5 oz) w. Mustard	560	28	44
Cream Cheese w. Olives (5 large)	340	14	46
Egg Salad w. Mayonnaise	570	29	49
Egg Salad Club w. Bacon, Mayo.	780	53	49
Grilled Cheese (5 oz)	540	30	44
Ham (4 oz); Cheese (4 oz), Mayo.	910	56	44
Lobster Salad (4 oz) w. Mayo.	530	25	45
Overstuffed Tuna Salad (7 oz)	870	39	75
Reuben (6 oz Beef/Pastrami, 2 oz Cheese,			
2 Tbsp Dressing)	920	60	28
Roast Beef (4 oz) w. Mustard	460	12	45
Roast Pork (4 oz) w. Apple Sauce	500	16	55
Shrimp Salad Club w. Bacon, Mayo.	800	57	48
Sloppy Joe w. Sauce (7 oz)	600	30	45
Steak Sandwich (5 oz cooked)	680	32	41
Triple Cheese (4 oz) Melt	720	45	46
Tuna (5 oz) Salad w. Mayo.	610	30	49
Turkey Breast (5 oz) w. Mayo.	460	18	44
Turkey Breast (5 oz) w. Mustard	360	7	44
Turkey Club w. Bacon, Mayo.	830	38	31
Vegetarian w. Avocado, Cheese	820	49	72
Subs: See *Subway* Page 240			

Wraps & Roll-Ups

	C	F	Cb
Average All Types			
(Meat/Chicken/Fish/Veges)			
Regular size, approx. 9 oz	500	25	48
Large, approx. 15 oz	830	40	80
Jumbo, approx. 22 oz	1400	70	134
Au Bon Pain: See Page 170			
Long John Silver: Page 212			
Taco Bell Fajita Wraps: Page 243			
Wendy's Pitas: Page 248			

Bagels

	C	F	Cb
Plain: unfilled, 3 oz	240	2	45
w. 2 Tbsp Cream Cheese	340	12	46
w. 2 oz Lox (Smoked Salmon)	320	4	45
Au Bon Pain: Page 170			
Einstein Bros Bagels: Page 197			

Croissants

	C	F	Cb
Unfilled: Medium 1 1/2 oz	180	10	20
w. Ham (2 oz), Salad	280	14	24
w. Ham (2 oz), Cheese (2 oz)	470	30	20
w. Chick (2 oz) Cheese (2 oz)	470	30	20
w. Turkey/Ham/Chse (2 oz ea.)	580	36	20
Au Bon Pain: Ham & Cheese	380	20	36
Spinach & Cheese	270	16	27

Vending Machines

	C	F	Cb
Brownie, frosted	180	9	24
Cheese Balls, 1 oz	150	8	16
Choc Chip Cookies, 4	130	7	19
Choc Milk, 8 fl.oz	225	9	26
Coca Cola Classic, 12 fl.oz	140	0	35
Diet Coke, 12 fl.oz	1	0	0
Corn Chips, 1 oz	160	10	15
Danish Pastry, 2 oz	220	10	25
Donut, plain, 1 3/4 oz	210	12	25
Fruit Pie, 4 oz	290	13	46
Granola/Cereal Bars	130	3	26
Hershey's, 1.55 oz bar	240	14	25
Hot Fries, 1 oz	140	10	11
Kellogg's Rice Krispies Treat	120	1.5	26
Lance: Captain's Wafers, 1 pkg	230	12	26
Big Town, 1 pkg	250	11	38
M & M's: Plain, 1.7 oz	240	10	34
Peanuts, 1.7 oz	250	13	30
Milk, whole, 8 fl.oz	150	8	12
Reduced Fat, 2%, 8 fl.oz	120	5	12
Milky Way, 2 oz	270	10	41
Onion Rings, 1 oz	120	6	16
Orange Juice, 8.75 fl.oz	120	0	28
Peanuts, roasted, 1 oz	165	14	6
Popcorn, plain, 1 oz	160	10	14
Pork Skins, 1 oz	160	10	0
Potato Chips, 1 oz	150	10	15
Reduced Fat, 1 oz	140	7	20
Pretzels, 1 oz	110	2	22
Raisins, 1/2 oz pkg	40	0	9
Reece's Peanut Butter Cups, 1.8 oz	280	17	28
Snickers, 2.1 oz bar	280	14	35
Tortilla Chips, 1 1oz	150	8	22

Fast-Food Chains & Restaurants

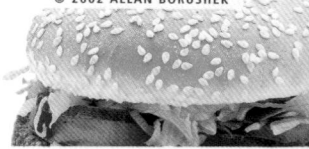

- **Cal** Calories
- **Fat** Fat (grams)
- **%Fc** Percent Fat Calories
- **S.Fat** Saturated Fat (grams)
- **Chol** Cholesterol (milligrams)
- **Sod** Sodium (milligrams)
- **Pro** Protein (grams)
- **Carb** Carbohydrates (grams)

© 2002 ALLAN BORUSHEK

Arby's®

	Cal	Fat	%Fc	S.Fat	Chol	Sod	Pro	Carb
Breakfast Items								
Biscuit: w. Butter	280	17	55%	4	0	780	5	27
w. Bacon	360	24	60%	7	10	220	9	27
w. Ham	330	20	55%	5	30	830	12	28
w. Sausage	460	33	65%	9	25	300	12	28
Croissant (Plain)	220	12	49%	7	25	230	4	25
w. Bacon	340	23	60%	13	30	520	10	28
w. Ham	310	20	58%	11	50	1130	13	29
w. Sausage	440	32	65%	15	45	600	13	29
Sourdough: w. Bacon	420	10	21%	2.5	10	960	16	66
w. Ham	390	6	14%	1	30	1570	19	67
w. Sausage	520	19	33%	5	25	1040	19	67
French-Toastix, no syrup	370	17	41%	4	0	440	7	48
Maple Syrup	130	0	0%	0	0	45	0	32
Roast Beef Sandwiches								
Arby's Melt w. Cheddar	340	15	39%	5	70	890	16	36
Arby-Q®	360	14	35%	4	70	1530	16	40
Beef 'N Cheddar	480	24	45%	8	90	1240	23	43
Big Montana®	630	32	46%	15	155	2080	47	42
Giant Roast Beef	480	23	43%	10	110	1440	32	42
Junior Roast Beef	310	13	38%	4.5	70	740	16	34
Regular Roast Beef	350	16	41%	6	85	950	21	34
Super Roast Beef	470	23	44%	7	85	1130	22	47
Sub Sandwiches: French Dip	410	18	39%	8	100	1680	28	42
Hot Ham 'N Swiss	530	27	46%	8	110	1860	29	45
Italian	780	53	61%	15	120	2440	29	49
Philly Beef 'N Swiss	700	42	54%	15	130	1940	36	46
Roast Beef	760	48	57%	16	130	2230	35	47
Turkey	630	37	53%	9	100	2170	26	51
Other Sandwiches								
Chicken Bacon 'N Swiss	610	33	49%	8	110	1550	31	49
Chicken Breast Fillet	540	30	50%	5	90	1160	24	47
Chicken Cordon Bleu	630	35	50%	8	120	1820	34	47
Grilled Chicken Deluxe	450	22	44%	4	110	1050	29	37
Hot Ham 'N Swiss	340	13	34%	4.5	90	1450	23	35
Roast Chicken Club	520	28	48%	7	115	1440	29	38
Market Fresh Sandwiches								
Roast Beef & Swiss	810	42	46%	13	130	1780	37	73
Roast Chicken Caesar	820	38	42%	9	140	2160	43	75
Roast Ham & Swiss	730	34	42%	8	125	2180	36	74
Roast Turkey & Swiss	760	33	39%	6	130	1920	43	75
Market Fresh Salads (no dressing)								
Caesar Salad	90	4	40%	2.5	10	170	7	8
Caesar Side Salad	45	2	40%	1	5	95	4	4
Chicken Finger Salad	570	34	54%	9	65	1300	30	39
Grilled Chicken Caesar Salad	230	8	31%	3.5	80	920	33	8
Turkey Club Salad	350	21	54%	10	90	920	33	9

	Cal	Fat	%Fc	S.Fat	Chol	Sod	Pro	Carb
Light Menu								
Garden Salad	70	1	13%	0	0	45	4	14
Grilled Chicken	280	5	16%	1.5	55	1170	29	30
Grilled Chicken Salad	210	4.5	19%	1.5	65	800	30	14
Roast Chicken Deluxe	260	5	17%	1	40	1010	23	33
Roast Chicken Salad	160	2.5	14%	0	40	700	20	15
Roast Turkey Deluxe	260	5	17%	0.5	40	980	23	33
Side Salad	25	0	0%	0	0	20	2	5
Sides: Cheddar Curly Fries w. Sauce	460	24	47%	6	5	1290	6	54
Chicken Finger 4-Pack	640	38	53%	8	70	1590	31	42
Chicken Finger Snack	580	32	50%	7	35	1450	19	55
Curly Fries, small	310	15	44%	3.5	0	770	4	39
Homestyle Fries, small	220	10	41%	2.5	0	430	3	32
Jalapeno Bites™	330	21	57%	9	40	670	7	30
Mozzarella Sticks	470	29	56%	14	60	1330	18	34
Onion Petals	410	24	52%	3.5	0	300	4	43
Potato Cakes (2)	250	16	58%	4	0	490	2	26
Baked Potato: Plain	355	0	0%	0	0	25	7	82
w. Butter & Sour Cream	500	24	43%	15	55	170	8	65
w. Broccoli 'N Cheddar	540	24	40%	12	50	680	12	71
Deluxe Baked Potato	650	34	47%	20	90	750	20	67
Desserts/Shakes								
Apple Turnover (Iced)	420	16	34%	4.5	0	230	4	65
Cheesecake (Plain)	320	23	65%	14	95	240	5	23
Cherry Turnover (Iced)	410	16	35%	4.5	0	250	4	63
Chocolate Chip Cookie	125	6	43%	2	10	85	2	16
Shakes: Chocolate, 14 oz	480	16	30%	8	45	370	10	84
Other flavours, average, 14 oz	470	15	29%	7	45	380	10	82
Condiments								
Arby's Sauce	15	0	0%	0	0	180	0	4
Au Jus Sauce	5	0	0%	0	0	385	0	1
BBQ Dipping Sauce	40	0	0%	0	0	350	0	10
BBQ Vinaigrette	140	11	70%	1.5	0	660	0	9
Bleu Cheese Dressing	300	30	90%	6	45	580	2	3
Bronco Berry Sauce™	90	0	0%	0	0	35	0	23
Buttermilk Ranch Dressing	360	39	98%	6	0	490	1	2
Reduced Calorie	60	0	0%	0	0	750	1	13
Caesar Dressing	310	34	98%	5	60	470	1	1
Croutons: Cheese & Garlic	100	6	54%	na	na	138	1	10
Seasoned	30	1	30%	0	0	70	1	1
BBQ Dipping Sauce	40	0	0%	0	0	350	0	10
German Mustard	5	0	0%	0	0	70	0	1
Horsey Sauce®	60	5	75%	0.5	5	150	0	3
Italian Dressing, Reduced Calorie	25	1	36%	1	0	1030	0	3
Mayonnaise	90	10	100%	1.5	10	65	0	0
Light Cholesterol Free	20	1.5	68%	0	0	110	0	1
Thousand Island Dressing	290	28	87%	4.5	35	480	1	9

Au Bon Pain®

	Cal	Fat	%Fc	S.Fat	Chol	Sod	Pro	Carb
Bagels: Plain, 5 oz	350	1.5	4%	0	0	660	14	72
Asiago Cheese, 4.2 oz	380	6	14%	3.5	15	690	17	66
Cheddar & Scallion, 4.2 oz	310	7	20%	4.5	20	650	14	47
Cinnamon Raisin, 5 oz	360	1.5	4%	0	0	540	12	77
Cranberry Walnut, 5oz	460	4	8%	0.5	0	590	15	93
Dutch Apple w. Walnut Streussel, 5 oz	350	5	13%	0	0	480	10	77
Everything, 4.2 oz	360	2.5	6%	0	0	710	14	72
Honey & Grain, 4.2 oz	360	2	5%	0	0	580	14	72
Jalapeno Double Cheddar, 4.2 oz	290	3.5	11%	2	10	600	12	53
Sesame, 4.2 oz	380	4	9%	0.5	0	540	15	70
Wild Blueberry, 4.5 oz	380	1.5	4%	0	0	570	14	80
Spreads: Plain Cream Cheese, 2 oz	180	18	90%	10	50	150	4	2
Plain Lite Cream Cheese, 2 oz	100	8	72%	5	20	280	6	4
Sundried Tomato Light, 2 oz	120	8	60%	5	20	320	6	6
Vanilla Hazelnut Light, 2 oz	150	11	66%	7	35	210	5	6
Sandwiches: Buffalo Chicken	640	20	28%	3.5	85	1650	40	76
Chicken Caesar (no dressing)	440	12	25%	5	70	900	37	43
Chicken Fo-Ca-cha-cha	870	30	31%	5	130	2280	74	90
Fields & Feta Wrap	560	17	27%	4	10	850	20	90
Fresh Mozzarella, Tomato & Pesto	650	30	42%	12	55	1090	30	70
Honey Dijon Chicken	730	18	22%	6	135	1990	57	85
Hot Roasted Turkey Club	950	50	47%	16	135	2240	50	80
Southwestern Tuna (no dressing)	760	46	54%	14	100	1030	40	48
Summer Turkey (no dressing)	430	4.5	9%	0	20	1380	35	62
Thai Chicken	420	6	13%	1	20	1320	20	72
Breads: Average. 1.75 oz slice	115	1.5	8%	0	0	300	5	22
Bread Rolls: Hearth, each	220	1.5	6%	0	0	410	10	43
Petit Pain, each	200	1	5%	0	0	570	7	40
Soups: Per 8 oz Serving								
Beef Barley	75	2	24%	0.5	15	660	6	10
Chicken Noodle	80	1.5	17%	0	15	670	8	10
Clam Chowder	270	20	67%	10	65	730	10	16
Cream of Broccoli	220	18	74%	9	40	770	5	14
Garden Vegetable	30	0	0%	0	0	820	2	8
Tomato Florentine	60	1	15%	0.5	5	1030	4	13
Vegetarian Chili	140	2.5	16%	0	0	1070	6	27
Salads: Per Serving (Container)								
Chicken Caesar	360	11	25%	6	65	910	36	28
Field Green, Gorgonzola & Walnut	400	34	77%	13	50	800	2	10
Garden Salad	160	1.5	8%	0	0	290	7	34
Mozzarella & Rst Red Pepper	340	18	48%	10	60	135	22	26
Oriental Chicken	270	4	13%	0.5	70	700	40	17
Tuna	490	27	50%	4.5	45	750	26	40
Cookies: Chocolate Chip	280	13	42%	8	40	85	3	40
English Toffee	220	12	49%	7	45	110	2	28
Oatmeal Raisin	250	10	36%	3.5	30	240	3	40
Shortbread	390	25	58%	15	65	190	3	40

	Cal	Fat	%Fc	S.Fat	Chol	Sod	Pro	Carb
Cakes & Bars:								
Apple Strudel	440	26	53%	8	0	780	5	48
Apple Coffee Cake	480	24	45%	12	100	285	6	60
Cherry Strudel	450	30	60%	12	0	730	5	45
Mochaccino Oreo Bar	405	24	53%	10	37	295	5	44
Pecan Roll, 6.8 oz roll	900	48	48%	15	50	480	1	110
Walnut Fudge Brownie	380	18	43%	10	100	150	5	56
Croissants: Per Croissant								
Hot: Ham & Cheese	380	20	47%	12	70	690	16	36
Spinach & Cheese	270	16	53%	10	40	330	10	27
Sweet Filled: Plain	270	15	50%	10	40	240	6	30
Almond	560	37	59%	15	105	250	12	50
Apple	280	10	32%	6	25	180	4	46
Chocolate	440	23	47%	15	30	230	7	53
Cinnamon Raisin	380	13	31%	8	35	290	7	50
Raspberry Cheese	380	20	47%	10	60	300	6	47
Muffins: Per Muffin								
Lowfat: Chocolate Cake	290	3	9%	0.5	20	630	4	68
Triple Berry	270	4	13%	0.5	25	560	5	60
Gourmet: Blueberry	410	15	33%	2.5	85	380	8	64
Carrot Nut	480	23	43%	5	55	650	8	60
Chocolate Chip	490	20	37%	7	35	560	8	70
Corn	470	18	34%	2.5	65	570	8	70
Pumpkin w. Streussel Topping	470	18	34%	3	60	550	8	74
Raisin Bran	390	10	23%	4	45	1030	10	65
Drinks: Cappuccino, 16 oz	150	6	36%	3.5	30	150	10	15
Iced Tea: Peach, 12 fl.oz	130	0	0%	0	0	20	0	33
Cafe Latte, 16 oz	150	6	36%	4	30	-	8	10
Mocha Blast, Iced, 10 oz	160	4	22%	3	20	-	-	-
Frozen Mocha Blast, 16 oz	320	3	8%	2	10	150	10	64

Applebee's®

	Cal	Fat	%Fc	S.Fat	Chol	Sod	Pro	Carb
Low Fat & Fabulous								
Asian Chicken Salad: Large	645	9.5	13%	na	na	na	32	108
Regular	370	5.5	13%	na	na	na	16	64
Blackened Chicken Salad: Large	410	5	11%	na	na	na	54	38
Regular	290	3	9%	na	na	na	38	28
Chicken Fajita Quesadilla	520	11	19%	na	na	na	42	62
Garlic Chicken Pasita	590	8	12%	na	na	na	39	89
Lemon Chicken Pasita	530	11	19%	na	na	na	29	78
Veggie Quesadilla	345	8	21%	na	na	na	22	46
Desserts, Sundaes								
Low Fat Brownie Sundae	415	2	4%	na	na	na	17	82
Low Fat Marble Cheesecake	260	2	8%	na	na	na	10	50
Low Fat Strawberry Shortcake	250	2	7%	na	na	na	10	48

Auntie Anne's®

	Cal	Fat	%Fc	S.Fat	Chol	Sod	Pro	Carb
Pretzels: With Butter								
Almond Crunch Pretzel	400	8	18%	5	20	400	9	72
Cinnamon Sugar Pretzel	450	9	18%	6	25	430	8	83
Garlic Pretzel	350	4.5	12%	3	10	850	9	68
Glazin' Raisin Pretzel	510	4	7%	2	10	480	11	107
Jalapeno Pretzel	310	4.5	13%	3	10	940	8	59
Original Pretzel	370	4	10%	2	10	930	10	72
Parmesan Herb Pretzel	440	13	27%	8	30	660	10	72
Sour Cream & Onion Pretzel	340	5	13%	3	10	930	9	66
Pretzels (without Butter): Deduct	50	5.5	-	4	20	20	0	0
Cool Drinks								
Auntie Anne's Lemonade, 22 fl.oz	180	0	0%	0	0	0	0	43
Kiwi-Banana Dutch Ice, 14 fl.oz	190	0	0%	0	0	30	0	44
Lemonade Dutch Ice, 14 fl.oz	315	0	0%	0	0	0	0	77
Mocha Dutch Ice, 14 fl.oz	400	10	23%	9	0	100	0	74
Orange Crème Dutch Ice, 14 fl.oz	280	0	0%	0	0	35	0	64
Pina Colada Dutch Ice, 14 fl.oz	220	0	0%	0	0	15	0	53
Raspberry Dutch Ice, 14 fl.oz	175	0	0%	0	0	30	0	40
Strawberry Dutch Ice, 14 fl.oz	220	0	0%	0	0	40	0	50
Wild Cherry Dutch Ice, 14 fl.oz	210	0	0%	0	0	25	0	48
Dipping Sauces: Caramel Dip	135	3	20%	1.5	5	110	1	27
Cheese Sauce	100	8	72%	4	10	510	3	4
Chocolate Flavored Dip	130	4	28%	1.5	2	65	1	24
Hot Salsa Cheese	100	8	72%	4	10	550	2	4
Light Cream Cheese	70	6	77%	4	25	140	3	1
Marinara Sauce	10	0	0%	0	0	180	0	4
Strawberry Cream Cheese	110	10	82%	6	35	105	2	4
Sweet Mustard	60	1.5	23%	1	40	120	0.5	8

Big Apple Bagels®

	Cal	Fat	%Fc	S.Fat	Chol	Sod	Pro	Carb
Bagels								
Apple Cinnamon	80	0.5	5%	0	0	na	3	16
Banana Nut	80	1	9%	0	0	na	3	15
Blueberry	75	0	2%	0	0	na	3	15
Cheddar Herb	85	1.5	18%	1	2	na	4	14
Cinnamon Rais.; Eight Grain; Honey Oat	80	0.5	5%	0	0	na	3	16
Plain	75	0.5	4%	0	0	na	3	15
Pumpernickel; Spinach; Strawberry	80	0.5	3%	0	0	na	3.5	15
Tom. Basil; Vegetable; Whole Wheat	75	0.5	4%	0	0	na	3	15
Cream Cheese: Plain	100	10	90%	6	na	na	2	1
Plain Lite	75	7	84%	4	na	na	3	1
Muffins								
Chocolate	85	2.5	26%	1	0	na	1.5	14
Chocolate, Fat Free	60	0	0%	0	0	na	1	15
Plain	85	2	21%	1	2.5	na	1.5	15
Plain, Fat Free	65	0	0%	0	0	na	1	15

Baskin-Robbins®

	Cal	Fat	%Fc	S.Fat	Chol	Sod	Pro	Carb
Hard Scooped Icecream: Per Regular Scoop								
Cherries Jubilee	240	13	49%	8	50	75	3	29
Chocolate: Regular Scoop	280	16	51%	10	55	110	4	31
Small Scoop	180	10	52%	6	35	65	3	20
Chocolate Chip	270	17	56%	11	60	85	4	26
Chocolate Chip Cookie Dough	300	17	51%	10	60	125	4	35
Chocolate Fudge	290	15	46%	10	41	180	4	34
Cookies 'N Cream	300	19	57%	12	55	140	4	29
French Vanilla	280	18	58%	13	90	90	4	25
German Choc Cake	310	15	43%	13	32	170	5	39
Gold Medal Ribbon	270	13	43%	8	50	170	3	35
Jamoca	250	15	54%	10	60	85	3	25
Jamoca Almond Fudge	280	16	51%	8	45	70	4	30
Mint Choc Chip	270	18	60%	11	60	85	4	26
Old Fashion Butter Pecan	290	20	62%	10	60	90	4	23
Peanut Butter 'N Chocolate	330	22	60%	10	50	170	6	29
Pink Bubblegum	270	14	47%	9	55	75	3	34
Pistachio-Almond	300	21	63%	10	55	80	6	23
Pralines 'N Cream	280	15	48%	8	50	135	3	33
Quarterback Crunch	290	17	53%	12	50	135	3	32
Reeses Peanut Butter	310	19	55%	11	55	125	5	30
Rocky Road	300	17	51%	9	50	105	5	34
Vanilla: Regular Scoop	250	16	52%	10	50	115	4	24
Small Scoop	160	10	58%	6	50	40	2	15
Very Berry Strawberry	220	10	41%	7	30	95	3	30
World Class Chocolate	280	16	51%	9	55	105	4	32
Lowfat Icecream: Regular Scoop								
Espresso 'N Cream	180	6	30%	2	11	135	6	39
No Sugar Added Icecream: Average	160	4	23%	3	10	110	6	27
Ices, Sherbets, Sorbets: Regular Scoop								
Ices: Daiquiri	130	0	0%	0	0	20	0	33
Sherbets: Rainbow/Orange	160	2	14%	1	5	50	1	34
Sorbets: Average all flavors	115	0	0%	0	0	10	0	29
Lowfat Yogurt (Hard): Regular Scoop								
Maui Brownie Madness	250	9	33%	3.5	20	130	4	38
Lowfat Yogurt (Soft Serve): Small Scoop								
Nonfat Frozen Yogurt	190	0.5	3%	0	5	120	7	39
Truly Free Yogurt, Cafe Mocha	140	0.5	4%	0	5	130	7	27
Shakes, Smoothies, Blasts: Regular (16 fl.oz)								
Shakes: Chocolate Icecream	750	43	52%	21	120	300	10	80
Vanilla Icecream	630	35	50%	22	170	220	10	69
Smoothies: Average all flavors	320	1	3%	0	5	160	7	70
Blasts: Cappuccino w/whipped crm	340	16	43%	10	70	120	6	44
Cones: Sugar Cone	60	3	45%	0	0	50	1	7
Cake Cone	25	0.5	18%	0	0	55	1	4
Waffle Cone: Large	120	1.5	11%	0	0	55	0	14
Fresh Baked	145	2	12%	0.5	13	5	2	30

Big Boy®

	Cal	Fat	%Fc	S.Fat	Chol	Sod	Pro	Carb
Sandwiches: Turkey	225	5	20%	2	75	835	22	24
Chicken w. Mozzarella	405	13	29%	6	76	420	42	26
Dinners: (w. Bread; No Dressing)								
Cajun & Salad	350	13	33%	4	65	610	38	20
Chicken Breast: w. Salad	350	13	33%	3	65	340	38	20
Chicken & Veg. Stir-fry (no bread)	560	14	23%	4	68	750	43	68
Fish: Cod Baked; Dijon, Salad	430	18	38%	4	68	570	44	21
Cod, Cajun, Salad	365	12	30%	4	68	460	43	20
Spaghetti Marinara & Salad	450	6	12%	3	8	760	15	87
Salad: Chicken Breast, Dijon	390	11	25%	2	65	415	42	31
Desserts: 'No-No' frozen dessert	75	0	0%	0	0	35	2	17
Yogurt, frozen, regular	70	0	0%	0	0	30	2	16
Shake	185	0	0%	0	2	130	8	36

Blimpie®

	Cal	Fat	%Fc	S.Fat	Chol	Sod	Pro	Carb
Cold Subs: Per 6" Sub on White								
Blimpie Best	410	13	29%	5	50	1480	29	47
Cheese Trio	490	23	42%	12	55	1120	25	48
Club Sub	370	11	26%	5	20	1180	23	48
Ham & Swiss	410	14	30%	7	50	1040	25	46
Ham, Salami & Provolone	480	20	37%	8	55	1370	24	49
Roast Beef	400	7	16%	3	65	1380	37	47
Tuna Sub	650	45	62%	6	55	860	18	49
Turkey Sub	330	7	19%	1.5	0	1190	19	48
Hot Subs: Grilled Chicken	400	9	20%	2	30	950	28	52
Grille Max	415	6	13%	1	5	820	18	72
Italian Meatball	500	22	40%	8	25	970	23	52
Mexi/Veggie Max	405	6	13%	1	0	1080	25	65
Roast Turkey Cordon Bleu	420	14	30%	6	60	1180	29	43
Steak & Cheese	550	26	43%	4	70	1080	27	51
Dressings: Fat Free Italian	20	0	0%	0	0	670	0	5
Blimpie Dressing, 1 fl. oz	120	8	60%	1	0	570	1	16
Blimpie Special Sub, 3/4 fl.oz	70	7	90%	1	0	0	0	2
Wraps: Zesty Italian	530	22	37%	7	45	1850	24	59
Chicken Caesar; Sth Western	610	31	46%	6	35	1770	26	56
Salads: Chef	150	6	36%	3	40	600	17	8
Coleslaw, 1/2 cup	180	13	65%	2	<5	230	1	13
Potato Salad, 2/3 cup	270	19	63%	3	10	560	2	19
Turkey Salad	90	0.5	0.1%	0	25	580	15	8
Soup: Chicken Noodle, 1 cup	140	3	19%	1	30	1190	8	20
Cookies: Oatmeal Raisin	190	8	38%	2	15	200	3	27
Donuts: 2.6 oz each	340	22	59%	6	0	340	5	28
Fudge Brownie: 1 brownie	245	11	40%	6	20	170	2.5	34
Muffin: Banana Nut	460	23	44%	3	55	440	8	55

Extra Listings: See www.CalorieKing.com

Menu Items	Cal	Fat	%FC	S.Fat	Chol	Sod	Pro	Carb
Biscuits, plain	380	18	43%	0	0	1300	8	60
Chicken & Noodles Entree	335	20	54%	4	67	915	21	18
Chicken Salad Platter w/fruit	600	39	59%	6	45	810	25	43
Chicken Stir-Fry	790	6	7%	1	70	2590	43	142
Hamburger plus bun	565	34	54%	13	126	370	38	23
Home Fries	225	11	44%	1	0	5	3	30
Pot Roast Sandwich	1155	46	36%	16	140	1655	57	125
Sausage Gravy	445	33	67%	18	30	1685	14	26
Sausage Patty	170	15	79%	6	20	355	9	0
Vegetable Stir-Fry	620	2.5	4%	0	0	2350	15	134
Wildfire Chicken Salad w/dressing	1660	98	53%	5	120	2530	58	125

Chicken	Cal	Fat	%FC	S.Fat	Chol	Sod	Pro	Carb
Breast	285	14	46%	na	65	530	26	12
Gizzards	385	20	47%	na	90	795	24	26
Leg	285	16	50%	na	50	540	26	9
Livers	340	19	50%	na	145	705	23	20
Thigh	355	24	61%	na	65	575	21	13
Wing	385	25	58%	na	80	655	23	17
Pasta								
Fettuccine Alfredo	1505	65	39%	na	50	3020	56	172
Meatballs	80	6	68%	na	20	230	5	2
Mostaccioli/Spaghetti: w. Meat Sce	835	15	16%	2	15	900	26	144
w/out Meat Sauce	790	10	11%	1	0	840	24	146
Ravioli: w. Meat Sauce	865	20	21%	na	17	935	30	138
w/out Meat Sauce	820	15	17%	na	0	880	27	139
Other Items								
Breadsticks	200	4	20%	na	11	215	5.5	36
Cheezy Potatoes	190	11	53%	6	20	580	6.5	18
Cole Slaw	130	10	65%	na	5	210	2	10
Corn Fritters	415	25	54%	na	4.5	550	5	42
Corn On The Cob	130	3	21%	na	1	25	3	22
French Fries	505	22	39%	na	1	235	5	44
Italian Sausage	105	10	86%	na	20	285	4	0
Liquid Margarine	100	11	99%	2	0	110	0	0
Mushrooms	290	16	50%	na	1	670	6	30
Potato Salad	95	4	38%	na	10	640	2	13
Sara Lee Chocolate Fudge Brownies	170	8	42%	2	5	125	2	22
Shrimp	275	10	32%	na	30	775	13	34
Sliced Roast Beef	50	2	36%	na	20	70	7	0

**For extra listings of Fast-Food Restaurants ~
Refer to www.CalorieKing.com**

Bojangles®

	Cal	Fat	%Fc	S.Fat	Chol	Sod	Pro	Carb
Cajun Spiced Chicken								
Breast	280	17	55%	3	75	565	18	12
Leg	265	16	55%	3	96	530	19	11
Thigh	310	15	44%	5	67	465	23	11
Wing	355	25	63%	5	94	630	21	11
Cajun Roast Chicken								
Breast, skin free	145	5	31%	1	84	560	24	0
Leg, skin free	160	8	45%	2	125	565	23	0
Thigh, skin free	215	15	63%	3	95	430	20	0
Wing, skin free	230	15	58%	3	117	615	22	3
Southern Style Chicken								
Breast	260	16	55%	3	76	700	16	12
Leg	255	15	53%	4	94	445	19	11
Thigh	310	21	61%	5	78	630	16	14
Wing	335	21	56%	5	86	685	17	19
Sandwiches/Snacks								
Buffalo Bites	180	5	25%	2	105	720	27	5
Cajun Filet: no Mayo	335	11	29%	5	45	400	22	41
w. Mayo	435	22	45%	7	55	505	22	41
Cajun Steak Sandwich	435	26	54%	8	55	985	18	39
Chicken Supremes	335	16	43%	6	58	630	21	26
Grilled Filet, no mayo	235	5	19%	3	51	540	23	25
w. Mayo	335	16	43%	5	61	645	23	25
Biscuit Sandwiches								
Bacon	290	17	53%	5	10	810	8	29
Bacon, Egg & Cheese	550	42	69%	14	160	1250	17	27
Biscuit (plain)	245	12	44%	3	2	665	4	29
Cajun Filet	455	21	42%	6	41	950	20	46
Country Ham	270	15	50%	4	20	1010	9	26
Egg	400	30	68%	6	120	630	8	26
Sausage	350	23	59%	7	20	810	9	26
Smoked Sausage	380	26	62%	9	20	940	10	27
Steak	650	49	68%	13	34	1130	14	37
Fixins'								
Bo Rounds	235	11	42%	4	13	330	3	31
Cajun Pintos	110	0	0%	0	0	480	6	18
Corn on the Cob	140	2	13%	0	0	20	5	34
Dirty Rice	165	6	33%	2	10	760	5	24
Green Beans	25	0	0%	0	0	710	0	5
Macaroni & Cheese	200	14	64%	5	26	420	7	12
Marinated Cole Slaw	135	3	20%	0	0	455	1	26
Multi-Grain Roll	150	3	18%	0	0	210	6	26
Potatoes, no Gravy	80	1	11%	0	0	380	2	16
Seasoned Fries	345	19	50%	5	13	480	5	39
Sweet Biscuits: Apple Cinnamon	330	13	35%	4	0	540	4	48
Bo Berry™	220	10	41%	3	0	410	3	29
Cinnamon	320	18	51%	4	0	560	4	37

	Cal	Fat	%Fc	S.Fat	Chol	Sod	Pro	Carb
Entrees								
1/4 Chicken: White meat w. skin, wing	280	12	39%	3.5	135	510	40	2
No skin or wing	170	4	21%	1	85	480	33	2
1/4 Chicken: Dark meat w. skin	320	21	59%	6	155	500	30	2
No skin	190	10	47%	3	115	440	22	1
1/2 Chicken w. skin	590	33	50%	10	280	1010	70	4
Chicken Pot Pie, 1 pie	750	46	55%	14	110	1530	26	57
Honey Glazed Ham (lean), 5 oz	210	8	34%	3	75	1460	24	10
Meat Loaf	290	17	53%	8	70	590	20	15
Meat Loaf & Brown Gravy	340	21	55%	8	70	870	21	18
Meat Loaf & Chunky Tom Sauce	310	17	49%	8	70	1010	21	21
Turkey: Breast, no skin	170	1	5%	0.5	100	850	36	1
w. Stuffing & Gravy	600	18	27%	3.5	75	2150	35	67
Soup								
Chicken Noodle, 6 oz	100	4.5	40%	1.5	30	500	6	8
Chicken Tortilla, 6 oz	170	8	42%	2.5	25	1060	8	18
Turkey Tortilla, 6 oz	160	7	39%	2	20	1090	9	18
Salads:								
Caesar Side Salad, 4 oz	200	17	77%	5	15	450	7	7
Caesar Entree, 11 oz	670	57	76%	11	40	1480	18	24
no dressing, 8 oz	230	12	47%	6	20	500	16	14
Chicken Caesar, 15 oz	810	60	66%	12	105	1840	43	25
Old Fashioned Potato Salad, 3/4 cup	200	12	54%	2	15	450	3	22
Sandwiches								
Chicken Salad	680	30	40%	5	120	1360	39	63
Chicken w. Cheese & Sauce	630	28	40%	8	90	930	37	61
No Cheese or Sauce	390	5	11%	1	55	810	31	60
Ham w. Cheese & Sauce	650	31	43%	9	85	1730	31	67
No Cheese or Sauce	410	8	17%	2.5	45	1390	25	65
Meat Loaf w. Cheese	690	27	35%	12	90	1480	36	83
Open Face	730	36	44%	14	95	2180	29	74
Turkey: Bacon Club	780	38	44%	14	145	1800	47	64
Open-Faced	720	20	25%	7	105	2850	41	93
Turkey w. Cheese & Sauce	620	25	36%	7	110	1300	39	64
No Cheese or Sauce	390	3.5	8%	0.5	60	1030	33	61
Side Dishes								
Corn, 3/4 cup	180	4	20%	0.5	0	170	5	30
Hot Cinnamon Apples, 3/4 cup	250	4.5	16%	0.5	0	45	0	56
Macaroni & Cheese, 3/4 cup	280	11	35%	6	30	890	13	33
Mash Potatoes & Gravy, 3/4 cup	230	9	35%	5	25	780	4	32
Rice Pilaf, 2/3 cup	180	5	25%	1	0	600	5	32
Savory Stuffing, 3/4 cup	310	12	35%	2	0	1140	6	44
Creamed Spinach, 3/4 cup	260	20	69%	13	55	740	9	11
Baked Goods								
Brownie	310	10	29%	1	5	150	3	51
Toll House Choc Chip Cookie	390	19	44%	6	15	350	4	51
Corn Bread, 1 loaf	200	6	27%	1.5	25	390	3	33

Burger King®

	Cal	Fat	%Fc	S.Fat	Chol	Sod	Pro	Car
Burgers:								
Whopper® Sandwich	680	39	51%	12	80	940	29	53
without Mayonnaise	530	22	37%	9	70	840	29	53
Whopper® w. Cheese Sandwich	780	47	54%	17	105	1390	34	55
without Mayonnaise	620	30	43%	14	90	1280	33	54
Double Whopper® Sandwich	920	57	56%	20	150	1020	48	53
without Mayonnaise	760	40	47%	17	135	920	48	53
Double Whopper® w. Cheese	1020	65	57%	25	170	1460	53	55
without Mayonnaise	860	48	50%	23	160	1350	53	54
Whopper JR® Sandwich	410	23	50%	7	50	520	18	32
without Mayonnaise	330	14	38%	6	45	470	18	32
Whopper JR® w. Cheese Sandwich	460	27	53%	10	6	740	21	33
without Mayonnaise	370	18	44%	9	55	680	21	30
Bull's-Eye® BBQ Deluxe Sandwich	400	23	51%	7	50	420	18	30
without Mayonnaise	310	14	41%	7	45	370	17	30
Hamburger	340	14	37%	6	45	530	18	30
Double Hamburger	480	26	48%	11	85	580	31	30
Cheeseburger	370	18	44%	9	55	750	22	31
Double Cheeseburger	570	34	54%	17	110	1020	35	32
Bacon Cheeseburger	410	21	46%	10	65	900	25	31
Bacon Double Cheeseburger	610	37	55%	18	120	1170	38	32
Chicken & Fish Sandwiches								
BK Big Fish® Sandwich	710	38	48%	14	50	1200	24	67
BK Broiler® Chicken Sandwich	550	25	41%	5	105	1110	30	52
without Mayonnaise	390	8	18%	2	90	1010	29	51
Chicken Sandwich	660	39	53%	8	70	1330	25	53
without Mayonnaise	460	17	33%	5	55	1190	25	54
Chicken Club Sandwich	740	44	53%	10	85	1530	30	55
without Mayonnaise	530	21	36%	6	65	1390	30	54
Chicken Tenders® Sandwich	450	27	54%	5	30	680	14	37
without Mayonnaise	290	10	31%	3	20	570	14	36
Chicken Tenders®: 4 pieces	170	9	47%	3	25	420	11	10
5 pieces	220	12	49%	3	30	530	14	13
6 pieces	250	14	50%	4	35	630	16	15
8 pieces	340	19	50%	5	50	840	22	20
Dipping Sauces (1 oz): Barbecue	35	0	0%	0	0	400	0	9
Honey Flavored	90	0	0%	0	0	0	0	23
Honey Mustard	90	6	60%	1	10	150	0	9
Ranch	120	13	97%	2	5	85	0	2
Sweet & Sour	40	0	0%	0	0	65	0	10
French Fries (Salted): Small, 2.6 oz	230	11	43%	3	0	630	3	29
Medium, 4 oz	360	18	45%	5	0	690	4	46
Large, 5.6 oz	500	25	45%	7	0	940	6	63
King Size, 7 oz	600	30	45%	8	0	1140	7	76
Onion Rings: Child's, 3.2 oz	320	16	45%	4	0	460	4	40
Medium, 4 oz	360	18	45%	5	0	690	4	46
King Size, 5.6 oz	550	27	44%	7	0	800	8	70

Sides/Condiments:	Cal	Fat	%FC	S.Fat	Chol	Sod	Pro	Carb
Ketchup, 1/2 oz	15	0	0%	0	0	180	0	4
American Cheese, 2 slices, 25g	100	8	72%	5	20	440	5	1
Bacon, 3 pieces, 8g	40	3	60%	1	10	150	3	0
Bull's Eye® BBQ Sauce, 1/2 oz	20	0	0%	0	0	130	0	5
Land O'Lakes Whipped Blend, 5g	25	3.5	97%	1	0	30	0	0
Jalapeno Poppers®, 4 pces	230	13	50%	5	20	790	7	22
Mozzarella Sticks, 4 pieces	290	16	49%	6	20	670	12	25
Breakfast: Biscuit, 3 oz	300	15	45%	3.5	0	830	6	35
Biscuit w. Egg	390	22	50%	5	150	1020	11	37
Biscuit w. Sausage	510	35	61%	10	30	1190	13	35
Biscuit w. Sausage, Egg, Cheese	650	46	63%	14	190	1600	20	38
Croissan'wich®: w. Sausage/Cheese	410	29	63%	11	40	830	14	24
w. Sausage/Egg/Cheese	500	36	65%	13	190	1020	19	26
French Toast Sticks (5), 4 oz	390	20	46%	4.5	0	440	6	46
Hash Brown Rounds: Small, 2.6 oz	240	15	56%	4	0	450	2	23
Large, 4.5 oz	390	25	57%	7	0	760	3	38
Mini-Minis: 4 Rolls w/out Icing	440	23	47%	6	25	710	6	51
Vanilla Icing only, 1 oz	110	3	25%	1	0	40	0	20
Grape/Strawberry Jam	30	0	0%	0	0	0	0	7
Desserts: Dutch Apple Pie, 4 oz	340	14	37%	3	0	470	2	52
Hershey's® Sundae Pie, 2.8 oz	310	18	52%	13	10	135	3	33
Beverages: Sprite, medium	220	0	0%	0	0	na	0	55
Coca-Cola®, medium	230	0	0%	0	0	na	0	56
Tropicana® Orange Juice, 10 fl.oz	140	0	0%	0	0	2	0	33
Reduced Fat Milk, 2% Fat, 8 fl.oz	130	5	35%	3	20	120	8	12
Chocolate Shake: Small, 10.7 oz	340	6	16%	4	25	210	10	62
Small, syrup added	400	6	14%	4	20	360	10	77
Medium, 14 oz	440	6	16%	4	35	270	13	80
Medium, syrup added	500	8	14%	5	25	440	13	95
Strawberry Shake: Med., syrup added	500	7	13%	5	25	350	12	95
Small, syrup added	390	6	14%	4	20	270	9	76
Vanilla Shake: Medium, 14 oz	430	8	17%	5	25	340	12	79
Small, 10.7 oz	330	6	16%	4	20	260	9	61

Carvel® Icecream

Soft Serving Icecream	Cal	Fat	%FC	S.Fat	Chol	Sod	Pro	Carb
Chocolate: Regular	420	22	47%	13	55	220	9	48
Vanilla: Regular	440	22	45%	13	90	240	11	46
No Sugar Added: Regular	285	6.5	20%	4.5	33	190	11	55
Large	365	8.5	21%	5.5	42	240	14	70
No Fat (average all flavors): Regular	265	0	0%	0	0	100	6	58
Sherbet, all flavors: Regular	310	2	5%	1	11	100	4.5	68
Blue Ribbon Cakes: Average, 4 oz	220	11	45%	6	25	125	4	27
Flying Saucers: Chocolate; Vanilla	240	10	37%	5	30	180	5	33
I' Love/Piece of Cake: 4 oz	260	13	45%	8	30	140	5	31
Sheet Cake; Small Round: 4 oz	210	11	47%	7	25	120	4	25

Captain D's® Seafood

	Cal	Fat	%Fc	S.Fat	Chol	Sod	Pro	Car
Platters								
Broiled Shrimp	720	8	10%	1	155	1760	32	131
Broiled Chicken	800	10	11%	2	82	1650	46	131
Broiled Fish	735	7	9%	1	49	1645	36	131
Broiled Fish & Chicken	775	10	12%	1	66	1650	41	131
Lunches								
Broiled Shrimp	420	7	15%	1	155	1725	25	64
Broiled Chicken	505	9	16%	2	82	1615	40	65
Broiled Fish	435	7	14%	1	49	1610	28	65
Broiled Fish & Chicken	480	8	15%	1	66	1610	34	68
Stuffed Crab	95	7	69%	na	na	250	8	1
Sandwiches								
Broiled Chicken	450	19	38%	na	105	860	40	29
Side Items								
Baked Potato	280	0	0%	0	0	20	6	64
Breadstick	115	4	32%	0	0	210	3	16
Cole Slaw	165	12	64%	na	16	245	3	12
Corn on the Cob	250	2	8%	na	0	15	8	60
Cheese, 1 oz	55	4.5	75%	na	14	205	3	0.5
Crackers (4)	50	1	18%	na	3	145	1.5	8
Cracklins, 1 oz	220	17	70%	na	0	740	1.5	16
French Fries	300	10	30%	na	0	150	3	50
Fried Okra	300	16	48%	na	0	445	7	34
Green Beans, seasoned	45	2	39%	na	4	750	2.5	5
Hushpuppy	125	4	29%	na	0	465	2.5	20
Rice	125	0	0%	0	0	10	3	28
Salad	85	0	0%	0	0	na	0	21
Vegetable Medley	35	1	25%	0	0	115	1	5
White Beans	125	0.5	4%	na	2	100	8	22
Salad Dressings: Per Serving								
Blue Cheese	105	12	99%	na	14	100	0.5	0.5
French	110	11	85%	na	7	185	0	4
Light Italian	15	0.5	28%	0	0	na	0	3
Ranch	90	10	98%	na	15	230	<1	0.5
Sour Cream, Imitation	30	3	93%	3	0	na	0	0.5
Sauces: Cocktail, 1 oz	35	0.5	11%	na	0	250	0.5	7
Sweet & Sour	50	0	0%	0	0	5	0	13
Tartar	75	7	84%	na	10	160	<1	3
Desserts								
Carrot Cake	435	23	47%	na	32	415	8	49
Cheesecake	420	31	66%	na	141	480	7	30
Chocolate Cake	305	10	30%	na	20	260	4	49
Pecan Pie	460	20	39%	na	4	375	5	64

	Cal	Fat	%Fc	S.Fat	Chol	Sod	Pro	Carb
Breakfast								
Bacon, 2 Strips	45	4	80%	1.5	10	150	3	0
Breakfast Burrito	550	32	52%	11	495	980	29	36
Breakfast Quesadilla	370	17	41%	5	240	910	16	38
English Muffin w. Margarine	210	9	38%	2	0	300	5	28
French Toast Dips, no Syrup	370	20	48%	2.5	0	430	6	42
Sausage, 1 Patty	190	18	85%	6	40	480	7	2
Scrambled Eggs	180	14	70%	3	455	110	13	1
Sunrise Sandwich, no Bacon/Sausage	360	21	30%	8	245	470	13	28
Sandwiches								
Famous Star® Hamburger	590	32	49%	9	70	910	24	50
Super Star® Hamburger	790	47	54%	15	130	980	41	51
Hamburger	280	9	29%	3.5	35	480	14	36
Western Bacon Cheeseburger®	660	30	41%	12	85	1410	31	64
Double Western Bacon Cheeseburger®	920	50	49%	21	155	1770	51	65
Charbroiled BBQ Chicken Sandwich™	290	3.5	11%	1	60	840	25	41
Charbroiled Chicken Club Sandwich™	470	23	44%	7	95	1110	31	37
Charbroiled Santa Fe Chicken S'wich™	540	31	52%	8	95	1210	28	37
Ranch Crispy Chicken Sandwich	660	31	42%	7	70	1180	24	71
Bacon Swiss Crispy Chicken S'wich	760	38	45%	11	90	1550	31	72
Charbroiled Sirloin Steak Sandwich	550	24	39%	4.5	80	1080	30	52
Carl's Catch Fish Sandwich™	530	28	47%	7	80	1030	18	55
American Cheese, large	60	5	75%	3.5	15	260	3	1
Swiss-style Cheese	50	4	72%	2.5	15	230	4	0
Great Stuff Potatoes								
Plain, no margarine	290	0	0%	0	0	20	6	68
Bacon & Cheese	640	29	41%	9	40	1660	21	75
Broccoli & Cheese	530	21	35%	5	15	940	11	76
Sour Cream & Chives	430	14	29%	4	10	180	7	70
Bakery/Desserts: Per Serving								
Blueberry Muffin	340	14	37%	2	40	340	5	49
Bran Raisin Muffin	370	14	34%	2	45	410	6	61
Cheese Danish	400	23	52%	6	15	390	5	49
Chocolate Cake	300	12	36%	3	30	350	3	48
Chocolate Chip Cookie	350	18	46%	7	20	330	3	46
Strawberry Swirl Cheesecake	290	17	53%	9	55	230	6	30
Side Orders: Per Serving								
Breadstick, 1	35	0.5	12%	0	0	60	1	7
Chicken Stars, 6 pieces	260	16	55%	4.5	40	480	13	14
CrissCut Fries®, 5 oz	410	24	53%	5	0	950	5	43
French Fries, small, 3 oz	290	14	43%	3	0	180	5	37
Hash Brown Nuggets, 4 oz	330	21	57%	4.5	0	470	3	32
Onion Rings, 5 oz	430	22	46%	5	0	700	7	53
Zucchini, 5 oz	320	19	53%	5	0	860	6	31
Salads: Per Serving (no dressing)								
Charbroiled Chicken Salad-to-Go™	200	7	31%	3	75	440	25	12
Garden Salad-to-Go™	50	2.5	50%	1.5	5	60	3	4

Chick-Fil-A®

	Cal	Fat	%FC	S.Fat	Chol	Sod	Pro	Car
Chick-Fil-A Sandwiches								
Chicken	290	10	31%	2	50	870	24	30
Chicken Deluxe	300	10	30%	2	50	870	25	30
Chicken (no bun/pickles)	160	8	45%	2	45	690	20	1
Chargrilled Chicken:	280	3	10%	1	40	640	27	36
Deluxe	290	3	9%	1	40	640	28	38
No bun, no pickles	130	3	21%	1	30	630	27	0
Club (no dressing)	390	12	28%	5	70	980	33	38
Chicken Salad (on whole wheat)	320	5	14%	2	10	810	25	42
Soup: Hearty Breast of Chicken	110	0	0%	0	45	760	16	10
Strips, Nuggets								
Chick-n-Strips (4-count)	230	8	31%	2	20	380	30	10
Nuggets (8-pack)	290	14	43%	3	60	770	28	12
Salads								
Chick-n-Strips Salad	290	10	31%	2	20	430	32	20
Chargrilled Chicken Garden	170	3	16%	1	25	650	26	10
Chicken Salad Plate	290	5	16%	0	35	570	20	40

Chili's®

	Cal	Fat	%FC	S.Fat	Chol	Sod	Pro	Car
Guiltless Grill								
Chicken Pita	600	9	14%	3	45	3010	39	90
Chicken Platter	565	9	14%	3	60	3285	38	83
Chicken Salad w. Dressing	270	5	17%	1	45	1475	29	27
Chicken Sandwich	525	8	14%	2	45	2925	44	70
Veggie Pasta	680	13	17%	4	125	760	34	102
w. Chicken	785	15	17%	5	165	1195	53	106

Church's Fried Chicken®

	Cal	Fat	%FC	S.Fat	Chol	Sod	Pro	Car
Fried Chicken								
Breast	200	12	54%	3	65	510	19	4
Leg	140	9	58%	2	45	160	13	2
Thigh	230	16	63%	4	80	520	16	5
Wing	250	16	58%	4	60	540	19	8
Tender Strip	80	4	45%	1	15	140	6	5
Side Items								
Apple Pie	280	12	39%	3	5	340	2	41
Biscuit	250	16	58%	3	5	640	2	26
Cajun Rice	130	7	48%	2	5	260	1	16
Cole Slaw	92	6	59%	1	0	230	4	8
Corn on the Cob	140	3	19%	1	0	15	4.5	24
French Fries	210	11	47%	3	0	60	3	29
Okra	210	16	69%	3	0	520	3	19
Potatoes & Gravy	90	3	30%	1	0	520	1	14

Chuck E. Cheese®

	Cal	Fat	%Fc	S.Fat	Chol	Sod	Pro	Carb
Appetizers								
Blended Pizza Sauce	35	0	0%	0	0	380	1	7
Buffalo Wings	220	15	61%	3.5	110	560	20	1
Lamb Wesson French Fries, cooked	285	10	32%	2.5	0	435	5	43
Sargento Mozzarella Sticks	380	24	57%	7	40	380	13	26
Sandwiches								
Grilled Chicken Sub	740	39	47%	12	110	1080	41	57
Ham & Cheese	770	41	48%	9	85	1490	39	60
Hot Dog	430	29	61%	13	50	710	15	27
Italian Sub	770	47	55%	16	80	1560	35	52
Pizza								
BQ Chicken, medium	410	13	29%	7	50	640	22	51
Beef, medium	410	17	37%	9	35	605	18	43
Cheese, medium	330	10	27%	6	20	460	15	43
Pepperoni, medium	370	14	34%	7	30	620	17	43
Sausage, medium	385	15	35%	8	30	660	18	44
Salad Dressings								
Kraft Catalina	35	0	0%	0	0	320	0	8
F Bleu Cheese	170	18	95%	3	15	120	1	1
F Lite Ranch	80	8	90%	1	5	240	1	2
F Olive Oil & Vinegar	90	9	90%	1	0	170	0	2
F Thousand Island	110	10	82%	2	10	170	0	4
Birthday Items								
" Chocolate Cake w/Whip Cream	210	11	48%	8	21	200	2	25
" White Cake w/Whip Cream	210	11	48%	8	25	165	2	26
Breakfast								
Kellogg's Snack Um's: Cinn. Blast	140	5	32%	1	0	210	2	24
Froot Loops; Rice Krispy, average	125	1	8%	1	0	205	2	26
CB Banana Loaf Cake	350	11	28%	4.5	30	320	5	50
CB Cinnamon Crumb Pound Cake	385	17	40%	3	38	235	4	55
Desserts								
CB Brownie	380	18	42%	4.5	20	145	4	46
CB Choc Chunk Cookie	410	19	42%	6	20	390	5	56
CB Original Krispy Treat	340	9	24%	2	0	250	3	50

CinnaMonster®

	Cal	Fat	%Fc	S.Fat	Chol	Sod	Pro	Carb
Cinnamon Roll								
Caramel Pecan	210	8	34%	4	25	585	4	30
Original	220	6	25%	3	50	220	5	25

Feedback **welcome**

Please send comments to: Allan Borushek
POB 1616, Costa Mesa CA 92628
Email: allan@calorieking.com

Cousins Subs®

	Cal	Fat	%FC	S.Fat	Chol	Sod	Pro	Car
Cold Italian 7½" Subs								
Cappocolla & Cheese/Genoa	570	35	55%	9	55	1600	32	30
Cousins Special	670	44	59%	13	70	1640	38	33
Genoa & Cheese	660	44	60%	15	75	1580	37	30
Regular	610	40	59%	12	65	1500	35	30
Cold 7½" Subs								
BLT (no mayo or cheese)	340	14	37%	5	40	1420	20	34
Club Sub (no mayo or cheese)	340	10	26%	7	110	2050	36	29
Cold Veggie (no mayo or cheese)	290	11	34%	5	10	250	21	27
Ham (no mayo or cheese)	310	9	26%	3	55	1440	30	30
Ham & Cheese	620	40	58%	6.5	90	1750	35	30
Provolone (Cheese) Sub	650	45	62%	21	80	1550	31	30
Roast Beef (no mayo or cheese)	360	8	20%	3	25	1570	41	30
Seafood with Crab	550	34	56%	11	30	1620	25	38
Tuna	750	54	65%	16	90	1400	30	32
Turkey Breast (no mayo or cheese)	320	9	25%	3	70	1980	32	30
Hot 7½" Subs								
Cheese Steak	470	17	33%	6	40	1540	33	46
Double	630	23	33%	8	55	2060	44	62
Chicken Breast (no mayo or cheese)	320	6	17%	2	10	1370	37	30
Gyro, regular	550	23	38%	8	30	1200	28	57
Hot Veggie (no mayo or cheese)	360	14	35%	6	15	320	26	33
Italian Sausage	800	56	63%	20	45	2200	44	51
Meatball & Cheese	660	41	56%	16	90	1610	42	30
Pepperoni Melt	700	46	59%	18	130	1900	41	30
Philly Cheese Steak	510	23	41%	15	45	1430	32	43
Steak (no mayo or cheese)	425	8	17%	4	40	1360	28	51
For mayonnaise add: 235 Cals; 26g Fat; 9g Sat.Fat; 30mg Cholesterol								
Mini 4" Subs: Italian Special	400	26	59%	8	40	970	22	20
Provolone (Cheese)	480	33	62%	15	59	1140	23	22
Ham (no mayo or cheese)	210	5	21%	2	35	960	20	20
Meatball & Cheese	380	23	54%	9	50	930	34	17
Seafood w. Crab	320	20	56%	6	17	940	14	22
Tuna	520	37	64%	11	62	965	21	22
Turkey Breast (no mayo or cheese)	170	4	21%	2	30	745	17	16
For mayonnaise add: 125 Cals; 14g Fat; 4.5g Sat.Fat; 16mg Cholesterol								
French Fries: Medium	400	19	43%	8	16	350	5	55
Large	525	24	41%	11	21	460	7	72
Extras: Hot Dog	275	16	52%	5	25	770	10	2
Italian/Wheat Bread, aver., half loaf	250	3	11%	1	5	450	8	46
Salads: Chef	190	8	38%	4	59	480	25	6
Garden	140	6	39%	0	0	180	15	
Italian	290	18	56%	7	56	540	26	
Seafood	175	6	31%	3	65	440	21	13
Side	80	2	23%	0	0	140	8	
Tuna	260	15	52%	4	45	480	26	
Cookies: Choc Chip; Cr'berry Walnut	210	11	48%	4	20	190	2	2

	Cal	Fat	%Fc	S.Fat	Chol	Sod	Pro	Carb
utterburgers: Bacon Deluxe	710	45	58%	17	165	1855	47	30
heese, Single	385	19	43%	7	75	1205	24	32
eluxe, Single	415	22	49%	7	75	935	24	30
ouble	460	21	42%	6	110	1155	36	32
ouble Cheese	590	33	50%	13	145	1825	43	32
ushroom & Swiss	570	33	52%	14	150	1335	43	25
ngle	320	13	36%	4	55	875	21	32
ourdough Melt	655	32	44%	13	145	1550	43	44
isconsin Swiss Melt	635	31	45%	13	145	1445	45	40
avorite Sandwiches: Chicken Filet	515	21	38%	5	55	850	25	54
hicken Tenders	465	25	49%	4	80	1040	35	28
rilled Chicken Breast	310	9	27%	3	60	1090	27	35
rilled Ham & Swiss	405	20	44%	9	80	1720	24	32
orwegian Cod Filet	605	10	14%	10	70	1230	26	52
illy Ribeye Steak	345	13	36%	7	50	1270	20	34
ork Tenderloin	530	17	29%	5	60	975	30	65
oast Beef	405	15	35%	5	80	1015	38	27
acked Turkey	315	9	27%	3	55	1500	21	33
urkey Sourdough BLT	525	20	35%	8	100	2500	34	44
arden Fresh Salads: Chef	405	20	46%	7	235	1920	34	17
rilled Chicken Caesar	410	20	44%	4	225	1285	37	21
rilled Chicken Cashew	525	33	57%	8	80	1370	37	28
aco: w. Shell	1130	89	71%	31	80	1645	28	59
w/out Shell	490	36	67%	20	80	1385	22	24
ossed Salad, small	105	6	50%	2	15	395	4	7
eafood & Chicken: Shrimp Boat	520	27	47%	3	90	1485	50	50
eckerBasket Chicken	1050	64	55%	17	355	1970	40	40
orwegian Cod	510	27	48%	6	75	1170	37	37
ies, Rings & Things: Dinner Roll	90	1	10%	0	0	170	3	16
heese Curds	600	40	60%	17	100	na	25	35
hili Cheddar Fries	620	32	47%	16	45	na	15	64
ole Slaw, small	210	15	66%	2.5	25	na	1	16
ench Fries, regular	355	15	37%	7	0	395	4	48
ashed Potatoes & Gravy, small	100	2.5	22%	0.5	2	300	2.5	17
nion Rings	395	23	54%	4	0	805	6	40
ozen Custard: Cake Cone, Single	340	19	50%	11	115	100	6	37
Dish, Single	310	18	53%	11	115	85	6	31
Waffle Cone, Single	410	19	42%	11	115	165	6	52
esserts: Lemon Ice	210	0	0%	0	0	5	6	52
ramel Cashew, small	575	33	51%	14	115	280	11	60
t Fudge Sundae, small	405	21	48%	14	115	130	7	47
d Fashioned Soda, Chocolate	445	19	38%	11	115	195	6	64
spberry Cooler	480	0	0%	0	0	10	0.5	116
ot Beer Float	465	16	32%	10	100	140	5	77
oothie, Raspberry	615	17	25%	10	105	90	6	107
oothie, Vanilla	555	17	28%	10	105	85	6	92
rtle, small	625	42	60%	15	115	255	8	54

Dairy Queen® Brazier®

	Cal	Fat	%Fc	S.Fat	Chol	Sod	Pro	Ca
Burgers/Sandwiches								
Chicken Breast Fillet Sandwich	430	20	42%	4	55	760	24	37
Chili 'n' Cheese Dog	330	21	57%	9	45	1090	14	22
DQ® Homestyle: Hamburger	290	12	37%	5	45	630	17	29
Cheeseburger	340	17	45%	8	55	850	20	29
Double Cheeseburger	540	31	52%	16	115	1130	35	30
Bacon Double Cheeseburger	610	36	53%	18	130	1380	41	31
Ultimate Burger	670	43	58%	19	135	1210	40	29
Grilled Chicken Sandwich	310	10	29%	2.5	50	1040	24	30
Hot Dog, regular	240	14	53%	5	25	730	9	19
Sides: Chkn Strip Basket w. Gravy	1000	50	45%	13	55	2510	35	102
Onion Rings	320	16	45%	4	0	180	5	39
The Great Steakmelt™ Basket	770	38	44%	13	75	2290	32	7
French Fries: Medium	440	23	47%	4.5	0	1110	5	5
Icecream Cones/Soft Serve								
DQ® Vanilla Soft Serve, 1/2 cup	140	4.5	29%	3	15	70	3	2
DQ® Choc. Soft Serve, 1/2 cup	150	5	30%	3.5	15	75	4	2
Vanilla Cone, medium	330	9	25%	6	30	160	8	5
Chocolate Cone, medium	340	11	27%	7	30	160	8	5
Dipped Cone, medium	490	24	44%	13	30	190	8	5
Novelties: Buster Bar®	450	28	56%	12	15	280	10	4
Chocolate Dilly® Bar	210	13	56%	7	10	75	3	2
DQ® Fudge Bar, No Sugar Added	50	0	0%	0	0	70	4	1
DQ® Sandwich	200	6	27%	3	10	140	4	3
DQ® Vanilla Orange Bar, NAS	60	0	0%	0	0	40	2	1
Lemon DQ Freez'r®, 1/2 cup	80	0	0%	0	0	10	0	2
Starkiss®	80	0	0%	0	0	10	0	2
Blizzards®								
Choc. Chip Cookie Dough, medium	950	36	34%	19	75	660	17	14
Choc. Sandwich Cookie, medium	640	23	32%	11	45	500	12	9
Chocolate Sundae, medium	400	10	23%	6	30	210	8	7
DQ® Treatza Cake® 1/8 cake:								
DQ® Frozen 8" Round Cake	370	13	32%	8	25	280	7	5
DQ® Treatza Pizza™, 1/8 pizza:								
Heath® DQ	180	7	35%	3.5	5	160	3	2
M & M's® DQ	190	7	33%	4	5	160	3	2
Royal Treats®: Banana Split	510	12	21%	8	30	180	8	9
Peanut Buster® Parfait	730	31	38%	17	35	400	16	9
Strawberry Shortcake	430	14	29%	9	60	360	7	7
Frozen Yogurt								
Cup of Yogurt, medium	230	0.5	2%	0	5	150	8	4
DQ® Nonfat Frozen Yogurt, 1/2 cup	100	0	0%	0	0	70	3	2
Heath Breeze®, medium	710	18	23%	11	20	580	15	12
Strawberry Breeze®, medium	460	1	31%	1	10	270	13	9
Yogurt Cone, medium	260	1	3%	0.5	5	160	9	4
Yogurt Strawberry Sundae, medium	280	0.5	2%	0	5	160	8	6
Misty® Slushes, medium	290	0	0%	0	0	30	0	

Del Taco®

	Cal	Fat	%Fc	S.Fat	Chol	Sod	Pro	Carb
Breakfast: Breakfast Burrito	250	11	40%	6	160	520	10	24
Bacon & Egg Quesadilla	450	23	46%	12	260	920	21	40
Egg & Cheese Burrito	450	24	48%	13	530	740	23	39
Macho Bacon & Egg Burrito™	1030	60	52%	20	790	1760	40	82
Steak & Egg Burrito	580	34	53%	16	560	1270	33	41
Tacos: Big Fat Chicken Taco™	340	13	34%	4	45	840	18	38
Big Fat Crispy Chicken Taco™	620	38	55%	9	60	1070	21	52
Big Fat Steak Taco™	390	19	44%	6	40	960	18	38
Big Fat Taco™	320	11	31%	5	35	680	16	39
Chicken Soft Taco	210	12	51%	4	30	520	11	16
Taco; Soft Taco	160	10	56%	4	20	150	7	11
Ultimate Taco	260	17	59%	8	50	470	14	13
Burritos: Combo Burrito™	530	22	37%	13	55	1680	28	61
Bean & Chse Red/Green Burrito, aver.	270	8	26%	5	15	1025	11	38
Chicken Works Burrito	520	23	40%	12	65	1620	26	57
Del Beef Burrito™	550	30	49%	17	90	1090	31	42
Del Classic Chicken Burrito™	560	36	58%	13	70	1100	24	41
Deluxe Combo Burrito™	570	25	39%	15	60	1700	29	64
Deluxe Del Beef Burrito™	590	33	50%	19	95	1110	32	45
Half Pound Red/Green Burrito	430	12	25%	9	20	1680	20	65
Macho Beef Burrito™	1170	62	48%	29	190	2190	60	89
Macho Combo Burrito™	1050	44	38%	21	115	2760	49	113
Spicy Chicken/Veggie Works Burrito	490	18	33%	11	25	1660	18	69
Steak Works Burrito	590	31	47%	16	70	1820	27	58
Quesadillas: Chicken	530	31	53%	21	104	1240	33	41
Regular	500	27	49%	20	75	860	23	39
Spicy Jack Chicken	570	30	47%	16	105	1300	32	40
Spicy Jack Regular	490	26	48%	17	75	920	23	38
Salads: Deluxe Chicken Salad™	730	34	42%	15	70	2360	33	75
Deluxe Taco Salad™	780	40	46%	18	80	2250	33	76
Tostada	200	9	41%	5	15	540	9	24
Burgers: Cheeseburger	330	13	35%	6	35	870	16	37
Double Del Cheeseburger™	560	35	56%	12	85	960	26	35
Del Cheeseburger™	430	25	52%	7	45	710	16	35
Nachos: Regular	360	24	60%	8	5	630	9	40
Macho Nachos®	1100	63	52%	24	55	2640	31	113
Sides: Beans 'n Cheese Cup	265	3	10%	2	5	1810	16	44
Rice Cup	140	2	13%	1	2	910	4	27
Fries: Chili Cheese, 10.5 oz	670	46	62%	15	45	880	17	50
Deluxe Chili Cheese™, 12 oz	720	49	61%	16	50	880	17	53
Large, 7 oz	490	32	59%	5	0	380	4	47
Regular, 5 oz	350	23	59%	4	0	270	3	34
Small, 3 oz	210	14	60%	2	0	160	2	20
Shakes: Chocolate, small (11.5 fl.oz)	520	12	21%	9	35	270	12	90
Vanilla; Strawb.,small, 11.5 fl.oz	420	7	15%	5	35	250	12	77
Chocolate, large, 15 fl.oz	680	16	21%	12	45	350	16	117
Vanilla; Strawb., large, 15 fl.oz	550	10	16%	6	50	320	16	97

Denny's®

	Cal	Fat	%Fc	S.Fat	Chol	Sod	Pro	Ca
Breakfast								
All American Slam	710	62	78%	20	685	1280	38	9
Cinnamon Swirl Slam	1125	78	62%	26	635	1375	38	68
Dagwood Breakfast Slam	1250	90	65%	38	800	3595	75	35
Denver Sam	1140	67	53%	19	795	3150	54	81
Farmer's Slam	1200	80	60%	24	705	3205	50	82
French Slam	1030	71	62%	20	775	1430	44	58
Grand Slam Slugger	790	46	52%	14	485	1440	32	58
Griddle Combo	830	60	65%	19	630	1020	35	40
Original Grand Slam	795	50	57%	14	460	2235	34	65
w. Syrup & Margarine	1030	60	52%	16	460	2385	34	101
Lumberjack Slam	1315	70	48%	18	480	1030	54	118
Scram Slam	740	62	75%	20	685	1295	40	14
Shamrock Slam	865	72	75%	23	515	1230	37	16
Slim Slam (no topping)	495	12	22%	3	35	1020	34	40
Breakfast Sides: Applesauce	60	0	0%	0	0	15	0	15
Bacon, 4 strips	210	18	77%	5	36	640	12	0
Bagel, 1 only	235	1	4%	0	0	495	9	40
Biscuit: Buttered	270	11	36%	4	0	790	5	40
w. Sausage Gravy	400	21	47%	6	10	1265	8	45
Cereal: Kellogg's Dry, average, 1 oz	100	0	0%	0	0	275	2	23
Country Fried Potatoes, 6 oz	515	35	61%	8	10	805	3	23
Cream Cheese, 1 oz	100	10	90%	6	30	90	2	
Egg: 1 only	120	10	75%	3	210	120	6	
Two Egg Breakfast	825	67	73%	17	540	1765	31	24
Egg Beaters (Egg Substitute)	70	5	63%	1	1	140	5	
Flour Tortillas and Salsa	290	8	0%	1.5	0	1030	6	50
Grits, 4 oz	80	0	0%	0	0	520	2	18
Ham, griller slice, 3 oz	95	3	29%	1	25	760	15	
Hashed Browns, 4 oz	220	14	57%	2	0	425	2	22
Covered, 6 oz	320	23	65%	7	30	605	9	21
Covered & Smothered, 8 oz	360	26	65%	7	30	790	9	24
Dble Covered & Smothered, 13 oz	460	26	51%	7	30	1215	12	48
Muffins: English, each	125	1	7%	0	0	200	5	24
Oatmeal (Quaker), 4 oz	100	2	18%	0	0	175	5	16
Oatmeal N' Fixins	460	6	12%	3	10	85	13	95
Sausage, 4 links	355	32	81%	2	65	945	16	
Sausage Gravy, 4 oz	125	10	71%	2	10	475	3	
Syrup: Blueberry/Strawberry, aver.	100	0	0%	0	0	35	12	2
Maple-flavored, 3 Tbsp	145	0	0%	0	0	25	0	4
Sugar-free	25	0	0%	0	0	70	0	
Toast, 1 slice dry	95	1	9%	0	0	165	3	
Toppings: Average, 3 oz	105	0	0%	0	0	15	0	24
Whipped Cream, dollop, 2 oz	25	2	78%	0	7	0	0	
Whipped Margarine, 1/2 oz	90	10	100%	2	0	120	0	
French Toast: Plain	505	24	43%	6	220	595	16	54
Cinnamon Swirl	1030	49	43%	21	280	675	23	12

	Cal	Fat	%Fc	S.Fat	Chol	Sod	Pro	Carb
melette (no extras):								
gs Benedict	695	46	60%	11	515	1720	34	34
am'n Cheddar	580	45	70%	8	670	1180	40	4
timate	585	47	72%	12	640	940	31	9
gge-Cheese	490	39	72%	13	645	535	26	10
affles: Plain	305	21	62%	3	145	200	7	23
w. Syrup & Butter	540	31	52%	5	145	345	7	59
uttermilk Hot Cakes								
Plain (3)	490	7	13%	1	0	1820	12	95
w. Syrup & Butter	725	17	21%	3	0	1965	12	130
illets:								
g Texas Chicken Fajita	1220	70	52%	19	520	1820	49	25
icken Fried Steak	1745	104	54%	28	605	2185	60	120
eat Lover's	1150	93	73%	26	460	2505	41	24
eak & Eggs (no extras)								
icken Fried Steak	430	36	75%	12	440	860	22	10
oons Over My Hammy	920	59	58%	24	580	2810	54	42
rk Chop	675	47	63%	13	570	1580	55	6
loin Steak	620	49	71%	18	570	630	43	1
noked Moons	840	53	57%	18	545	2260	47	42
Bone Steak	990	77	70%	31	655	1005	73	1
up								
icken Noodle	60	2	30%	0	10	640	2	8
ili w. Cheese topping	400	19	42%	8	55	1040	25	21
am Chowder	215	11	46%	9	5	905	5	22
eam of Broccoli	195	12	56%	9	0	320	2	15
eam of Potato	220	12	49%	9	0	760	4	23
lit Pea	145	5	31%	2	5	320	8	18
getable Beef	80	1	11%	1	5	320	6	11
ndwiches (no fries/sides)								
T	635	46	65%	8	55	1115	13	37
con Cheddar Burger	875	52	53%	19	165	1670	53	58
g Texas BBQ Burger	930	58	56%	24	165	2270	58	53
ffalo Chicken Burger	805	45	50%	9	75	2145	37	67
icken Burger	630	32	46%	7	80	1970	35	53
assic Burger	675	40	53%	15	105	1140	37	42
w. Cheese	840	53	57%	20	135	1595	47	43
ib Sandwich	720	38	48%	7	75	1665	32	62
uble Decker Burger	1245	80	58%	13	125	2200	55	82
rden Burger	665	33	45%	8	35	1050	18	75
rlic Mushroom Swiss Burger	870	51	53%	14	115	1530	48	58
lled Chicken	520	14	24%	3	70	1615	35	64
lled Chicken (Fit Fare®)	435	9	19%	3	80	2705	35	56
m & Swiss on Rye	495	30	54%	4	35	1535	22	34
eben	580	35	54%	6	70	2725	27	37
e Super Bird	620	32	46%	5	60	1380	35	48
rkey Breast w. Multigrain	475	26	49%	5	55	1105	28	39

	Cal	Fat	%FC	S.Fat	Chol	Sod	Pro	Ca
Salads (no dressing/bread unless indicated)								
Garden Deluxe Salad: w. Chicken Brst	265	11	38%	5	90	715	32	10
w. Buffalo Chicken Strips	515	35	61%	8	80	1200	33	26
w. Fried Chicken Strips	440	26	53%	6	75	1030	33	26
w. Salmon Fillet	340	9	24%	5	125	850	67	10
w. Turkey and Ham	320	11	31%	6	100	1705	43	12
Grilled Chicken Caesar w. Dressing	600	41	62%	10	100	1790	37	20
Side Caesar w. Dressing	360	26	65%	7	25	915	11	20
Side Garden Salad	115	4	32%	1	0	150	3	16
Dressings								
BBQ Sauce, 1.5 oz	50	1	19%	0	0	595	0	11
Blue Cheese, 1 oz	165	18	99%	3	20	205	1	
Caesar, 1 oz	135	14	95%	2	2	380	1	
French: Regular, 1 oz	105	10	85%	2	5	275	1	3
Guacamole, 1.5 oz	75	6	73%	2	0	265	1	4
Honey Mustard Fat-Free, 1 oz	40	0	0%	0	0	120	0	9
Italian Dressing: Reduced Calorie	70	8	100%	1	0	150	0	1
Marinara, 1.5 oz	50	2	38%	1	0	205	1	7
Ranch, 1 oz	100	11	98%	2	10	215	1	
Salsa, 2 oz	10	0	0%	0	0	220	0	2
Sour Cream, 1.5 oz	90	9	89%	6	20	25	1	2
Tartar, 1.5 oz	230	24	94%	3	15	185	0	5
Thousand Island, 1 oz	120	11	84%	2	15	170	0	5
Appetizers								
Buffalo Chicken Strips (5)	735	42	51%	4	95	1675	43	4.
Buffalo Wings (12)	855	54	57%	17	500	5550	92	
Chicken Strips (5)	720	33	41%	4	95	1665	47	56
Mozzarella Sticks (8)	710	41	52%	24	50	5220	36	49
Onion Rings	380	23	54%	6	5	2005	5	38
Sampler	1405	80	51%	24	75	5305	47	12
Entrees: Charleston Chicken	330	18	50%	4	65	995	25	16
Chicken Fried Steak	340	18	48%	8	25	945	16	2
Chicken Pot Pie Dinner	1065	55	46%	17	12	2915	41	10
Fried Shrimp Dinner	330	10	27%	2	135	775	17	18
Grilled Alaskan Salmon Dinner	210	4	17%	1	10	105	43	
Grilled Chicken Breast Dinner	130	4	28%	1	65	565	24	
Grilled Chicken Stir-Fry (no bread)	864	10	10%	1	65	3655	43	14
Mandarin Glazed Salmon (no bread)	615	20	29%	4	80	2035	53	5
Pot Roast Dinner w. Gravy	290	11	34%	5	85	930	42	
Roast Turkey & Stuffing w. Gravy	390	3	7%	1	115	2470	46	
Sirloin Steak Dinner	340	28	75%	8	685	345	18	
Steak & Shrimp Dinner	645	42	59%	14	150	1145	36	3
T-Bone Steak Dinner	860	65	68%	18	195	870	65	
Vegetable Stir-Fry (no bread)	430	9	19%	1	1	1755	12	7

For extra listings of Fast-Food Restaurants ~
Refer to www.CalorieKing.com

	Cal	Fat	%Fc	S.Fat	Chol	Sod	Pro	Carb
Sides								
Broccoli in Butter Sauce	50	2	36%	2	5	280	3	7
Carrots in Honey Glaze	80	3	34%	1	0	220	1	12
Corn in Butter Sauce	120	4	30%	2	5	260	3	19
Bread Stuffing, plain	100	1	9%	0	0	405	3	19
Fries: Unsalted	325	14	39%	6	0	130	5	44
Chili Cheese, 12 oz	815	44	49%	17	75	915	20	77
Seasoned	260	12	41%	3	0	555	5	35
Smothered Cheese, 9 oz	765	48	56%	17	80	875	27	69
Gravy, all types, average	15	0.5	30%	0	0	120	0	2
Green Beans w. Bacon	60	4	60%	2	5	390	1	6
Green Peas in Butter Sauce	100	2	18%	2	5	360	5	14
Grilled Mushrooms	15	0	0%	0	0	0	2	2
Potato: Baked, plain w. skin	220	0	0%	0	0	15	5	51
Mashed	105	1	9%	0	0	380	3	21
Vegetable Rice Pilaf	85	1	11%	0	0	325	2	16
Desserts								
Banana Royale	550	25	41%	15	65	185	6	80
Chocolate Layer Cake	275	12	39%	3	25	60	4	42
Hot Fudge Cake	620	30	44%	17	60	170	7	73
Lowfat Choc Chip Yogurt	110	2	16%	0.5	5	60	4	20
Rainbow Sherbet	120	1.5	11%	1	5	30	1	25
Pies, 1/6 slice: Apple	470	24	46%	6	0	470	3	64
Cheesecake, no topping	470	27	52%	13	90	280	6	48
Cherry	630	25	36%	6	0	550	3	100
Chocolate Peanut Butter	655	39	54%	19	25	320	15	64
Chocolate Silk	650	43	60%	26	165	220	10	60
Dutch Apple	440	19	39%	6	0	290	10	55
Hershey's Choc Chunks N' Chips	600	36	54%	25	10	270	6	58
Oreo® Cookies & Creme	690	30	39%	17	20	390	6	73
Pecan	600	28	42%	4	50	430	6	81
Pumpkin	235	7	27%	2	35	215	3	38
Dessert Toppings								
Blueberry, 2 oz	70	0	0%	0	0	10	0	17
Chocolate, 2 oz	320	25	71%	0	0	85	2	27
Fudge, 2 oz	200	10	45%	7	5	95	1	30
Strawberry, 2 oz	80	1	12%	0	0	10	1	17
Sundaes								
Single Scoop, no topping	190	14	67%	6	37	45	3	14
Double Scoop, no topping	375	27	65%	12	75	85	4	29
Banana Split	895	43	43%	19	80	175	15	112
Butterfinger® Hot Fudge	780	38	44%	25	71	335	10	106
Butterfinger® Blender Blaster	770	38	45%	23	108	345	13	97
Drinks								
Flavored Coffee, average	70	1	14%	1	2	5	0	15
Floats, Rootbeer/Cola	280	10	43%	6	40	110	3	47
Malted Milkshake, van./choc.	585	26	40%	16	100	280	12	82

Domino's® Pizza

	Cal	Fat	%Fc	S.Fat	Chol	Sod	Pro	Car
14" Hand Tossed Pizza: Per 2 Slices								
Cheese Pizza (Base)	515	15	27%	7	32	1080	21	75
With Topping: Beef	625	25	36%	11	53	1390	27	75
Cheddar Cheese	590	21	32%	11	50	1190	26	75
Italian Sausage & Mushroom	625	24	34%	10	54	1420	26	80
Pepperoni	615	24	35%	10	52	1445	26	75
X-tra Cheese & Pepperoni	680	29	38%	13	68	1675	30	76
Ham	550	17	28%	7	44	1375	26	75
Vegi	605	22	33%	10	47	1370	26	78
14" Thin Crust Pizza: Per 1/4 Pizza								
Cheese Pizza (Base)	380	17	39%	7	32	1170	17	43
With Topping: Beef	495	26	47%	11	53	1480	22	44
Cheddar Cheese	455	22	43%	11	50	1280	21	44
Pepperoni	480	25	47%	10	52	1535	21	44
X-tra Cheese & Pepperoni	550	30	49%	13	54	1765	25	45
Ham	415	18	39%	7	44	1465	21	44
Italian Sausage & Mushroom	500	25	45%	10	54	1515	22	48
Vegi	470	23	44%	10	47	1460	22	47
14" Deep Dish Pizza: Per 2 Slices								
Cheese Pizza (Base)	675	30	39%	11	41	1575	26	80
With Topping: Beef	785	40	46%	15	62	1885	31	80
Cheddar Cheese	745	36	43%	15	80	1685	30	80
Pepperoni	775	39	45%	14	61	1940	30	80
X-tra Cheese & Pepperoni	845	44	47%	17	77	2170	27	82
Ham	705	31	40%	11	54	1670	30	80
Italian Sausage & Mushroom	795	39	44%	15	64	1920	32	85
Vegi	765	36	42%	14	57	1865	31	83
14" Combination Toppings: Per Serving (Add to Cheese Pizza Base)								
America's Favorite	175	14	72%	6.5	37	580	10	4
Deluxe	110	9	73%	3.5	21	350	5	4
ExtravaganZZa	190	15	71%	6	37	700	10	4
Hawaiian	105	6.5	55%	3.5	26	465	8	3
Meatzza	240	19	71%	8.5	53	870	14	3
Pepperoni Extra	205	17	74%	8	44	730	11	2
6" Deep Dish: Per Pizza								
Cheese Pizza (Base)	600	27	42%	10	36	1340	23	6
With Topping: Beef	645	31	43%	12	44	1465	25	68
Cheddar Cheese	685	34	45%	15	58	1475	28	68
Pepperoni	650	31	43%	12	46	1525	25	68
Ham	610	28	41%	10	43	1495	25	68
Italian Sausage & Mushroom	650	30	42%	11	45	1475	25	70
Sides: Breadstick, 1 stk	115	4	31%	1	0	150	3	1
Cheesy Bread, 1 piece	140	6	39%	2	6	180	4	1
Barbeque Wings, each	50	2.5	44%	0.5	26	175	6	
Hot Wings, each	45	2	48%	0.5	26	355	5	0.1

	Cal	Fat	%Fc	S.Fat	Chol	Sod	Pro	Carb
12" Hand Tossed Pizza: *Per 2 Slices*								
Cheese Pizza (Base)	375	11	27%	5	23	775	15	55
With Topping: Beef	455	18	35%	8	38	990	19	55
Cheddar Cheese	435	16	33%	8	38	865	18	55
Pepperoni	450	18	36%	8	38	1050	18	55
X-tra Cheese & Pepperoni	500	22	40%	10	49	1215	21	56
Ham	400	12	27%	5	32	990	18	55
Italian Sausage & Mushroom	460	17	33%	7	39	1015	18	58
Vegi	440	16	33%	7	34	985	19	57
12" Thin Crust Pizza: *Per Slice (1/4)*								
Cheese Pizza (Base)	275	12	39%	5	23	835	12	31
With Topping: Beef	355	19	48%	8	38	1050	16	31
Cheddar Cheese	335	17	45%	8	38	925	15	31
Pepperoni	350	19	49%	8	38	1110	15	31
X-tra Cheese & Pepperoni	400	23	50%	10	49	1275	18	32
Ham	300	13	39%	5	32	1050	15	31
Italian Sausage & Mushroom	355	18	46%	7	39	1075	15	33
Vegi	340	17	45%	7	34	1045	16	34
12" Deep Dish Pizza: *Per 2 Slices*								
Cheese Pizza (Base)	480	22	40%	8	30	1125	19	56
With Topping: Beef	560	29	46%	11	45	1340	22	56
Cheddar Cheese	540	27	45%	11	45	1215	23	56
Pepperoni	560	29	46%	10	45	1400	22	56
Ham	505	23	41%	8	39	1340	22	56
Italian Sausage & Mushroom	560	28	45%	10	46	1365	22	59
Vegi	550	27	44%	10	41	1335	22	58
12" Combination Toppings: *Per Serving (Add to Cheese Pizza Base)*								
America's Favorite	135	11	73%	5	29	450	7	3
Deluxe	90	7	70%	3	17	290	4	2
ExtravaganZZa	155	12	70%	5	30	570	8	3
Hawaiian	75	4.5	54%	2.5	18	325	6	4
Meatzza	185	15	72%	6	42	690	11	2
Pepperoni Extra	150	12	72%	6	32	530	8	1
12" Toppings: *Per Serving (Add to Cheese Pizza Base)*								
Anchovies	35	1	39%	0	14	595	6	0
Bacon	100	9	77%	2	15	285	5	0
Banana Peppers	5	0	0%	0	0	135	0	1
Cheddar Cheese	55	4.5	74%	3	15	90	3	0
Xtra Cheese	50	4	71%	2	11	165	3	1
Green Peppers, Onions, Mushrooms	5	0	0%	0	0	1	0	1
Ham	25	1	37%	na	9	215	3	0.5
Italian Sausage	75	6	71%	na	16	240	3.5	2
Olives: Green	20	2	99%	0	0	385	0	2
Ripe	20	2	79%	0	0	110	0	1
Pepperoni	75	6.5	79%	na	15	275	3.5	0
Pineapple Tidbits	13	0	0%	na	0	1	0	3
Pre-Cooked Beef	80	7	80%	na	15	215	3.5	0

Donato's® Pizza

	Cal	Fat	%FC	S.Fat	Chol	Sod	Pro	Car
Pizza: Per Slice								
Chicken Vegy Medley	530	20	34%	7	50	1685	31	57
Classic Trio	720	41	51%	15	80	1915	33	56
Founders	745	42	51%	15	90	2595	36	58
Hawaiian	615	29	42%	9	50	1735	29	61
Mariachi Beef	620	31	45%	12	65	1895	30	58
Mariachi Chicken	600	27	40%	10	70	1900	35	57
Original	635	34	48%	12	65	1795	29	56
Serious Cheese	660	36	49%	15	65	1725	33	55
Serious Meat	885	53	54%	20	125	2535	46	57
Vegy	585	28	43%	9	35	1865	25	62
Works	745	41	50%	15	80	1920	34	61
Salads								
Garden/Lite Italian	270	15	50%	5	45	2615	16	18
Side Salad/Lite Italian	140	8	52%	3	20	1125	7	10
Subs								
Big Don/Italian	780	45	52%	13	85	2325	32	63
Big Don/Lite Italian	645	30	42%	11	85	2515	32	63
Ham & Cheese/Italian	660	31	42%	7	55	2020	32	64
Ham & Cheese/Lite Italian	530	54	92%	5	55	2210	32	64
Vegy/Lite Italian	445	12	24%	5	20	675	20	60

Dunkin Donuts®

	Cal	Fat	%FC	S.Fat	Chol	Sod	Pro	Car
Donuts: Each								
Apple Crumb Donut	230	10	40%	3	0	270	3	34
Apple N' Spice Donut	200	8	36%	1.5	0	270	3	29
Bavarian Kreme Donut	210	9	39%	2	0	270	3	30
Black Raspberry Donut	210	8	34%	1.5	0	280	3	32
Blueberry Cake Donut	240	10	38%	3	0	260	3	36
Boston Kreme Donut	240	9	34%	2	0	280	3	36
Butternut Cake Donut	300	16	48%	4.5	0	360	3	36
Caramel Apple Krunch Donut	300	14	42%	3	0	310	4	41
Chocolate Coconut Cake Donut	300	19	57%	6	0	370	4	31
Chocolate Frosted Cake Donut	300	16	48%	3	0	370	3	38
Chocolate Frosted Donut	200	9	41%	2	0	260	3	29
Chocolate Glazed Cake Donut	290	16	50%	3.5	0	370	3	33
Cinnamon Cake Donut	270	15	50%	3	0	360	3	31
Coconut Cake Donut	290	17	53%	5	0	360	3	33
Double Chocolate Cake Donut	310	17	49%	3.5	0	370	3	37
Dunkin' Donut	240	15	56%	3	0	340	3	25
Glazed Cake Donut	270	15	51%	3	0	360	3	33
Glazed Donut	180	8	40%	1.5	0	250	3	25
Jelly Filled Donut	210	8	34%	1.5	0	280	3	32
Jelly Stick Donut	290	12	37%	2.5	0	390	3	44
Kreme Filled (Choc./Vanilla)Donut	270	13	43%	3	0	260	3	35
Lemon Donut	200	9	41%	2	0	270	3	28

Dunkin Donuts® (Cont)

	Cal	Fat	%Fc	S.Fat	Chol	Sod	Pro	Carb
Donuts (Cont): Each								
Maple/Marble Frosted Donut	210	9	41%	2	0	260	3	29
Old Fashioned Cake Donut	250	15	54%	3	0	360	3	26
Powdered Cake Donut	270	15	50%	3	0	350	3	32
Sugared Cake Donut	250	15	54%	3	0	350	3	27
Strawberry Donut	210	8	34%	1.5	0	260	3	32
Strawberry/Vanilla Frosted Donut	210	9	39%	2	0	260	3	30
Sugar Raised Donut	170	8	42%	1.5	0	250	3	22
Toasted Coconut Cake Donut	300	17	51%	5	0	370	3	35
Whole Wheat Glazed Cake Donut	310	19	55%	4	0	380	4	32
Muffins: Each								
Apple Cinnamon Pecan	510	21	37%	6	70	590	8	74
Banana Nut	530	23	39%	6	75	540	10	72
Blueberry: Regular	490	17	31%	6	75	610	8	76
Reduced Fat	450	12	24%	9	65	590	8	77
Chocolate Chip	590	24	37%	10	75	560	9	88
Corn	500	16	29%	4.5	80	920	10	78
Cranberry Orange	470	15	29%	5	75	600	8	76
Honey Raisin Bran	490	16	29%	3.5	30	880	7	84
Lemon Poppyseed	580	19	30%	6	85	620	10	94
Omwich® Sandwiches								
Bagel Omwich®: Bacon Cheddar	600	21	32%	8	295	160	26	79
Pizza; Spanish, average	560	19	31%	6	270	1340	25	76
Biscuit Omwich®:								
Bacon Cheddar; Pizza, average	500	31	56%	10	280	1570	20	36
Egg/Cheese Sandwich	380	22	52%	8	180	1250	17	30
Sausage/Egg/Cheese Sandwich	590	42	64%	15	220	1620	25	31
Spanish Omwich	470	29	56%	9	285	1400	19	34
Croissant Omwich®: Bacon Cheddar	560	38	61%	13	295	1190	21	33
Pizza; Spanish Cheese, average	520	35	61%	11	275	910	18	33
English Muffin Omwich®:								
Bacon Cheddar	400	21	47%	8	295	1440	21	33
Ham/Egg/Cheese	320	12	34%	6	195	1340	22	31
Pizza; Spanish, average	360	18	45%	6	270	1160	18	33
Bagels: Each								
Bacon & Cheese	600	21	32%	7	300	1620	26	78
Berry Berry; Blueberry; Cinn. Raisin	340	3	8%	0.5	0	600	11	69
Garlic; Everything; Poppyseed	360	2.5	6%	0.5	0	710	12	67
Onion	330	4	11%	1	0	660	12	66
Plain	340	2.5	7%	0.5	0	680	12	67
Salt	340	2.5	7%	0.5	0	3030	12	67
Sesame	380	4.5	11%	0.5	0	720	12	74
Sundried Tomato	320	2.5	7%	0.5	0	700	13	66
Wheat	350	4.5	12%	1	0	640	13	67
Cream Cheese (Per Packet): Lite	130	11	76%	7	30	250	5	3
Average of other flavors	180	17	85%	11	50	310	3	3
Biscuit: Each	280	14	45%	4	0	850	6	32

	Cal	Fat	%Fc	S.Fat	Chol	Sod	Pro	Carb
Crullers: Each								
Glazed Cruller	290	15	47%	3	0	350	3	37
Glazed Chocolate Cruller	280	15	48%	3	0	360	3	35
Plain Cruller	240	15	56%	3	0	340	3	25
Powdered Cruller	270	15	50%	3	0	340	3	30
Sugar Cruller	250	15	54%	3	0	340	3	30
Cake Munchkins								
Butternut (3)	200	11	50%	3	0	240	2	25
Chocolate Cakes Glazed (3)	200	10	45%	2	0	250	2	26
Cinnamon (4)	250	14	50%	3	0	330	3	30
Coconut; Coconut Toasted (3)	200	12	54%	3.5	0	240	2	23
Glazed (3)	200	10	45%	2	0	250	2	27
Plain (4)	220	14	57%	3	0	310	2	22
Powdered; Sugared (4)	250	14	50%	3	0	310	2	29
Sugar Raised (7)	220	12	49%	2.5	0	290	4	26
Yeast Munchkin, Glazed (5)	200	9	41%	2	0	220	3	27
Yeast Munchkin, Jelly Filled (5)	210	9	39%	2	0	240	3	30
Yeast Lemon Filled (4)	170	8	42%	1.5	0	190	2	23
Fancies, Buns, Rolls, Fritters								
Apple Fritter	300	14	42%	3	0	360	4	41
Bismark Chocolate Iced Donut	340	15	40%	3.5	0	290	3	50
Bow Tie Donut	300	17	51%	3.5	0	340	4	34
Cinnamon Bun	510	15	26%	4	10	420	8	85
Coffee Roll: Regular	270	14	47%	3	0	340	4	33
Frosted (Choc./Maple/Vanilla)	290	15	47%	3	0	340	4	36
Eclair Donut	270	11	37%	2.5	0	290	3	39
Glazed Fritter	260	14	48%	3	0	330	4	31
Cookies: Per Cookie								
Chocolate varieties, average	220	11	47%	7	35	110	3	26
Oatmeal Raisin Pecan	220	10	41%	5	30	110	3	29
Peanut Butter, average	240	14	53%	6	30	140	5	24
Drinks: Dunkacinno	250	11	40%	3.5	10	240	2	34
Hot Chocolate, 10 oz	230	8	31%	2	0	310	2	38
Coffee/Coolatta®								
Coffee: w. Cream, 10 oz	410	22	48%	14	75	65	3	51
w. Milk, 10 oz	260	4	14%	2.5	15	75	4	52
w. 2% Milk, 10 oz	240	2	8%	1.5	10	80	4	52
w. Skim Milk, 10 oz	230	0	0%	0	0	80	4	52
Pina Coolatta®	270	3.5	12%	3	0	65	1	57
Vanilla Bean, 16 oz	450	7	14%	4	0	170	1	94
Other flavors	500	19	34%	15	0	160	2	82

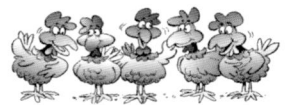

	Cal	Fat	%Fc	S.Fat	Chol	Sod	Pro	Carb
Bagels: Average all types, 4 oz	330	1	3%	0	0	500	11	70
Chocolate Chip Bagel, 4 oz	370	3	7%	2	0	500	11	76
Egg Bagel, 3½ oz	340	3	8%	1	35	510	11	69
Sesame Dip/Sunflower	370	5	12%	1	0	700	12	70
Cream Cheese: Plain, 2 Tbsp	70	7	90%	5	20	65	1	1
Plain Lite, 2 Tbsp	60	5	75%	3	15	85	1	2
Smoked Salmon, 2 Tbsp	60	5	75%	4	20	120	1	1
Flavors, average, 2 Tbsp	70	5	65%	5	15	50	1	5
Spreads: Fruit, 2 Tbsp	75	0	0%	0	0	20	0	19
Honey Butter, 1 Tbsp	90	8	80%	4	15	35	0	4
Peanut Butter, 2 Tbsp	190	15	71%	2	0	140	7	8
Sandwiches: BBQ Chicken	550	11	18%	2	50	1680	30	83
Baguette, Our Big Hero	920	39	38%	13	90	2640	45	98
Chicago Bagel Dog Asiago	740	34	41%	15	80	1360	29	78
Classic NY Lox & Bagel	660	27	37%	19	85	1150	26	79
Egg Santa Fe	650	24	33%	8	300	1210	30	78
Ham Deli	450	6	12%	2	45	1380	25	74
Holey Cow	900	50	50%	13	105	1450	36	77
Mediterranean Hummus	540	13	22%	4	15	880	18	89
Roast Beef Deli	460	4	7%	2	45	880	31	76
Roast Chicken & Smoked Gouda	520	11	19%	4	80	1380	37	68
Smoked Turkey Deli	420	1.5	3%	0	30	1270	25	75
The Veg-Out	490	13	24%	7	30	850	17	77
Tuna Salad Deli	500	7	13%	1.5	30	1060	32	77
Turkey Pastrami Deli	440	2	4%	0	40	1610	31	76
Turkey Pastrami Reuben Deli	660	19	26%	6	65	2590	39	83
Bagel Shtick: Asiago	450	9	18%	5	15	770	20	72
Cinnamon Sugar	570	24	38%	4	0	800	11	79
Everything	380	4.5	11%	0	0	1130	12	73
Sesame Bagel Shtick	420	8	17%	1	0	510	13	75
Bagel Chips: Plain, 1 oz serving	90	3	30%	0	0	330	2	13
Flavors, average, 1 oz	90	3	30%	0	0	330	2	15
Roll-Ups: Albuquerque Turkey	690	33	43%	14	80	1800	28	71
Baja Shaved Beef	720	36	45%	14	85	1490	30	67
Pacific Smoked Salmon	590	31	47%	18	100	1260	22	55
Cookies: Big Brownie	500	21	38%	4	30	280	4	70
Chocolate Chunk, 4 oz	600	28	42%	10	45	480	8	78
Oatmeal Raisin, 4 oz	550	21	34%	5	40	320	8	82
Muffins: Banana Nut	520	29	50%	5	95	430	9	59
Blueberry	460	24	47%	3	90	410	6	57
Chocolate Chip	240	13	49%	3	40	180	3	28
Lowfat Lemon Poppyseed	370	7	17%	1	0	560	8	69
Mocha Chocolate Chip	550	29	47%	8	95	430	7	66
97% Fat Free Apple Cinnamon	560	2	4%	0	0	85	8	77
Scones: All types, 5 oz	490	17	31%	8	45	500	9	75
Coffee: Cafe Latte, regular	140	5	32%	4	20	140	9	13
Cappuccino	90	3.5	35%	2	15	95	6	9

El Pollo Loco®

	Cal	Fat	%Fc	S.Fat	Chol	Sod	Pro	Carb
Flame Broiled Chicken: Breast	160	6	34%	2	0.1	390	26	0
Leg	90	5	50%	2	75	150	11	0
Thigh	180	12	60%	4	0.3	230	16	0
Wing	110	6	49%	2	80	220	12	0
Tortillas: 6" Corn	70	1	13%	0	0	35	1	14
6.5" Flour	90	3	30%	0	0	224	3	13
Burritos: Bean, Rice & Cheese	505	16	29%	6	17	1263	17	73
Chicken Lover's	475	19	36%	6	0.4	1373	29	47
Classic	580	22	34%	7	0.1	1595	31	66
Mexican Chicken Caesar	735	35	43%	8	79	1214	36	65
Southwest	625	27	39%	4	60	1795	30	69
Ultimate	635	23	33%	8	89	1237	39	66
Tacos: Chicken Soft Taco	225	12	46%	4	74	629	17	15
Taco Al Carbon	165	6	33%	2	68	21	13	14
Bowls: Flame Broiled Chicken Salad	355	13	33%	2	42	1079	25	39
Mexican Chicken Caesar Salad	735	35	43%	8	79	1214	36	65
Pollo Bowl	470	11	21%	2	42	1868	30	66
Smokey Black Bean Pollo Bowl	605	23	34%	7	54	1955	29	75
Southwest Chicken Salad	530	31	53%	5	52	1332	25	40
Specialties: Chicken Taquito	370	17	41%	-	25	690	15	43
Kids Dinosaur Chicken Bites	185	10	50%	2	64	345	12	11
Tortilla Chips, unsalted	425	24	51%	5	0	12	5	48
Tostada Salad, w/out shell & sour crm	305	11	33%	3	57	1175	29	28
Tostada, shell only	440	27	55%	4	0	610	7	42
Side Dishes: Cole Slaw	205	16	70%	3	11	358	2	12
Corn Cobbette	80	1	11%	0	0	10	3	18
French Fries	445	19	39%	5	0	605	6	61
Garden Salad	105	7	60%	3	15	99	5	7
Macaroni & Cheese	245	12	44%	4	22	950	10	24
Pinto Beans	185	4	19%	0	0	744	11	29
Potato Salad	255	14	49%	2	15	527	3	30
Smokey Black Beans	305	16	47%	6	13	731	7	35
Spanish Rice	130	3	21%	1	0	397	2	24
Dressings: Avocado Salsa	12	1	75%	0	0	204	0	2
Light Italian	25	1	36%	1	0	990	0	3
Ranch	350	39	100%	6	5	500	1	2
Southwest; Bleu Cheese	300	32	96%	6	18	443	0	2
1000 Island; Creamy Cilantro	270	27	90%	3	30	460	1	9
Condiments: Guacamole	30	2	60%	0	0	160	0	3
House/Spicy Chipotle Salsa	6	0	0%	0	0	96	0	2
Jalapeno Hot Sauce	5	0	0%	0	0	110	0	1
Light Sour Cream	45	3	60%	0	12	25	2	2
Pico de Gallo Salsa	11	0.5	41%	0	0	131	0	1.5
Desserts: Banana Split	715	28	35%	11	56	310	12	107
Churros	180	11	55%	3	5	221	3	18
Foster's Freeze without cone	180	5	25%	3	20	100	4	30
Smoothies, all types	365	7	17%	3	23	136	3	68

	Cal	Fat	%Fc	S.Fat	Chol	Sod	Pro	Carb
Soup; Bread								
Minestrone Soup	125	1	7%	na	1.5	910	1	23
Breadstick, dry	100	1	9%	na	0	180	4	18
Breadstick	170	8	42%	na	0	180	4	18
Salads: No Dressing								
Garden Salad	30	0	0%	0	0	20	2	6
Italian Chef Salad	260	21	72%	na	46	1445	15	13
Pasta Salad	600	26	39%	na	24	2020	19	68
Dressings: Per 1 oz								
Honey French	145	12	74%	na	0	205	0	9
House Italian	105	9.5	80%	na	0	510	0	5
Reduced Calorie Italian	65	4.5	62%	na	0	595	0	3
Ranch	155	17	99%	na	2.5	215	0	1
Thousand Island	130	13	90%	na	17	225	0	4
Pizza: Per Double Slice								
Cheese	465	15	29%	na	39	970	24	58
Combination	570	25	39%	na	60	1370	29	63
Pepperoni	525	22	37%	na	53	1225	26	61
Pasta: Per Serving								
Baked Spaghetti Parmesan	700	26	33%	na	60	770	38	76
Baked Ziti: Small	485	17	31%	na	35	575	23	56
Regular	745	26	31%	na	53	865	36	87
Cheese Ravioli: w. Tomato Sauce	475	15	28%	na	66	535	21	65
w. Meat Sauce	510	17	30%	na	72	795	20	65
Chicken Parmesan	465	9	17%	na	86	680	42	47
Fettucine Alfredo: Small	535	15	25%	na	14	170	17	80
Regular	800	22	25%	na	20	230	25	120
Fettucine Broccoli: Small	560	15	24%	na	14	190	20	85
Regular	825	23	25%	na	20	265	27	124
Small Spaghetti: w. Tomato Sauce	355	8	20%	na	0	230	12	62
w. Meat Sauce	370	8	19%	2	20	160	17	60
w. Meatballs	720	31	39%	na	61	725	27	80
Regular Spaghetti: w. Tomato Sauce	510	10	17%	na	0	245	16	93
w. Meat Sauce	555	12	19%	na	30	225	26	90
w. Meatballs	1020	42	37%	na	81	965	38	118
Lasagna: Regular	435	19	39%	na	144	965	21	41
Broccoli	425	18	38%	na	137	760	20	44
Sampler Platter	705	21	27%	na	82	730	26	97
Shrimp & Scallop Fettucine	650	20	27%	na	102	355	31	80
Desserts: Per Serving								
Cheesecake: Plain	335	26	70%	na	110	260	7	20
Turtle	370	27	65%	na	104	250	8	27
Lemon Ice, 12 oz	140	0	0%	0	0	10	0	36
Milk Chocolate Chunk Cookie	360	15	37%	na	30	345	6	54
Strawberry Topping, 1 oz	35	0	0%	0	0	37	0	8

Godfather's™ Pizza

	Cal	Fat	%FC	S.Fat	Chol	Sod	Pro	Carb
Original Crust: Per Slice								
Cheese Pizza: Mini, 1/4 pizza	130	3	21%	na	8	180	7	19
Medium, 1/8 pizza	230	5	19%	na	14	340	13	34
Large, 1/10 pizza	260	6	21%	na	18	395	15	36
Jumbo, 1/10 pizza	380	9	26%	na	27	580	22	53
Combo Pizza: Mini, 1/4 pizza	175	7	36%	na	16	380	10	21
Medium, 1/8 pizza	305	11	32%	na	27	660	17	36
Large, 1/10 pizza	340	12	32%	na	31	740	19	38
Jumbo, 1/10 pizza	505	18	32%	na	47	1095	29	56
Golden Crust: Per Slice								
Cheese Pizza: Medium, 1/8 pizza	210	10	31%	na	12	310	10	26
Large, 1/10 pizza	240	9	34%	na	14	365	12	28
Combo Pizza: Medium, 1/8 pizza	270	12	40%	na	22	560	13	28
Large, 1/10 pizza	305	14	42%	na	25	675	16	31

Golden Corral®

	Cal	Fat	%FC	S.Fat	Chol	Sod	Pro	Carb
Chicken								
Grilled	170	5	26%	na	100	520	32	0
Fried	370	19	46%	na	85	570	37	14
Shrimp, fried	250	12	43%	na	90	470	12	24
Steak								
Ribeye, 6 oz	450	35	70%	na	120	220	34	0
Sirloin, 5 oz	230	14	55%	na	90	270	27	0
Chopped, 4 oz	320	23	65%	na	100	160	28	0
Tips w. Onions	290	13	40%	na	120	260	30	8
Baked Potato	225	2	8%	na	0	60	5	46
Texas Toast	170	6	32%	na	0	230	5	26

Gretel's Pretzels®

	Cal	Fat	%FC	S.Fat	Chol	Sod	Pro	Carb
Pretzels								
Cinnamon/Sugar	195	3	14%	0.5	3	250	3	38
Original	170	3	16%	0.5	3	515	3	31
Poppy Seed	175	3.5	18%	0.5	3	250	3	31
Raisin Danish/Icing	350	2	5%	0.5	2	20	6.5	79
Sesame Seed	175	3.5	18%	0.5	3	250	3	31
Sweet Dough	115	0.5	3%	0.5	0	2.5	4	23

Haagen-Dazs®

~ See Page 30 of Icecream Section ~

	Cal	Fat	%FC	S.Fat	Chol	Sod	Pro	Carb
Breakfast Items								
Biscuits:								
Apple Cinnamon 'N' Raisin	250	8	29%	2	0	350	2	42
Bacon, Egg & Cheese	520	30	52%	10	210	1420	17	45
Biscuit 'N' Gravy	530	30	51%	10	15	1550	10	56
Chicken	590	27	41%	7	45	1820	24	62
Country Ham	440	22	45%	7	30	1710	14	44
Ham	410	20	44%	6	25	1200	13	45
Jelly	440	21	44%	6	0	1000	6	57
Made from Scratch® Biscuit	390	21	48%	6	0	1000	6	44
Omelet Biscuit	550	32	52%	12	225	1350	20	45
Sausage	550	36	59%	10	25	1310	12	44
Sausage & Egg	620	40	58%	13	225	1370	20	45
Steak Biscuit	580	32	49%	10	30	1580	15	56
Frisco Breakfast Sandwich (Ham)	450	22	44%	8	225	1290	22	42
Hash Rounds	230	14	55%	3	0	560	3	24
Hamburgers								
All Star	660	43	58%	14	100	1260	29	41
Bacon Swiss Crispy Chicken	670	44	59%	9	55	1600	24	45
Famous Star	570	35	55%	10	80	860	24	41
Frisco Burger	720	49	61%	15	95	1180	30	37
Hamburger	270	10	33%	4	35	550	13	30
Monster Burger®	1060	79	67%	29	185	1860	49	37
Monster Roast Beef	610	39	57%	18	105	1940	35	26
Six Dollar Burger®	950	62	58%	25	137	1685	38	58
Super Star	790	53	60%	17	145	970	40	41
Sandwiches								
Big Roast Beef™ Sandwich	410	24	52%	10	40	1140	24	26
Chicken Fillet Sandwich	480	23	43%	4	55	1190	24	44
Fisherman's Fillet™	530	28	47%	7	75	1280	25	45
Grilled Chicken Sandwich	350	16	41%	3	65	860	23	28
Hot Dog w. condiments	450	32	64%	12	55	1240	15	25
Hot Ham 'N' Cheese	300	12	35%	6	50	1390	16	34
Roast Beef Sandwich	310	16	46%	6	40	800	17	26
Fried Chicken								
Breast, each	370	15	36%	4	75	1190	29	29
Wing, each	200	8	36%	2	30	740	10	23
Thigh, each	330	15	41%	4	60	1000	19	30
Leg, each	170	7	37%	2	45	570	13	15
French Fries: Regular	340	16	42%	2	0	390	4	45
Large	440	21	43%	3	0	520	5	60
Monster	510	24	42%	3	0	590	6	67
Crispy Curls™: Medium	340	18	47%	4	0	950	5	41
Large	520	28	48%	5	0	1450	7	62
Monster	590	31	47%	6	0	1640	8	70

Hardee's® (Cont)

	Cal	Fat	%Fc	S.Fat	Chol	Sod	Pro	Carb
Sides								
Baked Beans, 5 oz	170	1	5%	0	0	600	8	32
Coleslaw	240	20	75%	3	10	340	2	13
Gravy, 1.5 oz	20	0	0%	0	0	260	1	3
Mashed Potatoes, small	70	0	0%	0.5	0	330	2	14
Salads: Side Salad, no dressing	25	0.5	18%	0	0	45	1	4
Garden Salad, no dressing	220	13	53%	10	40	350	12	10
Grilled Chicken Salad, no dressing	150	3	18%	1	60	610	20	10
Fat Free French Dressing	70	0	0%	0	0	580	0	17
Ranch Dressing	290	29	90%	4	25	510	1	6
Thousand Island Dressing	250	23	83%	3	35	540	1	10
Shakes/Drinks								
Chocolate Shake	370	5	12%	3	30	270	13	67
Vanilla Shake	350	5	13%	3	20	300	12	65
Orange Juice, 10 oz	140	0	0%	0	0	5	2	34
Desserts: Twist Cone	180	2	10%	1	5	120	4	34
Apple Turnover	270	12	40%	4	0	250	4	38
Peach Cobbler	310	7	20%	1	0	360	2	60

Harvey's®

	Cal	Fat	%Fc	S.Fat	Chol	Sod	Pro	Carb
Breakfast Items								
Pancakes	90	1	10%	na	8	na	2	17
Sausage	170	14	74%	na	12	na	9	3
Toast, plain	250	3	11%	na	1	na	8	48
Burgers								
Hamburger: Regular	360	14	35%	na	17	na	12	40
Double	530	26	44%	na	34	na	31	44
Super	480	19	36%	na	112	na	37	38
Cheeseburger	420	18	39%	na	30	na	22	41
Chicken Fingers, 1 serving	240	12	45%	na	57	na	15	18
Sandwiches: Chicken	420	16	34%	na	110	na	19	46
Western	350	10	26%	na	265	na	15	58
Sides: French Fries	480	24	45%	na	5	na	10	56
Hash Browns	150	9	54%	na	2	na	2	15
Hot Dog	330	15	41%	na	50	na	12	32
Onion Rings	290	14	43%	na	5	na	4	36
Muffins								
Blueberry	260	6	21%	na	1	na	4	45
Bran	300	13	39%	na	1	na	5	42
Apple Turnover, each	180	7	35%	na	7	na	1	28
Drinks: Apple Juice	80	2	23%	na	0	na	2	20
Orange Juice	80	1	11%	na	0	na	1	18
Shakes: Chocolate	320	11	31%	na	36	na	12	74
Strawberry; Vanilla	300	10	30%	na	36	na	11	69

Hot Dog On A Stick®

Menu Items:	Cal	Fat	%Fc	S.Fat	Chol	Sod	Pro	Carb
Fries	400	24	54%	4.5	0	35	5	41
American Cheese on a Stick	240	7	26%	7	30	730	8	21
Hot Dog on a Stick	250	14	50%	4	45	860	9	23
Muscle Beach Lemonade, regular	240	0	0%	0	0	20	0	58
Pepper Jack on a Stick	260	14	48%	8	35	600	10	23

I Can't Believe It's Yogurt®

	Cal	Fat	%Fc	S.Fat	Chol	Sod	Pro	Carb
Original Frozen Yogurt: Per Regular Serving (9 fl.oz)								
Awesome Amaretto	280	6	19%	4	20	230	6	51
Cookies 'N Cream	260	3	10%	1	5	200	7	54
French Vanilla	260	6	21%	4	45	200	7	47
Peanut Butter Bliss	310	12	35%	4	15	200	7	46
White Chocolate Mousse	280	7	23%	4	15	200	7	49
Nonfat Frozen Yogurt								
Average all flavors: Regular	220	0.5	2%	0	5	150	6	48
Small, 6.2 fl.oz	160	0	0%	0	0	100	4	32
Nonfat (w. NutraSweet)								
Average all flavors: Regular	190	0.5	2%	0	5	160	4	40
Small, 6.2 fl.oz	140	0.5	3%	0	5	110	4	29

In-N-Out Burger®

	Cal	Fat	%Fc	S.Fat	Chol	Sod	Pro	Carb
Burgers: Hamburger	390	19	44%	5	40	640	16	39
Cheeseburger	480	27	51%	10	60	1000	22	39
Double Double® (2 patties/2 sl. chse)	670	41	55%	18	120	1430	37	40
French Fries, 125g	400	18	41%	5	0	245	7	54
Shakes (15 oz)								
Chocolate	690	36	47%	24	95	350	9	83
Vanilla	680	37	49%	25	90	390	8	78
Strawberry	690	33	43%	22	85	280	8	91

Int'l House of Pancakes~ IHOP®

Pancakes: (Syrup/Butter extra)	Cal	Fat	%Fc	S.Fat	Chol	Sod	Pro	Carb
Buttermilk, 1 (2 oz)	110	3	25%	1	30	450	3	17
Short Stack, 3	330	9	25%	3	90	1350	9	51
Full Stack, 5	550	15	25%	5	150	2250	15	85
Buckwheat, 1 (2 oz)	110	4	33%	1	50	280	3	15
Country Griddle, 1 (2 oz)	120	3.5	26%	1	35	440	3	19
Harvest Grain 'N Nut, 1(2¼ oz)	180	9	45%	1.5	38	410	5	20
Crepes (Egg Pancakes), 1 (2 oz)	120	6	45%	1.5	80	230	3	14
Syrup: 1 Tbsp	50	0	0%	0	0	0	0	12
Whipped Butter, 1 Tbsp	80	9	100%	4.5	25	75	0	0
Waffles (Plain): Regular, 1 (3 oz)	310	15	44%	3.5	70	380	6	37
Belgian: Regular, 1 (4 oz)	390	19	44%	12	140	850	8	48

Jack in the Box®

	Cal	Fat	%FC	S.Fat	Chol	Sod	Pro	Carb
Breakfast								
Biscuit	190	9	43%	2.5	0	500	3	24
Breakfast Jack®	280	12	39%	5	190	750	17	28
French Toast Sticks	420	20	43%	4	5	420	7	53
Hash Browns	170	12	64%	2	0	250	1	14
Sausage Biscuit	380	27	64%	8	35	730	11	25
Sausage Croissant	660	48	65%	15	240	860	20	37
Sausage, Egg & Cheese Biscuit	510	36	64%	12	220	1050	19	27
Sourdough Breakfast Sandwich	450	24	48%	8	205	1040	21	36
Supreme Croissant	530	34	58%	10	225	1060	21	37
Ultimate Breakfast Sandwich	600	34	51%	10	410	1480	34	39
Country Crock Spread	25	3	100%	0.5	0	45	0	0
Grape Jelly, 1 packet	40	0	0%	0	0	5	0	10
Syrup	130	0	0%	0	0	5	0	30
Burgers								
Cheeseburger: Bacon Bacon	760	50	59%	17	135	1570	39	39
Bacon Ultimate	1020	71	63%	26	210	1740	58	37
Double	440	24	49%	11	80	1110	24	31
Ultimate	950	66	63%	26	195	1370	52	37
Hamburger	250	9	32%	3.5	30	610	12	30
Hamburger w. Cheese	300	13	39%	6	40	840	14	31
Jumbo Jack: Regular	550	30	49%	10	75	880	27	43
w. Cheese	640	38	53%	15	105	1340	31	44
Sourdough Jack	690	45	59%	15	105	1180	34	37
Sandwiches								
Chicken Fajita Pita	320	10	28%	4.5	55	850	24	34
Chicken Sandwich	400	21	47%	3	40	770	15	38
Chicken Supreme	830	49	53%	7	65	2140	33	66
Grilled Chicken Fillet	480	24	45%	6	65	1110	27	39
Jack's Spicy Chicken®	570	29	46%	2.5	50	1020	24	52
Sourdough Grilled Chicken Club	520	27	47%	6	80	1320	31	39
Snacks								
Bacon/Cheddar Potato Wedges	750	50	60%	16	45	1510	20	55
Chicken Breast Pieces: 5 piece	360	17	43%	3	80	970	27	24
Egg Rolls: 1 piece	150	8	48%	2	10	340	5	13
3 piece	440	24	49%	6	30	1020	15	40
Fish & Chips	780	39	45%	9	45	1740	19	86
Stuffed Jalapenos: 3 piece	230	13	51%	5	25	740	7	20
7 piece	530	31	53%	12	60	1730	16	46
Mexican Food: Monster Taco	270	17	57%	6	30	630	12	19
Salsa	10	0	0%	0	0	200	0	2
Taco	170	10	53%	3.5	15	390	7	12
Teriyaki Bowls								
Chicken	670	4	5%	1	15	1730	26	128
Soy Sauce	5	0	0%	0	0	480	1	1

	Cal	Fat	%Fc	S.Fat	Chol	Sod	Pro	Carb
Salads: No Dressing								
Garden Chicken	200	9	41%	4	65	420	23	8
Side	50	3	54%	1.5	10	75	2	3
Salad Dressings								
Blue Cheese	210	15	64%	2.5	25	750	1	11
Buttermilk House	290	30	93%	11	20	560	1	6
Low Calorie Italian	25	1.5	54%	0	0	670	0	2
Thousand Island	250	24	86%	4	35	570	1	10
Croutons	50	2	36%	1.5	0	100	1	8
Curly Fries								
Chili Cheese	650	41	57%	12	25	1760	14	60
Seasoned	410	23	50%	5	0	1010	6	45
French Fries: Regular	350	16	41%	4	0	710	4	46
Jumbo Fries	430	20	42%	5	0	890	4	58
Super Scoop	610	28	41%	6	0	1250	6	82
Onion Rings	450	25	50%	5	0	780	7	50
Condiments								
Cheese: American, 1 slice	45	4	80%	2	10	230	2	1
Swiss-style, 1 slice	40	4	90%	2	10	210	2	1
Dipping Sauce: Barbecue	45	0	0%	0	0	310	1	11
Buttermilk House	130	13	90%	5	10	240	0.5	3
Frank's Red Hot Buffalo	10	0	0%	0	0	840	0	2
Sweet & Sour	45	0	0%	0	0	160	0.5	11
Tartar	210	22	94%	3	30	340	1	2
Packet Sauce: Chinese Hot Mustard	10	0	0%	0	0	50	0	1
Hot Sauce	5	0	0%	0	0	110	0.5	1
Ketchup	10	0	0%	0	0	105	0	2
Mayonnaise	150	17	100%	2.5	15	120	0	0
Mustard	5	0	0%	0	0	55	0	1
Sour Cream	60	6	90%	4	20	30	1	1
Desserts								
Cheesecake	320	18	51%	10	65	220	7	32
Double Fudge Cake	300	10	30%	2	20	320	3	50
Hot Apple Turnover	340	18	48%	4	0	510	4	41
Icecream Shakes								
Cappuccino, regular	630	29	41%	17	90	320	11	80
Chocolate, regular	630	27	39%	16	85	330	11	85
Oreo Cookie Classic, regular	740	36	44%	19	95	490	13	91
Strawberry, regular	640	28	39%	15	85	300	10	85
Vanilla, regular	610	31	46%	18	95	320	12	73
Drinks								
Barq's Root Beer, regular	180	0	0%	0	0	40	0	50
Coca Cola, regular	170	0	0%	0	0	10	0	46
Dr Pepper; Minute Maid, regular	190	0	0%	0	0	25	0	49
Lowfat Milk (2%) 8 fl.oz	130	5	34%	3	25	85	9	14
Orange Juice, 10 fl.oz	150	0	0%	0	0	20	2	34
Sprite, regular	160	0	0%	0	0	40	0	41

Jamba Juice®

Smoothies: Per 24 fl.oz	Cal	Fat	%Fc	S.Fat	Chol	Sod	Pro	Carb
Aloha Pineapple™	430	2	4%	0	0	40	7	96
Banana Berry™	450	2	4%	0	0	30	5	103
Caribbean Passion®	415	2	4%	0	0	40	2	98
Chocolate Moo'd™	650	8	11%	4	10	30	15	131
Citrus Squeeze®; Orange-A-Peel™	420	2	4%	0	0	30	4	96
Coffee Moo'd™	595	6	9%	1	0	100	13	121
Coldbuster™	430	2	4%	0	0	100	5	97
Cranberry Craze®	395	2	5%	0	0	50	5	89
Jamba Powerboost™	455	2	4%	0	0	30	9	100
Kiwi-Berry® Burner	420	0	4%	0	0	30	3	100
Lime Sublime™	410	2	4%	0	0	20	3	95
Mango-A-Go-Go™	460	2	4%	0	0	20	2	109
Mocha Moo'd™	625	7	10%	2	10	20	14	126
Orange Berry Blitz™	375	2	5%	0	0	30	5	84
Orchard Oasis™	435	2	4%	0	0	30	2	102
Peach Pleasure®	440	2	4%	0	0	30	3	104
Peanut Butter Moo'd™	755	19	23%	4	0	20	23	124
Peenya Kowlada®	565	5	8%	1	0	30	8	123
Protein Berry Pizazz™	475	1	2%	0	0	20	25	91
Raspberry Refresher™	440	3	6%	0	0	40	3	101
Razzmatazz™	440	2	4%	0	0	40	3	102
Strawberries Wild™	415	1	2%	0	0	40	6	96

Note: Figures for saturated fat, cholesterol and sodium are author estimates.

Krispy Kreme®

Donuts:	Cal	Fat	%Fc	S.Fat	Chol	Sod	Pro	Carb
Cinnamon Apple Filled	280	13	42%	3	5	180	5	35
Cinnamon Bun/Twist	220	11	45%	3	0	160	5	26
Fudge Iced Cake	230	12	47%	3	15	280	3	28
Fudge Iced Creme Filled	340	18	48%	5	5	160	5	39
Fudge Iced Custard Filled	310	16	46%	4	5	170	4	39
Fudge Iced Glazed	280	14	45%	4	5	75	3	36
Fudge Iced Glazed Cruller	240	12	45%	3	10	160	2	31
Fudge Iced Sprinkles	220	10	41%	2.5	5	95	2	31
Glazed Blueberry	300	15	45%	3	5	200	2	37
Glazed Creme Filled	350	20	51%	5	5	135	3	39
Glazed Cruller	250	16	58%	4	5	190	2	24
Glazed Devil's Food	390	24	55%	5	5	250	2	41
Glazed Lemon Filled	280	14	45%	4	5	160	4	33
Glazed Raspberrry Filled	270	12	40%	3	5	170	4	37
Maple Iced Glazed	200	9	41%	2.5	0	100	3	28
Old Fashioned Sour Cream Cake	230	11	43%	2.5	10	300	3	30
Original Glazed	210	12	51%	3	5	65	2	22
Powdered Blueberry Filled	270	13	43%	4	5	170	5	33
Traditional Cake	200	11	50%	3	15	280	3	22

	Cal	Fat	%Fc	S.Fat	Chol	Sod	Pro	Carb
Original Recipe®								
Breast	400	24	54%	6	135	1115	29	16
Drumstick	140	9	58%	2	75	420	13	4
Thigh	250	18	65%	4.5	95	750	16	6
Whole Wing	140	10	64%	2.5	55	415	9	5
Extra Crispy™ : Breast	470	28	54%	8	160	874	39	17
Drumstick	195	12	55%	3	77	375	13	7
Thigh	380	27	64%	7	120	625	24	14
Whole Wing	220	15	61%	4	55	415	10	10
Hot & Spicy Chicken: Breast	505	29	52%	8	162	1170	38	23
Drumstick	175	10	51%	3	80	360	13	9
Thigh	355	26	66%	7	126	630	19	13
Whole Wing	210	15	64%	4	55	350	10	9
Other Entrees: Chunky Pot Pie	770	42	49%	13	70	2160	29	69
Crispy Strips: Colonels, 3 pieces	300	16	48%	4	60	1105	26	18
Spicy, 3 pieces	335	15	40%	4	70	1140	26	18
Popcorn Chicken: Small, 3.5 oz	360	23	57%	6	43	610	17	21
Large, 6 oz	620	40	58%	10	73	1050	30	36
Wings: Hot Wings, 6 pieces	470	33	63%	8	150	1230	27	18
Honey BBQ Wings, 6 pces	610	38	56%	10	193	1145	33	33
Sandwiches								
Original Recipe Chicken: w. Sauce	450	22	44%	5	70	940	29	33
without Sauce	360	13	33%	3.5	60	890	28	36
Honey BBQ Crunch Melt	560	26	42%	5	60	1010	33	48
Honey BBQ Flavored Chicken, w. Sce	310	6	17%	2	125	560	28	37
Triple Crunch Chicken: w. Sauce	490	29	53%	6	70	710	28	39
without Sauce	390	15	35%	4.5	50	650	25	36
Triple Crunch Zinger: w. Sauce	550	32	52%	7	65	630	26	39
without Sauce	450	18	36%	6	60	750	25	36
Tender Roast Chicken: w. Sauce	350	15	39%	3	75	880	32	26
without Sauce	270	5	17%	1.5	65	690	31	23
Twister	600	34	51%	7	50	1430	22	52
Side Dishes: Biscuit, 2 oz	180	10	50%	2.5	0	560	4	20
BBQ Baked Beans, 5.5 oz	190	3	14%	1	5	760	6	33
Coleslaw, 5 oz	240	14	50%	2	8	290	2	26
Corn on the Cob, 5.7 oz	150	1.5	9%	0.5	0	20	5	35
Macaroni & Cheese, 5.4 oz	180	8	40%	3	10	860	7	21
Mashed Potatoes w. Gravy, 4.8 oz	120	6	45%	1	1	440	1	17
Potato Salad, 5.6 oz	230	14	55%	2	15	540	4	23
Potato Wedges, 4.8 oz	280	13	42%	4	5	750	5	28
Desserts: Dble Choc Chip Cake, 2.7 oz	320	16	45%	4	55	230	4	41
Little Bucket Parfaits: Chocolate Crm	290	15	47%	11	15	330	3	37
Fudge Brownie	280	10	32%	3.5	145	190	3	44
Lemon Creme	410	14	31%	8	20	290	7	62
Strawberry Shortcake	200	7	32%	6	10	220	1	33
Colonels Pies: Apple Pie Slice, 4 oz	310	14	41%	3	0	280	2	44
Pecan Pie Slice, 4 oz	490	23	42%	5	65	510	5	66
Strawberry Creme Pie Slice, 2.7 oz	280	15	48%	8	15	130	4	32

Kenny Roger's Roasters®

	Cal	Fat	%FC	S.Fat	Chol	Sod	Pro	Carb
Chicken								
1/2 Chicken: No Skin or Wing	315	10	29%	3	220	880	56	1
w. Skin	515	28	49%	7	300	1130	65	2
1/4 Dark Meat: No Skin	170	7	37%	2	130	455	25	1
w. Skin	270	17	57%	4	165	525	29	1
1/4 White Meat: No Skin or Wing	145	2	12%	0.5	90	420	31	1
w. Skin	245	11	40%	3	136	605	35	1
Pies: Chicken Pot Pie	710	33	42%	11	70	1500	26	78
Pitas: BBQ Chicken	400	7	16%	1	110	1310	33	51
Chicken Caesar	605	35	52%	3	120	830	36	34
Roasted Chicken	685	35	46%	3	160	1620	47	42
Turkey: Sliced Breast	160	2	11%	0.5	80	590	34	0
Salads (No Dressing): Per Serving								
Chicken Caesar	285	9	28%	3	120	700	34	18
Pasta	230	12	47%	2	40	300	6	28
Roasted Chicken	290	10	31%	2	220	575	35	19
Side	25	0	0%	0	0	15	1	5
Sour Cream & Dill Pasta	230	16	63%	3	15	430	4	20
Tomato Cucumber	125	2	14%	1	0	795	1	10
Sandwiches: Turkey	385	12	28%	2	90	920	39	30
Side Dishes: Per Serving								
Cinnamon Apples	200	5	23%	3	15	5	0	41
Cole Slaw	225	16	64%	3	15	290	1	18
Corn: on the Cob	70	0.5	6%	0.5	0	10	2	14
Cornbread Stuffing	325	19	53%	3	5	765	7	34
Muffin	175	8	41%	1	0	210	2	24
Sweet Corn Niblets	115	0.5	4%	0.5	0	385	3	28
Creamy Parmesan Spinach	120	6	45%	3	10	550	10	10
Honey Baked Beans	150	1	6%	0.5	0	790	6	32
Italian Green Beans	115	8	63%	1	0	375	2	10
Macaroni & Cheese	200	6	27%	3	25	660	6	24
Potatoes: Baked Sweet	265	0	0%	0	0	25	4	62
Garlic Parsley	260	12	42%	5	15	870	3	37
Potato Salad	390	27	62%	3	0	630	3	34
Real Mashed	295	14	43%	3	2	480	4	39
Rice Pilaf	175	5	26%	0.5	0	145	3	43
Steamed Vegetables	50	0	0%	0	0	60	3	8
Zucchini & Squash Santa Fe	70	5	64%	0.5	0	210	1	8
Soup: Chicken Noodle, 1 bowl	90	2	20%	0.5	20	930	7	12
Chicken Noodle, 1 cup	55	1	16%	0.5	15	560	4	7

Kohr Bros®

	Cal	Fat	%FC	S.Fat	Chol	Sod	Pro	Carb
Frozen Custard: Per 1/2 Cup								
Chocolate	140	6	39%	4	25	75	4	18
Orange Sherbet	105	2	17%	1	8	35	1	21
Vanilla	130	6	42%	4	25	60	4	16

	Cal	Fat	%Fc	S.Fat	Chol	Sod	Pro	Carb
Original Skinless Flame Broiled Chicken								
Leg & Thigh	175	8	42%	2	54	365	21	3
Breast & Wing (skin on wing)	220	8	33%	2	27	495	34	3
Original Breast Meat	160	4	23%	1	23	400	28	2
Half Original Chicken (skin on wing)	390	16	37%	4	81	860	55	6
Rotisserie Chicken								
Leg & Thigh	300	18	54%	5	114	515	31	1
Breast & Wing	355	16	41%	4	140	675	49	1
Half Rotisserie Chicken	655	34	47%	9	254	1190	80	2
Fresh Roasted Carved Turkey								
Turkey Breast Sandwich	540	7	12%	0	118	800	49	68
1/2 Turkey Breast Sandwich	270	4	13%	0	60	400	25	34
1/4 lb Sliced White Meat	155	1	6%	0	95	60	34	0
1/4 lb Sliced Dark Meat	210	8	34%	3	96	90	32	0
Open-Faced Turkey S'wich: w. extras	670	21	28%	10	161	1395	51	69
Hand-Carved Turkey Dinner: w. extras	705	21	27%	10	160	1420	53	76
Turkey Pot Pie, 5.5 oz	905	45	45%	12	165	1380	42	83
Salads: Per Regular (no dressing)								
BBQ Chicken Salad, 15 1/2 oz	465	21	41%	8	121	740	40	30
Caesar Salad, 9 1/2 oz	170	8	42%	4	11	485	10	16
Chicken Caesar Salad, 12 oz	310	11	32%	4	83	545	36	16
Chinese Chicken Salad, 17 oz	295	8	24%	2	71	170	31	23
Koo Koo Roo House Salad, 16 oz	165	6	33%	2	7	360	9	21
Koo Koo Roo Slaw (side)	55	2	33%	0	0	230	1	10
Pesto Pasta Salad	170	5	27%	1	16	250	10	21
12 Vegetable Chopped Salad, 13 oz	80	1	12%	0	0	65	5	16
Soup: Ten Vegetable, 8 oz	120	3	22%	0	0	620	3	21
Sandwiches: BBQ Chicken	570	14	22%	7	115	1540	43	69
Original Chicken Breast	750	47	56%	9	128	1075	35	50
Chicken Caesar	730	37	46%	12	144	2140	51	49
Turkey Breast	540	7	12%	0	118	800	49	68
Dressings: Balsamic Viniagrette, 2 T.	90	9	90%	1	0	240	0	3
BBQ, 2 Tbsp	40	0	0%	0	0	280	0	10
Caesar, 2 Tbsp	160	18	95%	4	14	180	0	1
Chinese Chicken Salad, 2 Tbsp	110	8	65%	2	0	110	0	8
Chopped Salad, 2 Tbsp	100	7	63%	5	0	350	0	8
Cranberry Sauce, 1 oz	45	0	0%	0	0	14	0	11
Gravy, 2 oz	25	1	38%	0	0	310	1	3
Lahvash (flatbread), each	95	0	0%	0	0	145	4	20
Hot Sides								
Baked Yam	360	0	0%	0	0	25	5	86
Black Beans	140	2	13%	0	0	570	8	23
Confetti Rice	130	0	0%	0	0	165	3	29
Creamed Spinach	140	12	77%	6	38	395	3	9
Hand-Mashed Potatoes	185	5	24%	3	15	360	3	32
Macaroni & Cheese	270	11	37%	6	31	245	11	28
Roasted Garlic Potatoes	115	2	16%	1	3	165	2	22

Krystal®

	Cal	Fat	%Fc	S.Fat	Chol	Sod	Pro	Car
Breakfast								
Biscuit: Plain	260	15	52%	4	0	570	4	27
Bacon, Egg & Cheese	390	25	58%	8	225	870	12	28
Chik	340	17	45%	6	25	990	11	34
Sausage	440	32	65%	11	55	850	12	27
Country Breakfast	660	42	57%	14	590	1450	24	46
Hash Browns	190	13	62%	5	10	340	1	17
Sunriser	240	14	53%	5	255	460	12	14
Sandwiches								
Krystal: Regular	160	7	39%	3	20	260	7	17
Double	260	13	45%	6	40	550	13	24
Bacon Cheese	190	10	47%	4.5	25	430	10	16
Cheese	180	9	45%	4	25	430	9	16
Double Cheese	310	16	46%	7	65	800	16	26
Chik	240	11	41%	3.5	25	640	11	24
Chili Cheese Pup	210	12	51%	5	40	510	9	17
Corn Pup	260	19	66%	8	50	480	5	19
Plain Pup	170	9	48%	3.5	25	500	6	15
Fries								
Regular	370	18	44%	7	15	85	4	49
Chili Cheese	540	28	47%	13	45	800	13	59
Desserts/Drinks								
Chocolate Shake	380	11	26%	7	50	410	12	58
Krystal Chill	200	7	32%	3.5	25	1130	13	22
Apple Turnover	220	10	41%	3.5	0	300	3	31
Lemon Pie	360	10	25%	3.5	55	190	7	60

La Salsa Fresh Mexican Grill®

	Cal	Fat	%Fc	S.Fat	Chol	Sod	Pro	Car
Taco								
Mexico City Taco, Chicken	250	7	25%	2	50	130	17	27
Fish Taco (Sonora)	225	9	36%	4	45	440	15	21
La Salsa, Chicken w. Cheese	300	10	30%	4	55	220	17	35
Vegetarian w. Cheese	290	8	25%	3	5	285	12	39
Burrito								
Bean & Cheese	535	14	24%	6	10	920	16	27
Californian 'Veggie'	600	19	29%	8	20	800	20	87
El Champion Burrito (12", 2lbs)	1100	52	43%	18	200	1200	60	100
Burrito Grande	550	26	43%	9	95	530	30	50
Sides								
Cheese, 1/2 oz	60	5	75%	3	20	150	3	3
Black Beans (no cheese), 5 oz	290	1	3%	1	0	110	15	38
Rice, 3.5 oz	170	3	16%	0	0	230	3	31
1/2 Rice & 1/2 Beans (no cheese)	310	3	9%	0	9	250	9	44
Salsa, 2 Tbsp	15	0	0%	0	0	300	0	3

Pizza: Per Slice	Cal	Fat	%Fc	S.Fat	Chol	Sod	Pro	Carb
12" **Round:** Cheese	160	6	33%	3	15	320	8	22
Pepperoni	180	8	40%	3	20	420	9	21
12" **Square:** Cheese	140	5	32%	2	10	280	7	19
Pepperoni	160	6	34%	2.5	15	350	8	19
12" **Thin:** Cheese	120	6	45%	2.5	15	280	6	12
Pepperoni	150	8	48%	3.5	20	380	7	12
14" **Round:** Cheese	170	6	32%	2.5	15	360	8	23
Meatsa	220	10	41%	4	25	570	11	24
Pepperoni	200	8	36%	4	20	460	9	23
Supreme	230	10	39%	4	25	550	11	25
Veggie	190	7	33%	3	15	500	9	25
14" **Square:** Cheese	140	5	32%	2	10	280	7	19
Pepperoni	160	7	39%	2.5	15	350	8	19
14" **Thin:** Cheese	130	6	42%	2.5	15	320	6	13
Pepperoni	160	9	51%	3.5	20	420	7	13
16" **Round:** Cheese	230	8	31%	3.5	20	440	11	30
Pepperoni	260	11	38%	4.5	25	570	12	31
18" **Round:** Cheese	240	8	30%	3.5	20	470	12	32
Pepperoni	270	11	37%	4.5	30	600	13	32
Baby Pan! Pan!	310	15	44%	5.5	30	640	14	32
Pizza By The Slice: Cheese	290	10	31%	4.5	25	570	14	39
Pepperoni	340	14	37%	6	35	770	16	39
Sandwiches (Cold): Ham & Cheese	600	22	33%	9.5	55	1410	33	68
Italia	690	31	40%	13	75	1660	34	68
Tuna	820	39	43%	4.5	80	1330	45	71
Turkey	600	21	32%	9.5	55	1570	38	66
Veggie	580	24	37%	9.5	40	940	26	70
Sandwiches (Hot): Meatsa	960	53	50%	23	115	2240	48	72
Pepperoni	980	56	51%	26	125	2290	48	71
Supreme; Cheeser	900	49	49%	21	105	2040	42	74
Vegetarian	760	36	43%	17	65	1360	38	74
Salads: Antipasto	80	6	68%	2.5	15	340	5	4
Caesar	80	3	34%	1.5	5	190	5	7
Greek	60	3	45%	0	10	330	3	5
Tossed	50	0.5	9%	0	0	60	2	9
Dresssings (1 oz): Blue Cheese	230	24	94%	5	30	450	2	2
Buttermilk Ranch	270	29	97%	5	4	380	0	1
Caesar	230	25	98%	4.	55	360	1	1
Creamy Caesar; Golden Italian	220	23	94%	4	10	540	1	2
Fat Free Italian	25	0	0%	0	0	390	0	5
Honey French	220	18	74%	3	0	310	0	14
Thousand Island	220	21	86%	3	30	360	0	7
Italian Cheese Bread: 1 piece	110	5	41%	2	10	230	5	11
Crazy Bread: 1 stick, 1.2 oz	90	2.5	25%	0.5	0	120	3	14
Crazy Sauce: 4 oz	45	0	0%	0	0	250	1	9
Chicken Wings: 1 piece	50	4	72%	1	15	710	4	0
Cinnamon Stick	340	9	24%	1	0	440	8	57

Long John Silver's®

	Cal	Fat	%Fc	S.Fat	Chol	Sod	Pro	Carb
Sandwiches								
Ultimate Fish	480	25	47%	10	50	1400	19	46
Fish Sandwich	430	20	42%	5	35	1150	16	46
w. Cheese	480	25	47%	10	50	1390	19	46
Chicken Sandwich	340	14	37%	3.5	25	840	13	40
w. Cheese	390	19	44%	9	40	1090	16	40
Side Items								
Fries: Regular	250	15	54%	2.5	0	500	3	28
Large, 5 oz	420	24	51%	4	0	830	5	46
Cheese Sticks (3)	160	9	47%	4	10	360	6	12
Coleslaw, 4 oz	170	7	37%	0	0	310	2	23
Corn Cobbette: no butter	80	0.5	6%	0	0	0	3	19
w. butter	140	8	52%	1.5	0	0	3	19
Hushpuppy, 1 piece	60	2.5	38%	0	0	25	1	9
Rice, 4 oz	180	4	20%	0.5	0	560	3	34
Soup: Broccoli Cheese, 8 oz bowl	180	12	60%	4.5	15	1240	5	13
Clam Chowder: 1 cup	260	12	42%	5	35	1020	12	26
1 bowl	520	24	42%	10	70	2040	24	52
Salads								
Garden Salad	45	0	0%	0	0	25	3	9
Grilled Chicken Salad	140	2.5	16%	0.5	45	260	20	10
Ocean Chef Salad	130	2	14%	0	60	540	14	15
Side Salad, no dressing	20	0	0%	0	0	10	1	3
Dressing: Italian, 1 pkt	90	9	90%	1.5	0	290	0	2
Ranch, 1 pkt	170	18	95%	3	10	260	0	1
Ranch, Fat Free, 1 pkt	40	0	0%	0	0	290	0	9
Thousand Island, 1 pkt	120	10	75%	1.5	15	290	0	5
French, Fat Free, 1 pkt	40	0	0%	0	0	240	0	10
Chicken								
Battered Plank, 1 piece	140	8	52%	2.5	20	400	8	9
Fish								
Breaded Clams, 1 order	250	14	51%	3.5	35	560	9	25
Battered Shrimp, 1 piece	45	2.5	50%	1	15	125	2	3
Country Style Breaded Fish, 1 piece	200	10	45%	1.5	10	300	10	17
Crabcake, 1 cake	150	9	54%	2	15	180	4	12
Lemon Crumbed: Regular, 2 pces	240	12	45%	4	55	790	23	10
A-la-carte, 2 pces w. rice	480	17	32%	5	55	1490	27	52
Add-A-Piece (1) w.rice	150	7	42%	2	30	460	12	9
Fish Meal, 1 meal	730	29	36%	6	60	1720	31	89
Popcorn Shrimp, 1 serving	320	15	42%	2.5	85	1440	15	33
Condiments								
Honey Mustard Sauce, 1 pkt	20	0	0%	0	0	45	0	5
Ketchup, 1 pkt	10	0	0%	0	0	110	0	2
Malt Vinegar, 1 pkt	0	0	0%	0	0	15	0	0
Shrimp Sauce, 1 pkt	15	0	0%	0	0	180	0	3
Sweet & Sour Sauce, 1 pkt	20	0	0%	0	0	45	0	5
Tartar Sauce, 1 pkt	40	3.5	79%	0.5	5	105	0	2

	Cal	Fat	%Fc	S.Fat	Chol	Sod	Pro	Carb
Desserts: *Per Piece*								
Banana Split Sundae Pie	300	17	51%	9	15	130	4	34
Chocolate Créme Pie	280	17	55%	8	15	125	4	29
Double Lemon Pie	350	18	46%	10	40	180	6	41
Dutch Apple Pie	290	13	40%	4	0	250	2	44
Pecan Pie	390	19	44%	4	40	250	3	53
Pineapple Créme Cheesecake	310	17	49%	9	5	105	4	36
Strawberries N' Créme Pie	280	15	48%	8	15	130	4	32
Beverages: *Per Medium*								
Coca-Cola	270	0	0%	0	0	20	0	62
Diet Coke	0	0	0%	0	0	25	0	0
Dr Pepper	250	0	0%	0	0	60	0	69
H-C Pink Lemonade	260	0	0%	0	0	110	0	62
Minute Maid Lemonade	260	0	0%	0	0	110	0	69
Sprite	260	0	0%	0	0	55	0	62

Mazzio's Pizza®

	Cal	Fat	%Fc	S.Fat	Chol	Sod	Pro	Carb
Appetizers: *Per Serving*								
Garlic Bread w. Cheese, 2 slices	700	35	45%	7	15	1280	21	74
Meat Nachos	500	37	67%	17	15	1200	21	21
Sandwiches								
Ham & Cheese	790	39	44%	13	85	1900	40	71
BQ Beef & Cheddar	580	24	37%	11	95	1260	39	51
Chicken & Cheddar	570	24	38%	8	70	1350	33	56
Deluxe Submarine	810	43	48%	13	75	2240	39	68
Pizza: *Per Slice*								
Original Crust: Cheese	270	9	30%	3	17	660	12	37
The Works	345	14	37%	5	31	920	16	38
Pepperoni	305	12	35%	5	24	800	13	37
Sausage	35	14	38%	5	28	900	15	37
Deep Pan: Cheese	350	13	33%	5	15	620	17	42
Combo	410	18	40%	6	20	930	19	42
Pepperoni	380	17	40%	5	25	740	18	38
Sausage	430	21	44%	8	25	1040	21	41
Thin Crust: Cheese	220	12	49%	4	17	440	9	22
Pasta								
Chicken Parmesan	600	19	29%	3	50	1600	39	68
Fettuccine Alfredo, small	440	28	57%	16	55	680	14	34
Meat Lasagna, small	460	25	49%	10	85	1370	24	36
Spaghetti, small	290	10	31%	3	5	800	11	39

Feedback welcome

Please send comments to: Allan Borushek
POB 1616, Costa Mesa CA 92628
Email: allan@calorieking.com

McDonald's®

	Cal	Fat	%Fc	S.Fat	Chol	Sod	Pro	Carb
Sandwiches/Burgers								
Big Mac®	590	34	52%	11	85	1090	24	47
Big N' Tasty®	540	32	53%	10	80	970	24	39
with Cheese	590	37	56%	12	95	1210	27	40
BBQ Chicken Sandwich	340	8	21%	2	25	1180	18	48
Cheeseburger	330	14	38%	6	45	830	15	36
Chicken McGrill®	450	18	36%	3	60	970	26	46
Plain (no mayo)	340	7	19%	1.5	50	890	26	45
Crispy Chicken Deluxe™	550	27	44%	4.5	50	1180	23	54
Filet-O-Fish®	470	26	50%	5	50	890	15	45
Hamburger	280	10	32%	4	30	590	12	35
Quarter Pounder®	430	21	44%	8	70	840	23	37
with Cheese	530	30	51%	13	95	1310	28	38
Sourdough Crispy Chicken	580	29	45%	8	70	1400	26	54
Sourdough Supreme Burger	660	40	55%	16	110	1900	31	44
French Fries: Small	210	10	43%	1.5	0	135	3	26
Medium	450	22	44%	4	0	290	6	57
Large	540	26	43%	4.5	0	350	8	68
Super Size	610	29	42%	5	0	390	9	77
Breakfast Menu								
Bacon, Egg & Cheese Biscuit	480	31	58%	10	250	1410	20	31
Biscuit, 2.7 oz	240	11	41%	2.5	0	640	4	30
Breakfast Burrito	290	16	50%	6	170	680	13	24
Breakfast Sourdough	560	33	53%	11	260	1270	22	41
Egg McMuffin®	290	12	37%	4.5	235	790	17	27
English Muffin, 2 oz	140	2	13%	0	0	210	4	25
Ham, Egg & Cheese Bagel	550	23	38%	8	255	1490	26	58
Hash Browns, 2 oz	130	8	55%	1.5	0	330	1	14
Hotcakes: Plain, (3)	340	8	21%	1.5	20	630	9	58
w. Margarine, 2 pats	420	17	36%	3	20	750	9	56
w. Margarine, 2 pats & Syrup (1)	600	17	26%	3	20	770	9	104
Sausage Biscuit	410	28	61%	8	35	930	10	30
with Egg	490	33	61%	10	245	1010	16	31
Sausage McMuffin®	360	23	58%	8	45	740	13	26
with Egg	440	28	57%	10	255	890	19	27
Sausage Patty	170	16	85%	5	35	290	6	0
Scrambled Eggs (2), 3^{1}/2 oz	160	11	62%	3.5	425	170	13	1
Spanish Omelette Bagel	690	38	50%	14	275	1570	27	60
Steak, Egg & Cheese Bagel	700	35	45%	13	290	1290	38	57
Chicken McNuggets®/Sauces								
Chick McNuggets®4 Pces	190	11	52%	2.5	35	360	10	13
6 Pieces	290	17	53%	5.5	55	540	15	20
9 Pieces	430	25	52%	5	80	810	23	29
BBQ/Sweet 'N' Sour Sce (1 pkg), 1 oz	45	0	0%	0	0	200	0	10
Honey (1 pkg), ^{1}/2 oz	45	0	0%	0	0	0	0	12
Honey Mustard (1 pkg), ^{1}/2 oz	50	4.5	81%	0.5	10	85	0	3
Hot Mustard Sauce (1 pkg), 1 oz	60	3.5	53%	0	5	240	1	7

	Cal	Fat	%FC	S.Fat	Chol	Sod	Pro	Carb
McSalad Shaker™ Salads/Dressings								
Chef Salad	150	8	48%	3.5	95	740	17	5
Garden Salad	100	6	54%	3	75	120	7	4
Grilled Chicken Caesar Salad	100	2.5	23%	1.5	40	240	17	3
Croutons (1 pkg)	50	1	18%	0	0	105	1	9
Caesar Dressing (1 pkg)	150	13	78%	2.5	10	400	1	5
Fat-Free Herb Vinaigrette (1 pkg)	35	0	0%	0	0	260	0	8
Honey Mustard Dressing (1 pkg)	160	11	62%	1.5	15	260	1	13
Ranch Dressing (1 pkg)	170	18	95%	2.5	15	460	1	3
Red French Reduced Calorie (1 pkg)	130	6	42%	1	0	360	0	18
Thousand Island Dressing (1 pkg)	130	9	62%	1.5	15	350	1	11
Light Mayonnaise (1 pkg)	45	4.5	90%	0.5	10	100	0	1
Muffins/Danishes: Apple Danish	340	15	40%	3	20	340	5	47
Cheese Danish, 3.7 oz	400	21	47%	5	40	400	7	45
Cinnamon Roll, 3.4 oz	390	18	42%	5	65	310	6	50
Lowfat Apple Bran Muffin, 4 oz	300	3	9%	0.5	0	380	6	61
Desserts/Sundaes/Cookies/Shakes								
Baked Apple Pie, 2³/4 oz	260	13	45%	3.5	0	200	3	34
Chocolate Chip Cookie, 1 pkg	280	14	45%	8	40	170	3	37
Fruit 'n Yogurt Parfait: w. granola	380	5	12%	2	15	240	10	76
no granola	280	4	13%	2	15	115	8	53
McDonaldland® Cookies, 1 pkg	230	8	31%	2	0	250	3	38
McFlurry™: Butterfinger®	620	22	32%	14	70	260	16	90
M&M®	630	23	33%	15	75	210	16	90
Nestlé Crunch®	630	24	34%	16	75	230	16	89
Oreo® Cookie	570	20	32%	12	70	280	15	82
Nuts (Sundae/Topping), 1/4 oz	40	3.5	79%	0	0	55	2	2
Vanilla Reduced Fat Icecream Cone	150	4.5	27%	3	20	75	4	23
Root Beer Float, 16 fl.oz	310	7	20%	5	30	105	6	57
Shakes: average all, small, 14 fl.oz	360	9	23%	6	40	220	11	59
Sundae: Hot Caramel Sundae	360	10	25%	6	35	180	7	61
Hot Fudge Sundae, 6.3 oz	340	12	32%	9	30	170	8	52
Strawberry Sundae	290	7	22%	5	30	95	7	50
Drinks: Orange Juice, 6 fl.oz	80	0	0%	0	0	20	0	20
1% Lowfat Milk, 8 fl.oz ctn	100	2.5	23%	1.5	10	115	8	13
Coca-Cola Classic (25% Ice):								
Small, 16 fl.oz	150	0	0%	0	0	15	0	40
Medium, 21 fl.oz	210	0	0%	0	0	20	0	58
Large, 32 fl.oz	310	0	0%	0	0	30	0	86
Super Size, 42 fl.oz	410	0	0%	0	0	40	0	113
Diet Coke: Medium, 21 fl.oz	0	0	0%	0	0	30	0	0
Sprite(25% Ice): Small, 16 fl.oz	150	0	0%	0	0	55	0	39
Medium, 21 fl.oz	210	0	0%	0	0	80	0	56
Large, 32 fl. oz	310	0	0%	0	0	115	0	83
Super Size, 42 fl.oz	410	0	0%	0	0	160	0	109
Hi-C Orange Drink: Small, 16 fl.oz	160	0	0%	0	0	30	0	44
Medium, 21 fl.oz	240	0	0%	0	0	40	0	64

Mimi's Cafe®

	Cal	Fat	%FC	S.Fat	Chol	Sod	Pro	C
Broiled 10 oz Halibut Steak	625	16	23%	na	95	na	69	5
Capellini w. Tomatoes & Basil	680	8	11%	na	0	na	21	13
EggBeater Fitness Omelette	655	8	11%	na	0	na	36	11
Half-A-Turkey Sandwich	410	6	13%	na	75	na	33	5
Maggie's Chicken and Fruit	545	9	15%	na	135	na	57	5
Roasted Turkey Breast	540	8	13%	na	210	na	65	5
Two "AA" Large Eggs	395	8	18%	na	0	na	19	6
Vegetable Lover's Salad	525	4	7%	na	0	na	15	10
Veggie Burger	480	11	21%	na	0	na	27	6

Mrs Field's Cookies®

Per 1 Cookie, 1.7 oz

	Cal	Fat	%FC	S.Fat	Chol	Sod	Pro	C
Butter; Butter Toffee	220	10	41%	6	40	140	2	3
Chewy Fudge	220	11	45%	7	25	60	2	3
Coconut Macadamia	210	9	38%	3.5	15	170	2	2
Debra's Special	210	9	38%	4.5	30	140	3	2
Milk Choc	230	11	43%	7	30	140	3	2
Milk Choc w. Walnuts/Macadamia	240	13	48%	7	30	135	3	2
Oatmeal Raisin	180	7	35%	4	26	165	2	2
Peanut Butter	230	12	47%	6	35	190	4	2
Pumpkin Harvest	200	10	45%	6	30	200	3	2
Semi-Sweet Chocolate	230	10	39%	7	30	130	2	3
w. Pecans/Walnuts	220	12	49%	6	20	115	2	2
Triple Chocolate	220	10	41%	7	30	140	3	3
White Chunk Macadamia	240	13	49%	7	30	125	3	2

Nibblers: Per 2 Cookies, 1 oz

	Cal	Fat	%FC	S.Fat	Chol	Sod	Pro	C
Debra's Special	100	4.5	40%	2	10	80	1	1
Milk Choc w. Walnuts	120	6	45%	3	10	65	1	1
Peanut Butter; Triple Choc	110	6	49%	2.5	15	95	2	1
Semi-Sweet Chocolate	110	5	40%	3	10	60	1	1
White Chunk Macadamia	120	7	53%	3.5	10	60	1	1

Mrs Winner's Chicken®

Menu Items

	Cal	Fat	%FC	S.Fat	Chol	Sod	Pro	C
Biscuit	245	5	18%	na	0.5	500	4	4
Chicken: Baked Chicken Fillet	120	2	15%	na	35	360	10	0.
Breaded Chicken Sandwich	205	10	44%	na	35	1000	19	1
Chicken Fillet Sandwich	380	7	17%	na	30	540	12	4
Chicken Salad	585	8	12%	na	5	875	9	3
Chicken Salad Sandwich	315	6	17%	na	4	600	10	3
Coleslaw	190	16	76%	na	4	560	1	
Potato Fries	225	9	36%	na	4	220	6	2
Seafood Salad	555	9	15%	na	5	760	5	4
Steak Sandwich	540	11	18%	na	20	650	11	4

Nathan's Famous®

	Cal	Fat	%Fc	S.Fat	Chol	Sod	Pro	Carb
amburgers: Regular	435	23	48%	10	77	280	25	32
Double Burger	670	41	55%	18	154	460	44	32
Super Burger	535	32	54%	9	86	525	27	34
andwiches: Chicken Salad	155	4	23%	1	49	345	20	9
eaded Chicken Sandwich	510	25	44%	4	56	930	23	48
arbroiled Chicken S'wich	290	6	19%	1	53	860	24	35
eese Steak Sandwich	485	26	48%	10	73	580	26	37
let of Fish S'wich	405	15	33%	2	32	715	20	46
strami Sandwich	325	12	33%	4	48	1015	21	34
rkey Sandwich	270	2	7%	0	27	1460	28	34
atters: Fried Clam	1025	51	45%	7	49	1825	23	119
Chicken, 2 piece	1095	66	54%	14	212	1415	54	72
4 pieces	1790	109	55%	23	425	2370	102	99
Fillet of Fish	1455	74	46%	10	147	1840	61	137
Fried Shrimp	795	34	38%	5	83	1435	23	100
ench Fries	515	26	46%	4	0	60	9	62
ank Nuggets (7)	360	24	61%	6	46	745	9	25
ankfurter	310	19	55%	8	45	820	13	22

Olive Garden®

	Cal	Fat	%Fc	S.Fat	Chol	Sod	Pro	Carb
nch: Capellini Pomodora, 13 oz	380	10	24%	2.5	5	1030	13	60
icken Giardino, 13 oz	360	10	25%	3.5	50	900	23	47
guine alla Marinara, 11 oz	330	6	16%	0.5	0	710	10	57
rimp Primavera, 11 oz	400	6	14%	2.5	125	820	26	60
nner: Chicken Giardino, 21 oz	550	10	16%	4	85	1000	42	70
pellini Pomodora, 21 oz	620	16	23%	4	10	1620	22	98
guine alla Marinara, 26 oz	530	10	17%	1	0	1100	17	94
rimp Primavera, 19 oz	730	12	15%	4.5	255	1580	50	105
xtras: Minestrone Soup, 6 fl.oz	100	1	9%	0	0	550	4	17
eadstick, plain, 1 stick	140	1.5	10%	0	0	270	5	26

Papa John's Pizza®

r Slice: $^1/_8$ Large Pizza (14")	Cal	Fat	%Fc	S.Fat	Chol	Sod	Pro	Carb
iginal: All the Meats	410	18	40%	7	35	1040	20	42
eese; Garden	300	10	30%	3	20	550	14	37
pperoni	310	13	38%	5	25	760	15	35
usage	340	13	34%	6	25	810	15	40
e Works	370	17	41%	6	30	840	18	37
in Crust: All the Meats	330	20	55%	9	40	920	15	23
eese; Garden Special	240	12	45%	6	20	540	10	23
pperoni	270	15	50%	7	24	580	10	22
usage	270	15	50%	7	30	730	12	22
e Works	320	20	56%	8	35	760	14	24
eese Sticks, (2)	160	6	34%	1.5	10	290	7	20

Panda Express®

	Cal	Fat	%FC	S.Fat	Chol	Sod	Pro	Carb
Chicken: Black Pepper, 5 oz	210	10	43%	2	50	570	16	11
Orange Chicken, 5 oz	310	13	35%	2.5	65	420	17	31
Chicken w. Mushrooms, 5 oz	170	9	47%	1.5	35	570	12	9
Chicken w. String Beans, 5 oz	180	9	45%	1.5	35	620	12	12
Spicy Chicken w. Peanuts, 5 oz	510	29	49%	5	95	1250	35	28
Beef: Beef & Broccoli, 5 oz	180	11	55%	2.5	15	910	8	13
Pork: Sweet & Sour Pork, 4 oz	310	20	58%	7	75	250	21	8
Sweet & Sour Sauce, 2 oz	60	0	0%	0	0	150	0	16
Vegetables: Mixed Vegetables, 5 oz	80	3	38%	0	0	450	1	11
Soups: Hot & Sour Soup, 12 oz	110	4	27%	0.5	0	890	8	13
Egg Flower Soup, 12 oz	80	0	0%	0	0	640	3	18
Chow Mein & Rice: Per 8 oz Serve								
Vegetable Fried Rice	410	19	41%	3	110	440	8	47
Steamed Rice	220	0	0%	0	0	5	5	48
Lo Mein	270	10	33%	1.5	35	1090	7	37
Vegetable Chow Mein	300	10	30%	2	0	610	8	43
Egg Rolls: 2 rolls, 3 oz	190	6	32%	1	0	490	4	30

Perkin's® Family Restaurant

	Cal	Fat	%FC	S.Fat	Chol	Sod	Pro	Carb
Entrees: Chicken Dinner	620	13	19%	na	136	1360	60	60
Fish Dinner	470	7	13%	na	133	1390	33	60
Fruit Cup	50	0.5	9%	na	0	10	1	12
'Lite & Healthy'	105	2	17%	na	0	495	4	15
Omelettes: Country Club	930	79	76%	na	1154	1135	47	6
Deli Ham & Cheese	960	79	74%	na	864	1830	53	8
'Everything' Omelette	695	54	70%	na	814	870	45	9
Granny's Country Omelette	940	82	79%	na	810	785	43	7
w. 9 oz Hash Browns	1245	90	65%	na	810	870	48	57
Salads: Chef's, Mini	215	11	46%	na	55	645	23	7
Muffins: Banana Nut	585	29	45%	na	92	700	9	75
Blueberry	505	23	41%	na	88	670	7	71
Carrot	560	23	37%	na	81	780	7	88
Choc Choc Chip	545	26	43%	na	83	630	10	73
Cranberry Nut	560	28	45%	na	88	670	9	71
Oat Bran: Regular	515	16	28%	na	0	590	10	87
98% fat-free	495	1	2%	na	5	800	12	111
Pancakes: Buttermilk, (3)	440	12	25%	na	24	990	13	70
Harvest Grain: w. Low-Cal Syrup (5)	475	3.5	7%	na	0	1640	11	93
Short Stack (3)	270	2	7%	na	0	1020	7	56
Pies (Per Slice): Apple Pie	520	26	45%	na	0	460	3	72
Cherry Pie	570	24	38%	na	0	700	4	84
Coconut Cream Pie	440	21	43%	na	5	490	6	56
French Silk Pie	550	34	57%	na	53	480	4	59
Lemon Meringue Pie	395	15	34%	na	0	530	2	63
Peanut Butter Brownie	455	27	53%	na	29	435	9	4

Peter Piper™ Pizza

	Cal	Fat	%Fc	S.Fat	Chol	Sod	Pro	Carb
Pizza (Per Slice): Bacon, 1/8 large	330	12	33%	4	27	440	17	39
Beef, 1/8 large	295	8	24%	4	20	480	16	39
Black Olive, 1/8 large	280	7	23%	3	18	480	14	40
Cheese, 1/8 large	270	6	20%	3	18	270	14	39
Extra Cheddar, 1/8 large	300	9	27%	5	27	330	16	39
Green Pepper, 1/8 large	270	6	20%	3	18	270	14	39
Ham, 1/8 large	275	6	20%	3	21	330	15	39
Jalapeno, 1/8 large	270	6	20%	3	18	335	14	39
Mushroom, 1/8 large	205	5	22%	2	13	200	11	30
Onion, 1/8 large	270	6	20%	3	18	270	14	39
Pepperoni, 1/8 large	310	9	26%	5	24	555	15	39
Pineapple; Tomato, 1/8 large	275	6	20%	3	18	270	14	40
Sausage/Salam, 1/8 large	300	8	24%	5	25	520	16	39
Express Lunch, 1/2 pizza	360	12	30%	6	28	720	20	42

1-Potato-2®

	Cal	Fat	%Fc	S.Fat	Chol	Sod	Pro	Carb
Per Baked Potato (No Skin)								
Ultra-Lites: Chicken Stir-Fry	330	3	8%	1	21	1290	23	62
Chicken Fajita; Carribean Chicken	270	1.5	5%	0.5	21	555	16	49
Chick, Mushroom, Rst Red Pepper	245	2	7%	0.5	21	715	13	45
Crab & Broccoli DeLite	335	2.5	7%	1	35	740	21	57
Vegie & Herb Cheese	240	1.5	6%	1	5	425	13	44
Lite: Chicken Caesar & Broccoli	375	12	29%	3	31	845	21	50
Herb Roasted Vegetable	260	6	21%	1	1	210	6	48
Fresh Mex Chicken; Spinach Souffle	320	9	25%	4	60	570	15	45
Gourmet: Bacon & Cheese	660	47	64%	18	61	920	20	39
Bacon Double Cheeseburger	765	54	64%	21	88	1290	30	40
BBQ Chick, Cheddar, Bacon	685	43	56%	17	90	1765	31	44
Broccoli & Cheese	545	36	59%	14	42	575	16	45
Chicken Broccoli & Chedd.; 3 Cheese	590	37	56%	15	63	820	23	45
Chicken Caesar & Broccoli	710	51	65%	10	36	1375	16	53
Crab, Broccoli & Cheese	595	35	53%	14	55	1230	25	45
Mexican	670	46	62%	17	70	1070	18	50
Philly Steak & Cheese	675	40	53%	6	69	1410	34	45
Potato Skins (with Sour Cream)								
Bacon 'n Cheddar, 9 oz	975	53	49%	25	98	1340	29	100
Southwestern, 11 oz	910	46	45%	22	84	1425	27	105
Fresh Cut Fries: Small, 13 oz	615	39	57%	7	0	320	5	60
Topped Fries: Nacho Cheese	840	54	58%	11	13	625	10	80
Fresh Fries 'n Chicken Tenders	920	50	49%	9	48	895	26	92
Soups: Baked Potato Soup, 13 oz	640	26	37%	11	52	1630	20	81
Brocolli & Chse Potato Soup, 13 oz	665	29	39%	13	58	1435	21	80
Country Skillets: Idaho "Nachos"	1010	60	53%	20	82	840	30	88
BBQ Chick, Cheddar & Bacon	890	57	58%	16	63	760	24	70
Bacon, Ranch & Cheddar	1090	74	61%	20	71	940	19	87

Pick Up Stix®

	Cal	Fat	%FC	S.Fat	Chol	Sod	Pro	Ca
California Rolls	200	8	36%	na	10	320	5	2?
Beef Dishes: House Special	875	52	53%	na	130	840	50	4?
Mongolian	350	20	53%	na	50	240	20	2?
Szechwan	340	20	52%	na	50	275	20	2?
and Broccoli	510	27	48%	na	65	390	28	3?
Bowls								
Teriyaki Chicken	1155	22	17%	na	230	3000	83	148
Teriyaki Vegetable	450	1.5	3%	na	0	1,355	12	96
Buddah's Feast: Dark	105	0.5	4%	na	1	145	3	1?
Light	80	0.5	6%	na	0	60	3	1?
Chicken Dishes: Cashew	360	16	40%	na	75	265	20	34
Garlic	285	12	38%	na	75	195	19	2?
House	755	34	40%	na	215	800	50	5?
Kung Pao	440	22	44%	na	110	370	29	33
Lemon Twisted	260	3	9%	na	55	160	21	3?
Orange Peel	535	15	26%	na	80	715	21	78
Sweet n Sour	475	22	41%	na	25	160	12	6?
w/Vegetables	195	3	13%	na	55	185	21	20
Chow Mein								
Beef	350	10	25%	na	70	180	15	5?
Chicken	355	9	22%	na	85	175	16	5?
House Special	360	9	23%	na	90	190	16	5?
Shrimp	310	5	16%	na	100	200	12	5?
Vegetable	270	3	12%	na	55	150	9	5?
Fried Rice: Beef	505	16	29%	na	135	960	18	68
Chicken	475	13	25%	na	145	575	18	7?
Egg	420	8	17%	na	110	550	11	7?
House	480	14	26%	na	150	590	18	7?
Shrimp	430	10	20%	na	155	595	15	7?
Vegetable	390	8	19%	na	110	550	11	6?
Rice: White	205	0.5	2%	na	0	2	4	4?
Salad								
Chicken Salad w/out Dressing	470	20	38%	na	80	445	40	3?
Chinese Chicken Salad w/Lime Dress.	675	20	27%	na	80	1330	40	3?
Chinese Chicken Salad w/Orig. Dress.	650	22	31%	na	80	930	42	7?
Shrimp								
Black Bean	190	5	22%	na	110	260	13	2?
Garlic	185	5	22%	na	110	250	13	2?
Orange Peel	310	5	13%	na	105	755	13	5?
Szechwan	180	5	24%	na	110	290	13	2?
w/Vegetables	170	5	24%	na	105	170	12	1?
Soup: Hot & Sour	290	5	14%	na	110	535	18	2?
Wonton	290	13	39%	na	50	395	16	2?
Vegetables: Szechwan	105	1	10%	na	1	180	3	2?

*For extra listings of Fast-Food Restaurants ~
Refer to www.CalorieKing.com*

	Cal	Fat	%Fc	S.Fat	Chol	Sod	Pro	Carb
Pan Pizza: Per Medium Slice								
Beef Topping	330	18	49%	7	20	690	14	29
Cheese	290	14	43%	6	10	590	12	28
Chicken Supreme	270	12	40%	4	15	580	13	29
Ham	260	12	42%	4	15	610	11	28
Italian Sausage	340	20	53%	7	25	720	13	29
Meat Lover's®	360	21	53%	7	30	840	14	29
Pepperoni	280	14	45%	5	15	610	11	28
Pepperoni Lover's®	330	18	49%	7	20	760	14	29
Pork Topping	320	17	48%	6	20	730	15	45
Super Supreme	340	18	48%	6	25	780	13	29
Supreme	320	17	48%	6	20	670	13	29
Veggie Lover's®	270	12	40%	4	5	510	10	30
Personal Pan Pizza: Per Pizza								
Beef Topping	710	35	44%	14	45	1580	31	71
Cheese	630	28	40%	12	25	1370	28	71
Ham	580	23	36%	9	35	1450	27	70
Italian Sausage	740	39	47%	14	55	1640	31	71
Pepperoni	620	28	41%	11	30	1430	26	70
Pork Topping	700	34	44%	13	40	1670	31	71
Stuffed Crust: Per Large Slice								
Beef Topping	465	22	42%	10	30	1140	23	46
Cheese	445	19	38%	10	24	1090	22	46
Chicken Supreme	430	17	35%	8	32	1110	24	47
Ham	405	22	49%	12	39	1190	24	45
Italian Sausage	480	23	43%	10	35	1165	22	46
Meat Lover's®	545	29	48%	12	48	1430	26	46
Pepperoni	440	19	39%	9	27	1115	20	45
Pepperoni Lover's	525	26	45%	12	40	1415	26	46
Pork Topping	460	21	41%	10	29	1175	22	46
Super Supreme	505	25	45%	11	44	1370	25	46
Supreme	490	23	43%	10	33	1230	24	47
Veggie Lover's®	420	17	36%	8	19	1040	20	48
Thin 'n Crispy®: Per Medium Slice								
Beef Topping	270	15	50%	7	25	750	13	22
Cheese	200	9	41%	5	10	590	10	22
Chicken Supreme	200	7	32%	3.5	20	620	12	23
Ham	170	7	37%	3.5	15	610	9	21
Italian Sausage	290	17	53%	7	30	800	12	22
Meat Lover's®	310	19	55%	8	35	910	14	22
Pepperoni	190	9	43%	4	15	610	9	21
Pepperoni Lover's®	250	13	47%	6	20	760	12	22
Pork Topping	270	14	47%	6	25	820	13	22
Super Supreme	280	15	48%	5	25	840	13	23
Supreme	250	13	47%	6	20	710	12	23
Veggie Lover's®	190	7	33%	3	5	520	8	24

Pizza Hut® (Cont)

	Cal	Fat	%Fc	S.Fat	Chol	Sod	Pro	Car
Hand Tossed: Per Medium Slice								
Beef Topping	330	17	46%	8	25	880	16	29
Cheese	240	10	38%	5	10	650	12	28
Chicken Supreme	230	7	27%	3.5	15	650	13	29
Ham	260	10	35%	5	20	800	14	28
Italian Sausage	340	18.	48%	8	30	910	16	28
Meat Lover's®	320	17	48%	7	30	900	14	28
Pepperoni	280	13	42%	6	20	790	13	28
Pepperoni Lover's®	250	11	40%	4.5	15	730	11	27
Pork Topping	320	16	45%	7	25	920	16	29
Super Supreme	290	14	43%	6	25	850	13	29
Supreme	270	12	40%	5	20	730	13	29
Veggie Lover's®	220	8	33%	3	5	580	9	29
The Big New Yorker™: Per Slice								
Beef/Pork Topping	480	26	49%	11	40	1380	24	42
Cheese	380	17	40%	9	20	1140	19	41
Ham	340	13	34%	6	25	1160	18	41
Pepperoni	370	16	39%	7	20	1150	17	41
Italian Sausage	570	33	52%	14	55	1620	27	42
Supreme	450	23	46%	10	35	1350	22	43
Veggie Lover's®	450	22	44%	6	10	1340	18	52
The Edge: Per Square								
Chicken Supreme	90	3.5	35%	1.5	15	290	7	9
Meat Lover's®	160	11	62%	4.5	20	440	7	8
The Works	110	6	49%	2.5	10	270	5	9
Veggie Lover's®	70	3	39%	1.5	3	180	4	9
The Sicilian: Per Slice								
Beef Topping	260	11	38%	4.5	15	640	11	31
Cheese	290	13	40%	6	10	630	12	31
Chicken Supreme	270	11	37%	4	15	620	12	32
Ham	255	10	35%	5	14	745	11	30
Italian Sausage	335	18	49%	7.5	24	855	13	31
Meat Lovers	350	19	49%	7	25	830	14	31
Pepperoni	280	13	42%	5	15	630	10	31
Pepperoni Lovers	320	16	45%	7	20	780	13	31
Pork Topping	320	16	45%	6	20	750	13	31
Super Supreme	340	18	48%	6	20	780	13	32
Supreme	310	15	44%	6	15	690	12	32
Veggie Lovers	270	11	37%	4	15	620	12	32
Twisted Crust: Per Large Slice								
Cheese	450	16	32%	8	15	1210	20	58
Pepperoni	440	15	31%	6	20	1230	18	58
Supreme	470	18	34%	8	25	1280	20	59
Sandwiches: Ham & Cheese	550	21	34%	7	22	2150	33	57
Supreme Sandwich	640	28	39%	10	28	2150	34	62
Dessert Pizza: Apple, 1 slice	250	4.5	16%	1	0	230	3	48
Cherry, 1 slice	250	4.5	16%	1	0	220	3	47

Pizza Hut® (Cont)

	Cal	Fat	%Fc	S.Fat	Chol	Sod	Pro	Carb
sta: Cavatini Pasta	480	14	26%	6	8	1170	21	66
vatini Supreme Pasta	560	19	31%	8	10	1400	24	73
aghetti w. Marinara Sauce	490	6	11%	2	0	730	18	91
aghetti w. Meatballs	850	24	25%	10	17	1120	37	120
aghetti w. Meat Sauce	600	13	20%	5	8	910	23	98
des: Breadsticks, 1 serving	130	4	28%	1	0	170	3	20
eadstick Dipping Sce, 1 oz	30	0.5	15%	0	0	170	0.5	5
arlic Bread, 1 slice	150	8	48%	2	0	240	16	3
t Buffalo Wings (4)	210	12	51%	3	130	900	22	4
ild Wings (5)	200	12	54%	3.5	150	510	23	0
uce: Marinara (container)	60	1	15%	0	0	490	2	12
Ranch (container)	440	48	98%	8	20	840	2	4

Pizzeria Uno®

	Cal	Fat	%Fc	S.Fat	Chol	Sod	Pro	Carb
in Crust Pizza: 9" Individual								
getarian: w. Cheese	850	22	23%	12	55	1660	46	127
No Cheese	620	5	7%	1	0	1100	20	124
oup: Tomato Garden Veg.	125	1	7%	0	0	900	2.5	25
ght Lunch w. Soup	745	6	7%	1	0	2000	23	150
ntrees								
eggie Burger Meal	610	15	22%	1	0	1800	15	104
mato Basil Chicken	570	8	13%	1.5	55	1280	42	83
sty Pasta Marinara	380	3.5	8%	0.5	0	800	13	75
alads: Special House	90	1	10%	0	0	860	4	17
ght Lunch w. Salad	710	6	8%	1	0	1960	24	141
sta Green Salad	410	9	20%	1	0	700	14	69
eggie Dip Platter	460	11	22%	2	0	770	14	77

Popeye's®

	Cal	Fat	%Fc	S.Fat	Chol	Sod	Pro	Carb
hicken								
hicken Breast: Mild/Spicy	530	31	53%	11	195	1380	46	18
hicken Leg: Mild/Spicy	200	12	54%	4	108	500	17	7
hicken Thigh: Mild/Spicy	390	29	67%	10	150	887	25	12
hicken Wing: Mild/Spicy	220	15	61%	5	90	510	14	10
des								
scuit, 2 oz	225	12	48%	4	1	429	3	25
ajun Rice	180	7	35%	3	60	436	8	23
nnamon Apple Pie, 3 oz	250	10	36%	3	3	292	3	37
leslaw	235	17	65%	3	14	260	1	20
rn on the Cob	255	4	14%	1	0	24	7	48
ench Fries, 4.5 oz	380	18	43%	7	11	924	5	50
ashed Potatoes: no Gravy	95	2	19%	1	2	384	1	17
w. Gravy	120	4	30%	1	7	570	3	18
nion Rings, 4 oz	380	20	47%	8	15	270	7	43
ed Beans & Rice	340	19	50%	6	18	696	7	33

Quincy's® Family Steak House

	Cal	Fat	%FC	S.Fat	Chol	Sod	Pro	Carb
Steak: Chopped, 8 oz	500	42	76%	20	89	350	31	0
Country Style Steak w. Gravy	530	25	42%	7	54	1160	32	44
Cowboy Steak, 14 oz	580	33	51%	15	176	1310	61	0
Filet w. Bacon	340	17	45%	7	125	310	48	2
N.Y.Strip Steak, 10 oz	450	26	52%	13	148	155	53	1
Porterhouse Steak	680	46	61%	23	154	345	67	0
Ribeye, 10 oz	450	29	58%	13	116	155	48	0
Sirloin: Large	370	20	49%	9	119	390	46	2
Regular	285	16	51%	7	71	320	34	0
Sirloin Junior	195	10	46%	5	69	200	25	0
Sirloin Tips	205	8	35%	3	63	790	27	4
Smothered Strip Steak	620	41	60%	16	148	240	55	12
T-Bone, 13 oz	520	35	61%	18	118	265	51	0
Soups: Chili with Beans	235	11	42%	2	15	920	13	21
Clam Chowder	180	9	45%	1	0	835	3	21
Cream of Broccoli	170	10	53%	1	0	770	2	18
Vegetable Beef	90	2	20%	1	0	325	5	14
Entrees: Grilled Chicken	125	2	14%	0.5	55	540	25	1
Homestyle Chicken Filet	220	9	37%	2	25	680	13	21
Grilled Salmon	230	4	16%	1	109	110	46	1
Sth Breaded Shrimp	545	31	51%	6	135	820	19	47
Steak & Shrimp	680	39	52%	12	170	820	48	33
Roasted Herb Chicken	875	65	67%	17	340	1240	70	4
Roasted BBQ Chicken	940	65	62%	17	340	1550	70	21
Grilled Trout	300	12	36%	3	115	520	41	2
Sandwiches: No Mayo/Extras								
Bacon Cheeseburger	665	41	55%	17	87	1000	37	33
Grilled Chicken Sandwich	325	4	11%	1	55	1185	33	39
Philly Cheese Steak	590	30	46%	11	87	1685	37	38
Smothered Steak	430	15	31%	6	69	850	34	36
Spicy BBQ Chicken	370	5	12%	1	55	1610	34	45
Breads: Banana Nut	165	7	38%	1	5	195	2	22
Biscuit	270	15	50%	4	11	610	5	29
Cornbread	140	5	32%	1	0	340	3	19
Yeast Roll	160	4	23%	<1	0	285	1	29
Sides: Baked Potatoes	370	0	0%	0	0	25	8	86
Corn on the Cob	140	1	6%	20	0	540	5	33
Rice Pilaf	105	2	17%	0	0	270	2	20
Desserts: Banana Pudding	240	12	45%	9	10	240	3	30
Brownie Pudding Cake	310	5	15%	1	0	395	4	66
Chocolate Chip Cookie	60	3	45%	1	5	35	1	8
Apple Cobbler	255	8	28%	2	5	285	1	49
Cherry Cobbler; Peach Cobbler	300	8	24%	2	5	185	1	55
Frozen Yogurt	135	2	13%	1	5	85	5	25
Sugar Cookie	60	3	45%	1	5	30	1	8
Fudge Topping	105	4	34%	1	0	75	1	15
Pineapple Topping	80	0	0%	0	0	20	0	20

Rally's Hamburgers®

	Cal	Fat	%Fc	S.Fat	Chol	Sod	Pro	Carb
Burgers/Sandwiches								
Rallyburger	435	22	46%	7	63	1175	20	35
with Cheese	490	27	50%	13	78	1375	23	35
Big Buford	745	48	58%	20	151	1860	41	35
Chicken Fillet Sandwich	400	15	34%	4	42	790	21	43
Chili w. Cheese & Onion: 7 oz	360	22	55%	9	74	1145	23	20
13 oz size	670	41	55%	17	137	2125	43	37
Super Barbecue Bacon	595	31	47%	12	88	1710	29	49
Super Double Cheeseburger	760	48	57%	26	154	1735	41	37
French Fries								
Regular	210	11	47%	4	7	295	3	26
Large	320	16	45%	5	10	440	5	39
X-Large	425	21	44%	7	13	585	7	52
Shakes								
Vanilla, small	320	11	31%	6	38	200	9	49
Other flavors, small	410	12	26%	7	38	260	10	73

Rax®

	Cal	Fat	%Fc	S.Fat	Chol	Sod	Pro	Carb
Sandwiches								
Regular Rax	340	22	58%	7	54	710	16	31
Deluxe	520	35	61%	12	69	785	18	34
BBC (Beef Bacon & Cheddar)	715	51	64%	20	102	1455	28	36
Grilled Chicken	525	33	57%	8	69	995	24	32
Jr. Deluxe	370	25	61%	10	42	510	11	25
Barbeque Beef	400	20	45%	7	40	1030	13	43
Mushroom Melt	600	37	56%	13	104	1690	30	35
Turkey Bacon Club	680	46	61%	15	76	1900	29	37
Turkey	485	32	59%	8	50	1285	17	32
Cheddar Melt	345	23	60%	12	41	540	10	26
Philly Melt	540	32	53%	16	78	1295	28	35
Potatoes								
Plain	210	0	0%	0	0	10	0	50
Cheese/Broccoli	280	6	19%	3	4	620	7	50
Cheese	270	6	20%	3	4	620	7	47
Cheese/Bacon	400	19	43%	14	82	875	7	50
Butter	305	11	32%	9	0	30	0	50
Sour Cream Topping	260	4	14%	3	0	30	4	50
Soups								
Cream of Broccoli	170	10	53%	1	0	770	2	18
Chili w. Beans	235	11	42%	2	15	920	13	21
Salads								
Grilled Chicken Caesar	160	5	28%	3	50	1150	23	6
Caesar Side Salad	40	2	45%	1	5	330	2	3
Side Salad	40	4	90%	1	0	90	0	2
Gourmet Garden	220	9	37%	3	5	840	23	12

Red Lobster®

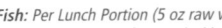

Fish: Per Lunch Portion (5 oz raw wt.)
(For **Dinner Portion** of 10 oz, double the figures.)
Prepared with No Added Fat
Add extra for butter sauce. [1 tsp = 30 cals; 3g fat (90%); 30mg sodium]

	Cal	Fat	%Fc	S.Fat	Chol	Sod	Pro	Carb
Catfish	170	10	53%	3	85	50	20	0
Cod (Atlantic)	100	1	9%	0	70	200	23	0
Flounder	100	1	9%	0	70	95	21	1
Grouper	110	1	8%	0	65	70	26	0
Haddock	110	1	8%	0	85	180	24	2
Halibut	110	1	8%	0	60	105	25	1
Lemon Sole	120	1	8%	0	65	90	27	1
Mackerel	190	12	57%	4	100	250	20	1
Monkfish	110	1	8%	0	80	95	24	0
Norwegian Salmon	230	12	47%	3	80	60	27	2
Ocean Perch (Atlantic)	130	4	28%	1	75	190	24	1
Pollock	120	1	8%	0	90	90	28	1
Rainbow Trout	170	9	48%	3	90	90	23	0
Red Rockfish	90	1	10%	0	85	95	21	0
Red Snapper	110	1	8%	0	70	140	25	0
Sockeye Salmon	160	4	23%	1	50	60	28	2
Swordfish	100	4	36%	1	100	140	17	0
Tilefish	100	2	18%	1	80	60	20	0
Yellowfin Tuna	180	6	30%	2	70	70	32	0
Shellfish								
King Crab Legs 16 oz	170	2	11%	0	100	900	32	6
Snow Crab Legs, 16 oz	150	2	12%	1	130	1630	33	1
Calamari, breaded, fried, 5 oz	360	21	53%	6	140	1150	13	30
Langostino, 5 oz	120	1	8%	0	210	410	26	2
Maine Lobster, 18 oz	240	8	30%	2	310	550	36	5
Rock Lobster, 1 tail, 13 oz	230	3	12%	1	200	1090	49	2
Calico Scallops, 5 oz	180	2	10%	0	115	260	32	8
Deep Sea Scallops, 5 oz	130	2	14%	0	50	260	26	2
Shrimp, 8-12 pces., 7 oz	120	2	15%	0	230	110	25	0
Steaks/Chicken								
Sirloin, 8 oz	350	15	39%	na	150	110	51	0
Strip Steak, 7 oz	690	64	83%	na	140	70	29	0
Hamburger, 1/3 lb	320	23	65%	na	105	70	27	0
Filet Mignon, 8 oz	350	16	41%	na	140	105	47	0
Rib Eye Steak, 12 oz	980	82	75%	na	220	150	56	0
Skinless Chicken Breast, 4 oz	140	3	19%	na	70	60	26	0

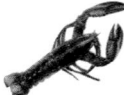

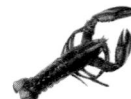
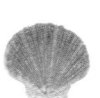
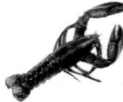

Round Table® Pizza

Large Pizza: Per Slice
(Thin = 1/8 whole; Pan = 1/6 whole)

		Cal	Fat	%Fc	S.Fat	Chol	Sod	Pro	Carb
Bacon Super Deli:	Thin	400	26	57%	9	50	780	18	32
	Pan	520	27	47%	9	50	760	24	52
Cheese:	Thin	320	12	34%	8	40	480	14	32
	Pan	420	14	31%	9	40	500	20	52
Chicken & Garlic Gourmet:									
	Thin	340	14	37%	7	50	560	18	34
	Pan	460	16	31%	8	50	620	22	54
Classic Pesto:	Thin	340	16	42%	7	30	420	14	36
	Pan	460	17	34%	8	30	480	18	54
Garden Pesto:	Thin	340	15	40%	7	30	400	14	36
	Pan	460	17	33%	8	30	460	18	56
Gourmet Veggie:	Thin	320	13	37%	6	30	400	14	36
	Pan	440	15	31%	7	40	460	18	56
Guinevere's Garden Delight:									
	Thin	300	11	33%	6	30	500	14	36
	Pan	400	12	28%	7	30	500	18	54
Italian Garlic Supreme:									
	Thin	400	21	47%	8	50	440	16	34
	Pan	500	21	38%	8	50	480	20	54
King Arthur's Supreme:									
	Thin	400	20	45%	8	50	680	18	36
	Pan	480	20	38%	8	50	640	20	54
Maui Zaui:	Thin	340	13	34%	7	40	700	18	36
	Pan	620	20	29%	12	60	980	30	74
Pepperoni:	Thin	340	16	42%	6	40	480	16	34
	Pan	440	16	33%	7	40	480	18	52
Roastin Toastin Garlic:									
	Thin	380	18	43%	8	50	620	18	36
	Pan	510	22	39%	10	52	705	24	56
Salute Chicken & Garlic:									
	Thin	300	11	33%	7	40	500	16	36
	Pan	400	12	27%	8	40	540	18	56
Salute Veggie:	Thin	280	9	29%	4	20	340	12	38
	Pan	380	10	24%	5	20	380	16	56
Sandwichess									
Chicken Club		800	38	43%	14	115	1510	39	72
Ham & Honey Mustard		760	33	39%	13	95	1630	36	76
Garden Vegetable		670	29	39%	10	55	990	25	75
Garlic Parmesan Twists (3)		430	15	31%	6	25	690	17	55
Turkey Pesto		830	40	43%	14	85	1200	42	71
Turkey Santa Fe		840	44	47%	16	95	1360	39	72

    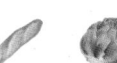

Roy Rogers®

	Cal	Fat	%Fc	S.Fat	Chol	Sod	Pro	Carb
Breakfast Items: Biscuit	390	21	48%	6	0	1000	6	44
Cinnamon 'N' Raisin Biscuit	370	18	44%	5	0	450	3	48
Sausage Biscuit	510	31	55%	10	25	1360	14	44
Sausage & Egg Biscuit	560	35	56%	11	170	1400	18	44
Bacon Biscuit	420	23	49%	7	5	1140	9	44
Bacon/Ham & Egg Biscuit	470	26	50%	8	150	1190	14	44
Ham & Cheese Biscuit	450	24	48%	8	25	1570	11	48
Ham, Egg & Cheese Biscuit	500	27	49%	10	170	1620	16	48
Sourdough Ham, Egg & Cheese	480	24	45%	9	185	1440	20	45
Big Country Breakfast: with Bacon	740	43	52%	13	305	1800	25	61
with Sausage	920	60	59%	19	340	2230	33	61
with Ham	710	39	49%	11	330	2210	24	67
3 Pancakes	280	2	6%	1	15	890	8	56
with 1 Sausage	430	16	33%	6	40	1290	16	56
with 2 Bacon	350	9	23%	3	25	1130	13	56
Bagel, all types, average	300	2	6%	0.5	0	520	10	60
Hashrounds	230	14	55%	3	0	560	3	24
Burgers								
Hamburger	260	9	31%	4	20	460	11	33
Cheeseburger	300	13	39%	7	25	690	13	34
1/4 lb Hamburger	430	18	38%	8	25	450	25	41
1/4 lb Cheeseburger	470	22	42%	10	30	680	27	42
Sourdough Bacon Cheeseburger	730	46	57%	18	65	1470	35	43
Sourdough Grilled Chicken	500	21	38%	6	45	1530	30	46
Bacon Cheeseburger	490	28	51%	13	35	800	30	29
Sandwiches: Roast Beef	260	4	14%	1	60	700	24	30
Chicken Fillet	500	24	43%	5	20	1050	19	49
Grilled Chicken	340	11	29%	2	30	910	25	32
Fisherman's Fillet (seasonal)	490	21	39%	5	15	1040	21	56
Chicken: Fried: Breast	370	15	36%	4	75	1190	29	29
Wing	200	8	36%	2	30	740	10	23
Thigh	330	15	41%	4	60	1000	19	30
Leg	170	7	37%	2	45	570	13	15
1/4 Roy's Roaster: White Meat	500	29	52%	9	240	1450	56	3
No Skin	190	6	28%	2	100	700	32	2
Dark Meat	490	34	62%	10	225	1120	43	2
No Skin	190	10	47%	3	110	400	24	1
Nuggets: 6 piece	290	18	56%	4	15	610	12	20
Salads: Grilled Chicken	120	4	30%	1	60	520	18	2
Garden	190	14	66%	9	40	280	12	3
Fries: Regular	350	15	39%	4	0	150	5	49
Large	430	18	38%	5	0	190	6	59
Baked Potato: w. Margarine	240	13	49%	2	0	220	3	27
Cornbread	310	17	49%	3	30	260	4	35
Coleslaw, 5 oz	295	25	76%	4	15	430	2	16
Desserts: Hot Fudge Sundae	320	10	28%	5	25	260	8	50
Strawberry Sundae	260	6	21%	3	15	95	6	44

Rubio's Baja Grill®

	Cal	Fat	%Fc	S.Fat	Chol	Sod	Pro	Carb
HealthMex®								
All HealthMex® items have less that 22% of calories from fat.								
Bean & Rice Burrito	340	7	19%	1	5	990	11	58
Burrito w. Chicken/Mahi Mahi	380	9	20%	2	30	960	30	48
Combo	690	13	17%	3	72	1735	51	93
Taco w. Chicken	180	3	15%	1	20	340	14	24
Taco w. Mahi Mahi	190	2	9%	0	35	260	18	25
Taco Combo: w. Chicken	480	8	15%	1	47	1195	33	68
w. Chicken & Mahi Mahi	490	7	13%	1	62	1115	37	69
w. Mahi Mahi	500	7	13%	1	77	1035	41	70
Tacos: Carne Asada	210	7	30%	1	20	520	12	25
Carnitas	290	14	43%	2	45	125	15	24
Fish Taco	280	14	45%	3	30	280	11	28
Fish Taco Especial	370	21	51%	5	45	380	15	29
Grilled Chicken	200	5	23%	1	20	260	14	24
Grilled Mahi Mahi Fish	300	14	42%	3	55	270	21	23
Shrimp	260	13	45%	2	90	430	12	23
Burritos: Bean & Cheese	490	20	37%	4	45	1000	20	57
Carne Asada	470	21	40%	1	45	1460	25	48
Carnitas	640	36	51%	10	100	540	33	47
Chicken	540	25	42%	8	70	1000	35	47
Especial: w. Carne Asada	690	39	51%	6	75	1680	29	56
w. Chicken	670	36	48%	6	75	1220	34	55
w. Carnitas	820	51	56%	8	120	990	36	55
Fish	590	30	46%	4	45	830	21	60
Mahi Mahi	640	31	44%	9	100	870	39	52
Shrimp	480	22	41%	8	130	1200	19	52
Combos: Baja Grill Combo	1100	45	37%	12	65	2440	50	129
Cabo Combo	1190	55	42%	25	160	2200	41	137
Pesky's Combo	1170	61	47%	15	90	1480	41	115
Baja Bowls: Grilled Chicken	260	6	21%	2	30	1440	19	35
Grilled Steak	270	8	27%	3	30	1710	16	36
Los Otros: Nachos Grande	1400	91	59%	18	145	1900	44	109
w. Steak	1520	97	57%	19	180	2650	58	110
w. Chicken	1500	94	56%	21	175	2200	63	110
Kid Pesky® Meals								
Beans	80	1	11%	0	5	200	5	13
Bean/Cheese Burrito	480	20	38%	8	45	810	20	55
Cheese Quesadilla	520	29	50%	9	80	820	22	41
Chips	350	18	46%	6	3	500	6	44
Fish Taco	280	14	45%	9	30	140	11	26
Rice	50	2	36%	0	7	335	1	7
Taquitos	320	17	48%	6	80	420	20	22
Churro, mini	65	4	55%	1	5	60	1	7

Note: Rubio's uses only skinless chicken breast & lean trimmed steak.
Canola oil is used – no lard or MSG. Saturated fat counts are author estimates only.

Sbarro's®

	Cal	Fat	%Fc	S.Fat	Chol	Sod	Pro	Carb
Baked Ziti, 1 serving	930	42	41%	21	115	954	44	90
Chicken Parmigiana, 2 pces, 7 oz	365	20	51%	5	73	743	31	13
Meat Lasagne, 1 serving	825	41	45%	22	119	1431	41	68
Spaghetti w/Sauce, 1 serving	910	23	23%	3	3	848	26	144
Pizza: Per Slice								
Cheeze	485	18	33%	10	60	1073	23	55
Pepperoni	590	27	41%	13	73	1423	29	55
Sausage	640	29	41%	14	86	1559	33	56
Supreme	600	25	37%	12	69	1583	30	59
Stuffed Pizza: Per Slice								
Spinach/Broccoli	825	40	43%	14	63	1536	33	85
Sausage Pepperoni	965	47	44%	19	120	2515	45	83

Schlotzsky's® Deli

	Cal	Fat	%Fc	S.Fat	Chol	Sod	Pro	Carb
Light & Flavorful Sandwiches								
Albacore Tuna, regular	565	17	27%	9	50	1795	37	70
Chicken Breast, regular	540	10	16%	3	30	2490	35	75
Dijon Chicken, regular	475	4.5	8%	2	30	1815	39	70
Pesto Chicken, regular	515	8.5	15%	5	30	1900	36	73
Santa Fe Chicken, small	445	14	28%	4	30	1755	29	52
Smoked Turkey Breast, regular	500	6.5	12%	1	30	2105	33	76
The Vegetarian, regular	510	16	28%	2	0	1230	20	71
Original Sandwiches: Per Regular Sandwich								
Cheese Original	830	43	45%	13	60	2005	38	75
Deluxe	1030	53	45%	16	80	3970	57	79
Ham & Cheese	770	32	40%	12	60	3350	44	78
The Original	800	38	45%	15	60	2315	36	75
Turkey	900	42	45%	12	50	3075	50	78
Specialty Deli: Per Regular Sandwich								
Albacore Tuna Melt	860	42	44%	14	60	2430	53	72
BLT	860	48	50%	20	60	1785	28	72
Chicken Club	865	37	38%	10	50	2480	52	78
Corned Beef	570	16	25%	8	80	2855	37	73
Corned Beef Reuben	840	36	40%	18	90	3560	47	76
Pastrami & Swiss	920	40	39%	18	80	4055	54	79
Pastrami Reuben	965	45	42%	10	50	3860	52	80
Roast Beef	650	20	30%	8	70	1795	42	72
Roast Beef & Cheese	870	37	40%	10	60	2510	56	75
Texas Schlotzsky's	850	41	45%	14	70	3290	44	78
The Philly	820	29	35%	8	40	2525	57	80
Turkey & Bacon Club	1000	53	45%	15	60	3080	56	73
Turkey Guacamole	760	30	35%	8	30	2870	35	85
Turkey Reuben	900	40	40%	10	50	3800	52	80
Vegetable Club	620	27	40%	7	0	1475	18	74
Western Vegetarian	630	30	40%	8	0	75	18	42

	Cal	Fat	%Fc	S.Fat	Chol	Sod	Pro	Carb
Leaf Salads: *(No dressing, croutons, chow mein noodles, crackers)*								
Caesar Salad	65	4.5	60%	1	0	175	5	2
Chicken Caesar Salad	145	5.5	34%	1	10	440	21	4
Chinese Chicken Salad	180	3.5	18%	1	10	265	18	14
Garden Salad	110	3	25%	0	0	120	4	14
Greek Salad	190	12	55%	3	10	595	9	14
Ham & Turkey Chef's Salad	250	13	45%	3	10	1490	23	14
Smoked Turkey Chef's Salad	230	10	40%	3	10	1340	23	14
Deli Salads: Cole Slaw, 1/2 cup	180	13	65%	3	10	310	1	13
Macaroni Salad, 3/4 cup	360	25	63%	6	20	660	4	25
Potato Salad: Choice, 2/3 cup	270	19	63%	1	0	560	2	19
w. Mustard & Egg, 2/3 cup	240	16	63%	3	210	570	2	18
Diced w. Egg, 2/3 cup	230	14	55%	3	210	640	3	19
Deli-Style Potato Chips, 1.5 oz	210	10	43%	0	0	220	3	25
Bread *(Regular Size)*								
Dark Rye/Sourdough Bun	330	1.5	5%	0	0	790	11	68
Jalapeno Cheese Bun	345	3	7%	2	10	870	11	69
Wheat Bun	330	2	5%	0	0	840	13	64
Soups: *8 oz Cup*								
*-Bean Medley	200	3	15%	0	0	2000	10	34
Boston Clam Chowder	440	10	25%	3	30	1820	10	26
Chicken Noodle (Old Fashioned)	180	4	15%	1	10	1680	10	24
Cream of Broccoli	380	7	50%	2	10	1860	6	24
Minestrone	140	2	15%	0	0	1740	6	26
Vegetable Vegetarian	100	0	0%	0	0	1420	6	20
Sourdough Crust Pizzas *(8")*								
Average all types	600	19	29%	8	80	3410	36	72
Desserts: *Per Serving*								
Cookies: Chocolate Chip/Chunk	160	7	40%	3	20	140	2	24
Oatmeal Raisin	170	5	26%	2	10	140	1	24
Peanut Butter	170	8	40%	3	20	190	2	21
Other Cookies, average	170	8	40%	3	20	160	2	22
Fudge Brownie Cake	410	25	35%	6	40	135	5	46
New York/Strawb. Swirl Cheesecake	310	18	55%	8	50	230	7	31
Kid Schlotzsky's *(no Cookie/Drink)*								
Ham & Cheese, small	440	18	35%	7	30	1340	22	47
Kid's Cheese Pizza	450	13	25%	4	20	395	18	66
Kid's Pepperoni Pizza	490	17	31%	10	40	520	19	66
Peanut Butter & Jelly, small	500	15	25%	4	0	750	14	78

Note: Figures for saturated fat and cholesterol are author estimates only.

7-Eleven®

	Cal	Fat	%Fc	S.Fat	Chol	Sod	Pro	Carb
Hot Dogs								
Big Bite w. Bun	550	34	55%	14	60	1340	16	24
Hot Dog Bun only	120	1.5	11%	na	na	210	4	22
Smokie Bite w. Bun	390	26	60%	9	60	1100	15	24
Spicy Bite w. Bun	550	40	65%	15	100	1700	23	24
Croissant: Egg, Ham & Cheese	380	20	47%	7	155	950	18	31
English Muffin								
w. Egg/Cheese/Canadian Bacon	265	21	52%	5	160	840	15	29
Biscuit: Sausage/Egg/Cheese	420	23	49%	9	170	1100	17	36
w. Sausage & Cheese	370	21	52%	8	30	970	10	36
Burritos								
Ramona: Beef & Bean	290	9	27%	4	76	290	17	37
Potato & Beef	340	14	37%	6	33	280	13	41
Bean & Cheese	340	13	34%	6	34	300	15	41
Reynoldos Jumbo Burritos:								
Beef & Bean	630	20	28%	5	10	1470	25	88
Beef & Potato	550	16	26%	5	15	1650	16	82
Bean & Cheese	680	25	33%	10	22	1335	26	88
Red Hot	600	20	30%	5	15	1810	22	83
Green	640	22	31%	7	22	1680	23	87
Chimichanga: Average all types	270	8	27%	1.5	0	580	13	37
Turkey Hoagies/Pitas/Subs								
Turkey Hoagie: Regular, 8.7 oz	320	13	37%	8	70	2100	13	35
Large, 13 oz	510	17	30%	11	90	2600	21	70
Pita: Smoked Turkey, 7.6 oz	410	18	40%	5	60	1400	26	37
Turkey & Cheddar, 8.7 oz	470	19	36%	5	60	1750	29	46
Sandwich: Grilled Smkd Turkey, 9.2 oz	645	18	25%	5	70	2000	35	85
Subs: Italian	480	20	38%	6	60	1700	26	50
Turkey Super Sub: 6" Sub, 8 oz	440	16	33%	3.5	40	1360	24	51
12" Sub, 16 oz	880	32	33%	7	80	2720	48	101
Fountain Drinks (Figures Assume 1/4 Ice)								
Coca-Cola/Pepsi/Dr.Pepper/7Up:								
Gulp, 16 oz	150	0	0%	0	0	15	0	38
Big Gulp, 32 oz	300	0	0%	0	0	30	0	75
Super Gulp, 44 oz	410	0	0%	0	0	40	0	102
Double Gulp, 64 oz	600	0	0%	0	0	60	0	150
Diet Coke/Diet Pepsi, 16 oz	1	0	0%	0	0	20	0	0
Slurpees: Average All Flavors,								
16 oz size	200	0	0%	0	0	15	0	50
22 oz size	275	0	0%	0	0	20	0	69
32 oz size	400	0	0%	0	0	30	0	100
44 oz size	550	0	0%	0	0	40	0	138
Café Coolers: Mocha, 12 oz	350	12	30%	11	0	170	1	63
French Vanilla, 12 oz	380	16	39%	15	0	230	1	58

	Cal	Fat	%Fc	S.Fat	Chol	Sod	Pro	Carb
Main Menu								
All-American Burger	690	32	42%	na	150	930	54	44
Bacon Cheeseburger	890	49	50%	na	195	1490	66	44
Baked White Fish	510	8.5	15%	na	94	2230	48	58
Baked Potato, Plain	310	0	0%	0	0	25	7	67
Cajun Whitefish	480	11	20%	na	73	885	40	56
Charbroiled Blackened Chicken	830	26	28%	na	97	2015	47	100
Charbroiled Chicken Breast	795	23	26%	na	97	1830	47	99
Chicken Alfredo	1705	78	41%	na	430	3145	85	170
Chicken Parmesan Sandwich	750	30	36%	na	99	2520	42	80
Chicken Stir Fry	1200	35	26%	na	103	4315	48	172
Corned Beef Reuben Sandwich	790	53	60%	na	180	4145	40	37
Fish Sandwich	830	17	18%	na	67	2600	44	126
French Fries, 4 oz	210	11	47%	5	0	440	3	25
Fried Chicken Sandwich	560	15	24%	na	66	3170	31	77
Fried Fish Platter	1050	39	33%	na	97	2050	49	123
Grilled Shrimp	720	20	25%	na	195	1400	39	96
Half O'Pound Burger	1350	53	35%	na	225	1885	89	130
Ham Steak Dinner (no veges)	670	26	35%	na	100	3210	48	60
Hot Roast Beef Sandwich w. Veg.	770	24	28%	na	98	2900	44	95
Italian Feast	1435	45	28%	na	262	4630	64	204
Mushroom Swiss Burger	970	58	54%	na	175	1125	64	49
Original Slim Jim Sandwich	1005	34	31%	na	98	4395	54	123
Patty Melt	945	60	57%	na	190	1275	50	40
Roast Beef Platter (no veges)	880	30	31%	na	135	3255	59	96
Shrimper's Feast	1035	39	34%	na	182	2130	39	128
Shrimp Stir Fry	875	19	20%	na	200	3975	41	131
Spaghetti	495	16	29%	4	55	390	24	63
Steak (6 oz), 6 Grilled Shrimp	1330	57	39%	na	250	2220	76	128
Steak (6 oz), 5 Fried Shrimp	1385	58	38%	na	248	2250	76	139
Turkey Club/Whole Wheat	950	53	50%	na	178	2690	71	47
Ultimate Grilled Cheese S'wich	895	46	46%	na	102	3000	42	77
Children's Menu								
All-American Jnr Burger	235	11	42%	4	30	545	14	20
Kid's: Chicken Dinner	245	13	48%	4	40	150	21	11
Fish 'N Chips w. Fries	335	17	46%	5	41	460	13	33
Fried Shrimp	195	12	55%	4	70	635	10	12
Spaghetti	250	8	29%	2	27	195	13	32
Desserts, Icecream, Sundaes								
Apple Pie: a la Mode	1205	53	40%	na	49	1115	12	174
w. NutraSweet	455	18	36%	na	0	415	4	64
Cheesecake, 1 slice, 4 oz	365	26	64%	na	62	190	5	23
Carrot Cake	500	26	47%	6	37	475	9	56
Hot Fudge Sundae	600	30	45%	na	80	230	10	75
Original Strawberry Pie	330	17	46%	4	0	250	2	45
Strawberry Sundae	610	27	40%	na	88	190	9	85
Walnut Brownie	575	34	53%	15	35	435	10	61

Shakey's®

	Cal	Fat	%Fc	S.Fat	Chol	Sod	Pro	Car
Pizzas (12"): Per Slice (1/10 Pizza)								
Cheese only: Thin Crust	135	5	33%	3	15	320	8	13
Thick Crust	170	5	26%	3	15	420	7	22
Homestyle Pan	305	14	41%	7	20	590	14	31
Onion/Olives/Mushrooms: Thin	125	5	36%	3	10	315	7	14
Thick Crust	160	4	23%	2	15	420	9	22
Homestyle Pan	320	15	42%	7	20	650	15	32
Sausage Pepperoni: Thin Crust	165	8	44%	5	15	395	9	13
Thick Crust	205	8	35%	5	20	425	11	22
Homestyle Pan	375	20	48%	11	25	680	17	31
Sausage Mushroom: Thin Crust	140	6	39%	3	15	335	8	13
Thick Crust	180	6	30%	3	15	420	10	22
Homestyle Pan	340	17	45%	8	25	680	16	31
Pepperoni: Thin Crust	150	7	42%	4	15	400	8	13
Thick Crust	185	6	29%	4	15	420	10	22
Homestyle Pan	345	15	39%	9	25	740	16	31
Shakey's Special: Thin Crust	170	9	48%	5	15	475	13	13
Thick Crust	210	8	34%	4	20	420	13	22
Homestyle Pan	385	21	49%	11	30	880	18	32
Other Items								
3-Piece Chicken & Potato	945	56	53%	18	na	2290	57	51
5-Piece Fried Chicken & Potato	1700	90	48%	30	na	5330	97	130
Hot Ham & Cheese Sandwich	550	21	34%	10	na	2135	36	56
Potato Wedges, 15 pieces	950	36	34%	10	na	3700	17	120
Shakey's Super Hot Hero	810	44	49%	15	na	2690	36	67
Spagh. w. Meat Sce/Garlic Bread	940	33	32%	10	na	1900	26	134

Note: Saturated fat figures are author estimates only.

Sizzler®

	Cal	Fat	%Fc	S.Fat	Chol	Sod	Pro	Carb
Hot Entrees								
Hamburger	625	33	48%	12	142	335	45	36
Dakota Ranch Steak: 6 oz	315	20	57%	8	100	255	30	0
8 oz	420	27	58%	11	135	340	37	0
9 1/2 oz	500	32	58%	13	160	400	47	0
Hibachi Chicken Breast								
w. Pineapple	195	3	14%	1	65	685	28	13
Lemon-Herb Chicken Breast	140	3	19%	1	65	380	27	0
Malibu Chicken Patty, each	310	19	55%	3	75	590	23	11
Salmon	250	12	43%	2	40	230	32	0
Santa Fe Chicken Breast	150	3	18%	1	65	350	30	0
Shrimp: Broiled	150	6	36%	0	218	375	23	0
Fried, 4 only	225	2	8%	0	118	705	18	35
Mini	150	1	6%	0	80	480	13	24
Shrimp Scampi	145	3	19%	1	150	385	27	0
Swordfish	315	14	40%	3	90	330	45	0

	Cal	Fat	%FC	S.Fat	Chol	Sod	Pro	Carb
Hot Bar: Broccoli Cheese Soup, 4 oz	140	9	58%	2	8	355	3	10
Chicken Noodle Soup, 4 oz	30	1	30%	0	7	495	2	4
Chicken Wings, 1 oz	75	4	48%	1	20	135	4	4
Clam Chowder, 4 oz	120	6	46%	0	6	510	3	11
Focaccia Bread, 2 pces	110	7	57%	1	0	135	2	9
Meatballs, 4 balls	155	11	64%	5	30	460	9	5
Minestrone Soup, 4 oz	35	0	0%	0	0	445	1	7
Pasta: Fettucine, 2 oz	80	1	11%	0	5	5	3	15
Spaghetti, 2 oz	80	0	0%	0	0	0	3	16
Potato Skins, 2 oz	160	8	45%	1	0	465	2	22
Refried Beans, 1/4 cup	60	1	15%	2	5	270	4	11
Saltine Crackers, 2 crackers	25	1	36%	0	2	75	1	4
Taco Filling, 2 oz	105	9	77%	4	16	230	2	3
Taco Shells, each	50	2	36%	0	0	20	1	7
Salads & Toppings								
Prepared Salads: Per 2 oz								
Carrot & Raisin	130	10	69%	2	10	105	1	10
Chinese Chicken; Teriyaki Beef	55	2	33%	0	10	120	4	6
Mediterranean Minted Fruit	30	0	0%	0	0	10	1	7
Mexican Fiesta	55	1	16%	0	0	100	2	10
Old Fashioned Potato	85	5	53%	1	10	230	1	10
Red Herb Potato	120	9	68%	1	10	270	1	9
Seafood	55	3	49%	1	7	255	3	4
Seafood Louis Pasta	65	2	28%	0	15	140	3	9
Spicy Jicama	15	0	0%	0	0	30	0	4
Tuna Pasta	135	10	67%	1	10	190	6	6
Dessert Bar: Chocolate Syrup, 1 oz	90	0	0%	0	0	15	0	21
Choc/Vanilla Soft Serve, 4 oz	135	4	27%	4	0	100	1	24
Strawberry Topping, 1 oz	70	0	0%	0	0	5	0	18
Whipped Topping, 1 Tbsp	10	1	90%	1	0	0	0	1
Sides: Cottage Cheese, 2 oz	50	1	18%	1	5	230	8	2
Eggs, 1 oz	45	3	60%	1	120	35	4	0
Garbanzo Beans, 1/4 cup	65	1	14%	0	0	255	3	11
Kidney Beans, 1/4 cup	50	0	0%	0	0	220	3	10
Olives, 1 oz	60	6	90%	1	0	180	1	1
Peaches, 1/4 cup	35	0	0%	0	0	5	0	9
Peas, 1/4 cup	30	0	0%	0	0	35	2	6
Real Bacon Bits, 1 Tbsp	30	2	60%	0	0	165	2	2
Turkey Ham, 1 oz	60	5	75%	2	19	375	4	0
Dressings (1 oz): Blue Cheese	110	12	98%	4	8	170	1	1
Honey Mustard	160	16	90%	2	10	110	0	4
Italian, Lite	15	0	0%	0	0	350	0	2
Japanese Rice Vinegar, Fat Free	10	0	0%	0	0	180	0	2
Parmesan Italian	100	10	90%	2	0	450	0	2
Ranch	120	12	90%	2	10	240	0	2
Ranch, Reduced-Calorie	90	8	80%	2	10	270	0	4
Thousand Island	145	15	93%	2	10	125	0	3

Skippers®

	Cal	Fat	%Fc	S.Fat	Chol	Sod	Pro	Carb
Chowder: Smoked Salmon	165	7	38%	2	20	75	13	14
Clam: 1 cup	100	4	32%	1	12	525	3	14
Entrees: Per Serving								
Chicken: Tenderloin Strip								
w. Fries, 5 pces	795	38	43%	13	77	800	44	69
'Lite Catch', 3 pces	305	15	44%	5	58	675	26	17
Chicken: Strips, Create A Catch	80	4	45%	2	15	150	8	4
Strips, Fish, Fries	805	40	45%	13	100	860	80	72
Strips, Shrimp, Fries	800	39	44%	13	97	1035	36	77
Clam: Strips w. Fries	1005	70	63%	20	14	570	22	90
Strips, Fish, Fries	870	54	56%	18	60	670	25	81
Cod: 3 pces. w. Fries	665	32	43%	10	38	1055	27	68
4 pces. w. Fries	760	36	43%	12	50	1390	34	74
5 pces. w. Fries	855	41	43%	14	62	1725	42	80
Fish Meal: 1 fillet w. Fries	560	28	45%	9	55	410	17	51
2 fillets w. Fries	735	38	47%	13	108	765	28	71
2 pces w. Salad, Lite Catch	410	23	50%	7	120	940	25	27
3 fillets, w. Fries	910	48	47%	16	160	1120	39	82
3 fillets + Salad, small	410	23	50%	7	120	940	25	27
'Create a Catch'	175	10	51%	3	53	360	11	11
Fish, Oysters, Fries	885	44	45%	16	80	810	25	95
Oyster w. Fries, 'Basket'	1040	51	44%	17	52	855	28	118
Salmon, baked	270	11	37%	2	70	505	39	1
Shrimp, Fish, Fries:	730	37	46%	12	105	945	24	77
Jumbo w. Fries, Basket	710	35	44%	11	73	910	20	79
Original w. Fries, Basket	725	36	45%	12	102	1120	20	82
Skipper's Platter Basket	1040	63	55%	20	110	1200	32	97
Sandwiches								
Chicken, 'Create a Catch'	605	32	48%	11	82	975	31	44
Fish: 'Create a Catch', regular	525	33	57%	9	86	1190	19	43
Double	700	73	94%	19	140	1550	30	54
French Fries	385	18	42%	4	2	50	6	50
Potato, baked	145	0	0%	0	0	5	4	32
Salads: Coleslaw	290	27	84%	4	50	330	2	10
Green, small, Lite Catch	60	3	45%	1	13	225	3	6
Shrimp & Seafood	170	3	16%	1	80	660	23	15
Side	25	0	0%	0	0	10	0	4
Salad Dressings & Sauces								
Blue Cheese	220	23	94%	10	8	240	1	4
Italian Gourmet	140	15	96%	3	0	200	0	2
Low Cal	15	1	53%	0	6	80	0	2
Ranch House	190	20	95%	4	0	300	1	2
Thousand Island	160	14	79%	3	6	415	0	8
Barbeque Sauce, 1Tbsp	25	1	36%	0	0	225	0	5
Cocktail Sauce, 1 Tbsp	20	0	0%	0	0	215	0	5
Tartar Sauce, 1Tbsp	65	7	97%	2	4	100	0	0
Drinks: Root Beer Float	300	10	30%	3	10	65	3	33

	Cal	Fat	%FC	S.Fat	Chol	Sod	Pro	Carb
Burgers: #1. Burger	575	36	56%	7	37	755	14	43
#2. Burger	480	25	47%	5	29	760	14	43
#1. Cheeseburger	645	42	58%	11	52	1105	18	44
#2. Cheeseburger	550	31	51%	9	44	1110	18	44
Bacon Cheeseburger	725	49	61%	13	67	1435	23	44
Super Sonic #1	930	66	64%	19	96	1475	28	45
Super Sonic #2	890	55	55%	17	88	1570	28	46
Jr. Burger	355	21	53%	6	45	1295	14	27
Toaster Sandwiches: BLT	580	41	63%	9	47	1305	19	42
Grilled Cheese	280	12	38%	5	15	830	12	39
Bacon Cheddar Burger	675	38	50%	11	59	1875	26	60
Chicken Club	675	29	38%	8	85	1460	39	75
Sandwiches: Country Fried Steak	750	47	56%	12	60	805	24	56
Breaded Chicken	580	23	35%	4	53	425	28	66
Grilled Chicken	345	13	34%	2	70	830	27	31
Chicken: Chicken Strip Dinner	750	32	38%	5	47	1975	32	86
Chicken Strip Snack	270	13	43%	2	35	760	19	22
Coneys								
Plain: Regular	260	16	55%	5	30	655	8	22
Extra Long	485	27	50%	10	50	1160	14	44
Cheese: Regular	365	24	59%	10	52	960	13	24
Extra-Long	665	42	57%	17	87	1650	23	47
Corn Dog	280	17	54%	5	15	480	6	23
Faves & Craves								
French Fries: Regular	195	11	51%	2	0	650	2	22
Large	250	13	47%	2	0	760	3	30
Super Sonic	360	18	45%	3	0	965	5	44
Ched 'R' Peppers®	255	12	42%	5	28	1055	8	29
Cheese Fries: Regular	265	17	58%	6	15	1000	6	23
Large	320	19	53%	6	15	1110	7	31
Chili Cheese Fries, regular	300	19	57%	6	22	950	8	24
Fritos® Chili Pie	610	44	65%	13	53	815	18	36
Mozzarella Sticks	380	19	45%	11	50	1300	20	35
Onion Rings: Regular	330	5	14%	1	0	310	8	66
Large	505	7	12%	1	0	485	12	102
Tater Tots: Regular	260	16	55%	3	0	1045	0	27
Cheese, regular	330	22	60%	7	15	1395	4	28
Chili Cheese, regular	365	25	61%	7	22	1350	5	28
Blasts, regular	640	27	38%	21	45	600	11	57
Slushes, regular, average all flavors	335	0	0%	0	0	16	0	84
Slush Floats/Flurry®, average, reg.	390	12	27%	12	30	260	6	44
Banana Split	465	11	21%	10	23	225	6	75
Hot Fudge Sundae	390	15	34%	15	27	255	6	40
Icecream Cone	285	11	27%	11	26	225	6	23
Drinks: Barq's Root Beer, large	335	0	0%	0	0	70	0	84
Coca-Cola, large	290	0	0%	0	0	25	0	72
Coca-Cola Float, large	545	17	28%	17	43	355	9	59

Souplantation®

	Cal	Fat	%Fc	S.Fat	Chol	Sod	Pro	Carb
Soups: Per 1 Cup								
Low Fat: Chicken Tortilla	100	3	27%	1	20	990	12	5
Chicken/Turkey Noodle	160	3	17%	2	20	480	15	17
Vegetable Medley	90	1	10%	0	0	520	2	14
Regular Soup:								
Chesapeake Corn Chowder	310	13	38%	5	20	720	12	43
Cream of Mushroom	290	21	65%	8	30	820	10	15
Irish Potato Leek	260	16	55%	8	35	680	5	23
Minestrone w. Italian Sausage	210	11	47%	4	20	890	13	14
Navy Bean w. Ham	340	10	26%	4	40	980	35	30
New England Clam Chowder	330	20	55%	10	80	630	18	21
Vegetarian Harvest	190	8	38%	2	0	990	5	23
Chili: House Chili	230	3	12%	2	15	560	15	26
Breads								
Buttermilk Corn	140	2	13%	0	10	270	3	27
Sourdough	150	0.5	3%	0	0	240	9	27
Focaccia: Garlic Parmesan	100	3	27%	0	0	170	2	15
Pizza /Tomarillo	140	6	39%	2	10	270	5	16
Fresh Tossed Salads: Per 1 Cup								
Antipasto Salad; BBQ, average	140	10	64%	3	15	350	5	6
Classic Caesar Salad	190	14	66%	2	10	280	5	10
Won Ton Chicken Salad	150	8	48%	1	10	220	6	12
Prepared Salads: Per 1/2 Cup								
Artichoke Rice	160	8	45%	1	3	780	3	21
Aunt Doris' Red Pepper Slaw	70	0	0%	0	0	480	1	18
Baja Bean & Cilantro	180	3	15%	0	0	190	9	29
BBQ Potato	160	8	45%	1	5	270	2	20
Carrot Raisin	90	3	30%	0	5	80	1	17
Chinese Krab	160	8	45%	1	3	260	5	19
Confetti Pasta w. Cheddar & Dill	160	9	51%	2	10	380	5	16
Dijon Potato w. Garlic Dill Vinegar	140	7	45%	1	0	260	3	16
Greek Couscous w. Feta Cheese	170	9	48%	1	4	480	6	19
Oriental Ginger Slaw w. Krab	70	3	39%	0	2	80	2	8
Southern Dill Potato	120	3	23%	2	5	300	4	20
Thai Noodle w. Peanut Sce	170	8	42%	1	0	310	5	17
Dressing & Croutons: Per 2 Tbsp								
Blue Cheese Dressing	140	14	90%	2.5	10	230	1	3
Blush Vinaigrette	120	12	90%	2	0	320	0	3
Creamy Cucumber Dressing	80	7	79%	1	0	290	0	4
Garden French Tomato	40	1.5	34%	0	0	270	0	7
Honey Mustard Dressing	150	13	78%	2	10	230	0	8
Fat Free	45	0	0%	0	0	160	0	10
Ranch House Dressing	130	13	90%	2	10	180	1	1
Fat Free	50	0	0%	0	0	180	1	2
Thousand Island Dressing	110	11	90%	1.5	5	250	0	3
Zesty Italian Dressing	160	18	100%	2.5	0	280	0	1
Fat Free	20	0	0%	0	0	340	0	5

Souplantation® (Cont)

	Cal	Fat	%FC	S.Fat	Chol	Sod	Pro	Carb
Hot Tossed Pastas: Per Cup								
Bruschetta	260	4	14%	2	10	450	10	41
Creamy	360	16	40%	8	45	510	12	43
Garden Vegetable: w. Meatballs	270	7	23%	3	10	460	11	42
w. Italian Sausage	300	10	30%	3	20	540	12	42
Italian Vegetable Beef	270	6	20%	2	10	470	10	43
Vegetarian Marinara w. Basil	260	4	14%	2	10	750	10	44
Muffins: Per Muffin								
Regular: Apple Raisin	150	7	42%	1	10	190	2	22
Apricot/Banana/Cherry Nut	150	7	42%	1	10	190	2	22
Carrot Pineapple w. Oat Bran	150	6	36%	1	10	230	3	23
Chocolate Varieties	170	8	42%	2	10	190	3	22
Georgia Peach Poppyseed	150	6	36%	1	10	210	2	20
Lemon	140	4	26%	1	10	190	2	19
Wild Maine Blueberry	140	5	32%	1	10	180	2	22
Zucchini Nut	150	7	42%	1	10	190	2	22
Desserts: Per 1/2 Cup								
Apple Medley	70	0	0%	0	0	5	1	18
Banana Royale	80	0	0%	0	0	5	1	20
Chocolate Chip Cookie, small	70	3	39%	1	5	90	1	10
Jello, flavored	80	0	0%	0	0	40	1	20
Rice Pudding	110	2	16%	1	10	50	3	20
Tropical Fruit Salad	75	0	0%	0	0	5	1	19
Vanilla Pudding	140	3	19%	0	10	160	4	24
Vanilla Soft Serving	140	4	26%	3	20	70	3	22
Chocolate Syrup, 2 Tbsp	70	0	0%	0	10	15	0	18
Granola Topping, 2 Tbsp	110	4	33%	2	0	14	2	16

Spaghetti Warehouse®

	Cal	Fat	%FC	S.Fat	Chol	Sod	Pro	Carb
Lunch: Minestrone Soup	80	1.5	17%	0.5	2	1040	4	12
Grilled Chicken Marinara	530	8	14%	1.5	96	400	46	65
Seafood Marinara	385	5	12%	1	48	400	19	65
Spaghetti: w. Tomato Sauce	425	5	11%	0.5	0	490	13	82
w. Marinara Sauce #12	440	5	10%	1	0	400	14	84
Spicy Marinara Sce Spaghetti	280	4	13%	1	2	280	9	52
Vegetable Primavera	340	4	11%	0.5	0	345	12	65
Dinner: Minestrone, 1 bowl	110	2	16%	1	3	1495	6	18
Grilled Chicken Marinara	640	10	14%	2	96	550	50	85
Grilled Halibut	880	14	14%	2	93	780	78	106
Grilled Marinated Chicken Breast	910	17	17%	3	145	825	74	116
Marinara Sauce #12	520	6	10%	1	0	390	17	99
Seafood Marinara	520	8	14%	1	77	605	27	86
Spaghetti w. Tomato Sauce	525	6	10%	1	0	650	17	101
Spicy Marinara Sce Spaghetti	330	6	16%	1.5	3	410	10	60
Vegetable Primavera	610	8	12%	1	0	660	21	116

Subway®

	Cal	Fat	%Fc	S.Fat	Chol	Sod	Pro	Carb
7 Under 6™ Sandwiches (6") ~ Figures based on Italian bread and following toppings:								
Lettuce, tomato, onion, green peppers, olives and pickles.								
Ham	260	4.5	16%	1.5	25	1260	17	39
Roast Beef	264	4.5	15%	1	20	840	18	39
Roasted Chicken Breast	310	6	17%	1.5	48	880	25	40
SUBWAY Club®	294	5	15%	1.5	33	1250	22	40
Turkey Breast	254	3.5	12%	1	20	1000	16	39
Turkey Breast & Ham	267	4.5	15%	1	26	1210	18	40
Veggie Delite®	200	2.5	11%	0.5	0	500	7	37
Breakfast Sandwiches (6"): Figures based on Italian bread.								
Bacon & Egg	305	15	44%	4	184	500	13	29
Cheese & Egg	302	15	45%	4.5	187	520	13	29
Ham & Egg	290	12	37%	3	189	700	15	30
Western Egg	285	12	38%	2.5	182	510	13	31
Classic Sandwiches (6") ~ Figures based on Italian bread and following toppings:								
Lettuce, tomato, onion, green peppers, olives, pickles, cheese, oil, vinegar, salt and pepper.								
BMT®	453	24	48%	8	56	1740	21	40
Cold Cut Trio™	415	20	43%	7	57	1670	19	40
Meatball	500	25	45%	10	56	1350	23	46
Seafood & Crab	378	16	38%	4.5	24	1270	14	46
Steak & Cheese	362	13	32%	4.5	37	1200	23	41
SUBWAY Melt®	384	15	35%	5	44	1720	22	40
Tuna	420	21	45%	5	42	1180	18	39
Deli Sandwiches (6"): Ham	194	3.5	16%	1	12	750	10	30
Roast Beef	206	4	17%	1	13	600	12	31
Tuna	310	15	44%	4	26	810	12	31
Turkey Breast	215	3.5	16%	1	13	700	12	31
Select Sandwiches (6") ~ Figures based on Italian bread and following toppings:								
Lettuce, tomato, onion, green peppers and select sauce.								
Asiago Caesar Chicken	390	15	35%	3	47	1000	22	41
Caesar Italian BMT®	530	31	53%	10	66	1840	22	41
Honey Mustard Melt	376	11	26%	5	44	1590	22	47
Honey Mustard Turkey w. Cucumber	275	3.5	11%	1	20	990	16	46
Horseradish Roast Beef	400	17	38%	3	27	880	18	42
Horseradish Steak & Cheese	468	22	42%	6	44	1110	22	43
Southwest Chicken	362	13	32%	2.5	43	960	21	40
Southwest Steak & Cheese	412	18	39%	6	44	1120	22	42
Wraps (6"): Asiago Caesar Chicken	413	15	33%	3	47	1320	22	46
Steak & Cheese	353	9	23%	4	37	1400	22	46
Turkey Breast & Bacon	310	7	20%	2.5	28	1510	18	45
Salad Dressings (2 oz): Fat-Free French	70	0	0%	0	0	390	0	17
Fat-Free Italian	20	0	0%	0	0	610	0	4
Fat-Free Ranch	60	0	0%	0	0	530	0	14
Select Sauces (1 Tbsp): Asiago Caesar	77	8	94%	1.5	7	160	1	1
Honey Mustard	20	0	0%	0	0	100	0	5
Horseradish	100	9	81%	1.5	5	130	0	2
Southwest	60	6	90%	1	5	130	0	1

	Cal	Fat	%FC	S.Fat	Chol	Sod	Pro	Carb
7 Under 6™ Salads: Figures include lettuce, tomato, onion, green peppers, olives and pickles.								
Ham	112	3	24%	1	25	1070	11	11
Roast Beef	114	3	24%	0.5	20	660	12	11
Roasted Chicken Breast	137	3	20%	0.5	36	730	16	12
SUBWAY Club®	145	3.5	22%	1	33	1070	17	12
Turkey Breast	105	2	17%	0	20	820	11	11
Turkey Breast & Ham	117	3	23%	0.5	26	1030	13	11
Veggie Delite®	50	1	18%	0	0	310	2	9
Classic Salads: Figures include lettuce, tomato, onion, green peppers, olives, pickles and cheese.								
BMT®	272	19	63%	7	56	1440	16	11
Cold Cut Trio	234	15	58%	6	57	1370	14	11
Meatball	320	20	56%	9	56	1050	17	17
Seafood & Crab®	197	11	50%	3.5	24	970	9	17
Steak & Cheese	182	8	40%	3.5	37	890	17	12
SUBWAY Melt®	203	10	44%	4.5	44	1410	17	11
Tuna	238	16	61%	4	42	880	13	10
Condiments & Extras								
Bacon, 2 strips	45	4	80%	1.5	8	180	2	0
Cheese: American , 2 triangles	40	3.5	77%	2	10	200	2	0
Cheddar , 2 triangles	60	5	75%	3	15	95	4	0
Provolone, 2 half circles	50	4	72%	2	11	125	4	0
Swiss, 2 triangles	53	4	70%	2.5	13	30	4	0
Mayonnaise: 1 Tbsp	110	12	98%	3	9	80	0	0
Light Mayonnaise, 1 Tbsp	46	5	98%	1	6	100	0	1
Mustard, 2 tsp	8	0	0%	0	0	115	0	2
Olive Oil Blend, 1 tsp	45	5	100%	1	0	0	0	0
Vinegar, 1 tsp	1	0	0%	0	0	0	0	0
Breads: 6" Asiago	220	5	20%	3	8	460	9	34
6" Country Wheat	206	2.5	11%	0.5	0	360	8	39
6" Hearty Italian	190	2	9%	0.5	0	350	7	36
6" Italian (White) Bread	178	2	10%	0.5	0	350	7	33
6" Parmesan Oregano	195	3	14%	0.5	4	400	8	34
6" Sesame Italian	210	4.5	19%	0.5	0	360	8	34
6" Sourdough	265	3	10%	1.5	0	460	10	49
6" Wheat Bread	186	1.5	7%	0.5	0	360	7	36
Deli Style Roll	150	2.5	15%	0.5	0	260	5	27
Wrap	200	2	9%	0.5	0	670	6	39
Cookies (each): Choc. Chip; M&M	210	10	43%	3.5	12	135	3	29
Chocolate Chunk	210	10	43%	3	12	150	2	30
Oatmeal Raisin	197	8	37%	2	14	180	3	29
Peanut Butter	220	12	49%	3	0	200	3	26
Sugar	222	12	49%	3	18	170	2	28
White Macadamia Nut	220	12	49%	3	13	140	2	27
Fruizle Express (small): Berry Lishus	113	0	0%	0	0	30	1	28
Peach Pizazz	103	0	0%	0	0	25	0	26
Pineapple Delight	133	0	0%	0	0	25	1	33
Sunrise Refresher	120	0	0%	0	0	20	1	29

Steak 'n Shake®

Steakburgers & Sandwiches	Cal	Fat	%Fc	S.Fat	Chol	Sod	Pro	Car
Steakburger	275	7	23%	2	60	425	18	33
with Cheese	355	13	33%	6	80	660	23	33
Super	375	12	29%	4	100	445	30	33
Super with Cheese	450	18	36%	8	120	680	35	33
Triple	475	17	32%	8	160	470	43	33
Triple with Cheese	625	30	43%	15	180	935	52	34
Ham Sandwich	450	22	44%	7	na	1860	29	37
Grilled Cheese Sandwich	250	13	47%	6	20	610	9	24
Grilled Chicken Sandwich	510	22	39%	5	85	1150	26	53
Other Items: Baked Beans	175	4	21%	1	0	655	9	27
Chef Salad	315	18	51%	5	120	1580	41	6
Chili & Oyster Crackers	335	14	38%	4	na	1160	16	37
Chili Mac & 4 Saltines	310	12	35%	3	na	1300	15	34
Chili 3 Ways & 4 Saltines	410	16	35%	4	na	1730	19	45
Cottage Cheese, 1/2 cup	95	4	38%	1	20	200	12	3
French Fries	210	10	43%	3	10	300	3	28
Lettuce/Tom/ Salad/1oz 1000 Island	170	15	79%	3	15	225	1	7
Desserts: Apple Danish	390	24	55%	6	30	350	6	35
Brownie	260	12	42%	4	10	165	3	39
Cheesecake	370	11	27%	6	60	295	7	61
with Strawberries	385	11	26%	5	60	295	7	65
Pies: Apple	405	18	40%	5	40	480	4	61
Cherry	335	14	38%	4	30	270	6	48
Apple, A La Mode	550	25	41%	9	80	525	4	76
Cherry, A La Mode	475	22	42%	7	70	315	6	63
Sundaes: Brownie Fudge	645	35	49%	15	30	260	7	81
Hot Fudge Nut	530	34	58%	14	60	120	5	51
Strawberry	330	22	60%	8	50	80	2	29
Vanilla Ice Cream	250	12	43%	6	40	70	1	23
Shakes & Drinks: Hot Chocolate	685	19	25%	6	50	670	17	129
Floats: Coca-Cola	515	17	30%	8	0	230	16	76
Orange	500	17	31%	8	0	225	16	74
Lemon	555	19	31%	9	0	250	18	82
Root Beer	530	17	29%	8	0	240	17	78
Freezes: Lemon	550	25	41%	10	0	215	15	69
Orange	515	24	42%	10	0	200	14	63
Shakes: Chocolate/Vanilla	610	38	56%	10	100	180	13	57
Strawberry	650	40	55%	11	100	190	16	62

(Cholesterol & Saturated Fat Figures - Estimates only)

Sweet Tomatoes®

~ Same Menu & Data as Souplantation (Page 238) ~

Starbucks ~ See Page 153

Sub Station®

	Cal	Fat	%Fc	S.Fat	Chol	Sod	Pro	Carb
andwiches: Ham/Turkey & Cheese	510	30	53%	na	na	1160	18	40
oast Beef/Turkey & Cheese	525	31	54%	na	na	1045	24	39
alami, Pepperoni, Turkey								
Bologna, Ham, Cheese	635	42	60%	na	na	1590	23	40

Taco Bell®

	Cal	Fat	%Fc	S.Fat	Chol	Sod	Pro	Carb
acos: Taco, regular	210	12	51%	4	30	330	9	18
aco Supreme®	260	16	65%	6	40	350	10	20
aja Chicken Taco	280	15	48%	4	40	680	14	21
oft Taco Beef	210	10	43%	4	30	570	11	20
oft Taco Chicken	190	7	33%	2.5	35	480	13	19
oft Taco Steak	280	17	55%	4	35	630	12	20
ouble Decker® Taco	380	17	40%	5	30	740	15	43
ouble Decker® Taco Supreme	420	21	45%	8	40	760	15	45
Gorditas								
heesy Gordita Crunch	560	33	53%	11	60	980	21	44
heesy Gordita Crunch Supreme	610	37	55%	13	70	990	22	47
ordita Baja™ Beef	360	21	53%	5	35	810	13	29
ordita Baja™ Chicken; Steak	340	18	48%	4	35	730	16	28
ordita Santa Fe™ Beef	380	23	54%	5	35	700	14	31
ordita Santa Fe™ Chicken; Steak	370	20	49%	4	40	610	17	30
ordita Supreme® Beef; Steak	300	14	42%	5	35	550	17	27
ordita Supreme® Chicken	300	13	39%	5	45	530	16	28
ordita Nacho Cheese Beef	310	15	44%	4	25	780	13	30
ordita Nacho Cheese Chkn; Steak	290	13	40%	3	20	695	16	28
Chalupas								
halupa Baja® Beef	420	27	58%	7	35	760	14	30
halupa Baja® Chicken; Steak	400	24	54%	6	40	670	17	27
halupa Santa Fe™ Beef	440	29	59%	7	35	660	14	31
halupa Santa Fe™ Chicken; Steak	420	26	56%	6	40	580	17	30
halupa Supreme® Beef	380	23	54%	8	40	580	14	29
halupa Supreme® Chicken	360	20	50%	7	45	490	17	28
halupa Supreme® Steak	360	20	50%	7	35	500	17	27
halupa Nacho Cheese Beef	370	22	54%	6	25	740	13	30
halupa Nacho Cheese Chkn; Steak	350	19	49%	4.5	20	650	16	29
pecialities: Tostada	250	12	43%	4.5	15	640	10	27
heese Quesadilla	440	28	51%	11	55	1100	19	39
hicken Quesadilla	540	30	50%	12	80	1270	28	40
nchirito® Beef	370	19	46%	9	50	1300	18	33
nchirito® Chicken; Steak	350	16	41%	8	50	1215	22	31
Meximelt®	290	15	47%	7	45	830	15	22
Mexican Pizza	390	25	58%	8	45	930	18	28
aco Salad w. Salsa & Shell	850	52	55%	14	70	2250	30	69
aco Salad w. Salsa, w/out Shell	400	22	50%	10	70	1510	24	31

CONTINUED NEXT PAGE

	Cal	Fat	%Fc	S.Fat	Chol	Sod	Pro	Carb
Burritos: Bean Burrito	370	12	29%	3.5	10	1080	13	54
Burrito Supreme Beef	430	18	38%	7	40	1210	17	50
Burrito Supreme Chicken/Steak	410	16	35%	6	45	1120	20	49
Chili Cheese Burrito	330	13	35%	5	25	900	13	40
Double Burrito Supreme Beef	510	23	41%	9	60	1500	23	52
Double Burrito Supreme® Chicken	460	17	33%	6	70	1200	27	50
Fiesta Burrito Chicken; Steak	370	12	29%	4	35	1000	17	48
7-Layer Burrito	520	22	38%	7	25	1270	16	65
Grilled Stuft Chicken; Steak	690	29	38%	8	70	1900	33	73
Nachos and Sides: Nachos, 3.5 oz	320	18	51%	4	3	560	5	34
Nachos Supreme®	440	24	49%	7	35	800	14	44
Nachos BellGrande®	760	39	46%	11	35	1300	20	83
Mucho Grande Nachos	1320	82	56%	25	75	2670	31	116
Pintos 'n Cheese, 4.5 oz	180	8	40%	4	15	640	9	18
Mexican Rice, 4.75 oz	190	9	43%	3.5	15	750	5	23
Cinnamon Twists, 1.25 oz	150	4.5	27%	1	0	190	1	27

Taco Time®

	Cal	Fat	%Fc	S.Fat	Chol	Sod	Pro	Carb
Burritos: Casita Burrito®, Beef	715	36	45%	na	55	1355	31	64
Crisp Burrito: Bean	340	13	34%	na	5	480	12	44
Beef	380	21	50%	na	35	700	19	29
Chicken	330	18	49%	na	50	480	21	21
Soft Combination Burrito: Beef	530	22	37%	na	45	1055	27	54
Chicken	465	15	29%	na	65	985	31	49
Soft Bean Burrito	455	14	28%	na	20	805	19	61
Soft Beef Burrito	600	30	45%	na	70	1305	35	46
Soft Chicken Burrito	475	16	30%	na	110	1165	43	37
Taco: Natural Soft Chicken	510	20	35%	na	70	1260	30	52
Crisp Taco: Beef	210	13	56%	na	30	350	12	13
Chicken	175	8.5	44%	na	40	310	14	11
Soft/Natural Soft Taco: Beef	560	28	45%	na	50	1200	25	55
Soft Taco: Chicken	475	22	42%	na	70	900	28	37
Wraps: Beef	860	42	44%	na	55	2025	34	90
Chicken	795	35	33%	na	75	1955	38	86
Veggie	735	34	42%	na	30	1605	23	89
Sth West Chicken	725	22	27%	na	70	2060	38	98
Specialties: Crustos®	460	27	53%	na	0	0	6	50
Mexi Fries®: Regular, 5.6 oz	440	28	58%	na	0	650	4.5	42
Mexican Rice, 2.3 oz	80	0.5	0.1%	na	0	260	2	18
Mexi-Meal: Beef (no dressing)	985	54	49%	na	70	1645	41	85
Mexi-Meal: Chicken (no dressing)	895	46	46%	na	100	1380	45	74
Quesadilla, Cheese (Kid's Meal)	290	14	44%	na	30	330	11	35
Salads: Beef Taco (no dressing), reg.	315	20	57%	na	45	575	19	15
Chicken Taco Salad (no dressing), reg.	250	13	47%	na	65	505	23	11
Tostada Delight® Salad, Beef	705	43	55%	na	55	1130	32	50
Sauce: Enchilada/Hot Sauce, 1 oz	6	0	0%	0	0	80	0.2	1.5

	Cal	Fat	%Fc	S.Fat	Chol	Sod	Pro	Carb
Tacos: Bravo	355	15	38%	5	26	655	15	39
Burger	280	11	35%	5	35	580	14	29
Crispy	195	12	55%	4	26	255	9	13
El Grande	480	29	54%	10	67	765	24	30
El Grande Chicken	330	18	49%	5	41	735	17	24
Softshell	230	10	39%	4	26	505	11	23
Softshell Chicken	175	5	25%	2	21	615	11	22
Burritos: Bean Burrito	380	12	28%	5	15	810	15	54
Beefy Burrito	440	20	41%	9	53	860	22	44
Chicken and Potato Burrito	455	19	37%	5	19	1345	15	56
Meat and Potato Burrito	510	23	40%	7	23	1235	15	58
Super Burrito	455	19	37%	7	34	910	19	51
Specialities								
Chicken Festiva Burrito	545	28	46%	7	37	1150	17	56
Chicken Festiva Salad (w. dressing)	685	50	65%	11	70	1425	21	39
Chicken Festiva Salad (no dressing)	360	19	47%	6	49	660	21	27
Potato Olés Bravo	585	36	55%	10	13	1810	9	55
Sierra Chicken Sandwich	510	28	49%	6	70	930	27	40
Super Nachos	925	62	60%	15	47	1450	24	70
Super Potato Olés	990	63	57%	19	47	3025	23	83
Taco Salad (with dressing)	715	45	56%	12	40	1795	21	55
Taco Salad (no dressing)	545	28	46%	9	40	880	20	50
Platters: Beef and Bean Chimi	745	34	41%	9	41	1770	26	82
Chicken Enchilada	710	33	42%	11	48	2310	28	72
Cheese and Chiles Chimi	800	43	48%	14	50	1915	27	74
Sides: Green Chili	225	12	48%	5	15	1235	10	20
Mexican Rice	250	5	18%	1	0	855	6	44
Nachos	455	32	63%	8	14	850	8	36
Potato Olés: Small (Kid's Meal)	305	18	53%	4	0	880	3	33
Regular	415	24	52%	6	0	1195	4	45
Large	545	32	53%	8	0	1570	5	60
Refried Beans	375	13	31%	5	15	990	20	46
Side Salad	290	24	74%	5	20	555	3	15
Texas Style Chili	375	22	52%	10	56	945	21	23
Desserts: Apple Grande	260	9	31%	3	7	240	5	40
Choco Taco	310	17	49%	10	20	100	3	37
Churros	160	11	63%	2	10	115	2	13
Dichos Cookies, 2	70	4	53%	0	0	10	2	6
Taco John's Cinnamon Mint Swirl	60	0	0%	0	0	5	1	14
Teddy Graham Cubs	60	2	30%	0	0	80	1	10

TCBY® Frozen Yogurt

~ See Page 31 - Icecream Section ~

Tim Horton's®

	Cal	Fat	%FC	S.Fat	Chol	Sod	Pro	Car
Bagels: Average all types	300	2	6%	0	0	520	11	59
Baked Goods: Butter Croissant	210	11	47%	6	30	370	5	25
Cheese Croissant	240	12	45%	5	20	370	6	27
Cherry Cheese Danish	380	23	54%	9	45	410	7	33
Southern Country Cranberry Biscuit	470	19	36%	5	0	1050	7	68
Beverages: Cafe Mocha	250	10	36%	4	0	330	3	34
Cappuccino Ice	430	23	48%	14	80	50	3	54
Coffee	80	4	45%	2	12	20	1	10
French Vanilla	130	5	35%	4	0	120	3	20
Fruit Punch	150	0	0%	0	0	10	0	38
Hot Chocolate	200	6	27%	2	0	370	2	44
Cakes: Black Forest	500	21	38%	14	0	790	4	75
Chocolot Fantasy	420	15	32%	7	35	630	5	72
Shadow, white & chocolate	430	19	40%	10	35	470	4	63
Cookies: Chocolate Chip	150	7	42%	3	20	140	2	21
Oatmeal Raisin	150	6	36%	2	15	140	2	22
Peanut Butter Chocolate Chunk	170	10	53%	4	15	150	3	18
Plain Macaroon	140	8	51%	7	0	60	1	14
Cream Cheese: Regular, average	150	13	78%	9	40	230	3	3
Plain Light	90	7	70%	5	20	200	4	3
Donuts								
Cake Donut: Chocolate Glazed	350	22	57%	7	10	340	3	35
Old Fashion Glazed	270	12	40%	4	15	260	3	39
Old Fashion Plain	220	12	49%	4	15	260	3	24
Filled Donut: Angel Cream	280	13	42%	4	0	280	4	36
Yeast: Apple Fritter	300	14	42%	5	0	280	5	40
Chocolate Dip	230	10	39%	3	0	270	4	33
Muffins: Blueberry Bran	300	9	27%	2	10	690	5	51
Carrot Whole Wheat	410	22	48%	2	10	580	5	52
Low Fat Carrot/Cranberry	260	2	7%	0	0	620	5	60
Wild Blueberry	330	11	30%	2	15	520	4	54
Pies: Apple	540	31	52%	6	0	230	4	62
Cherry	570	31	49%	6	0	320	4	70
Chocolate Cream	490	31	57%	16	10	170	2	52
Tarts: Fresh Strawberry	220	9	37%	2	0	140	1	36
Raisin Butter	330	11	30%	3	15	200	4	54
Sandwiches								
Albacore Tuna Salad	350	8	21%	1	15	1100	21	49
Black Forest Ham & Swiss	640	27	45%	9	75	1540	33	53
Chunky Chicken Salad	380	10	24%	1	45	770	23	50
Fireside Roast Beef	470	19	36%	3	35	1470	22	48
Garden Vegetable	460	24	47%	11	45	30	12	50
Harvest Turkey Breast	470	18	34%	2	30	1460	22	53
Soup: Chicken Noodle	100	3	27%	1	14	710	5	15
Cream of Mushroom	195	10	46%	3	5	950	4	21
Hearty Vegetable; Minestrone	130	2	14%	0	0	830	3	27
Vegetable Beef Barley	110	2	16%	0	9	840	5	18

Togo's® Eatery

	Cal	Fat	%Fc	S.Fat	Chol	Sod	Pro	Carb
Salads: Caesar Salad	470	30	57%	na	72	1190	30	22
Chef's Salad	385	19	44%	na	65	1585	26	26
Cobb Salad	485	24	44%	na	294	985	40	29
Garden Salad	255	10	35%	na	214	580	11.5	31
Mandarin Orange Chicken	300	10	30%	na	60	210	27	25
Oriental Chicken	320	14	39%	na	60	290	30	18
Taco Salad	945	59	56%	na	70	1625	29	76
Sandwiches: Per 6" sandwich on white roll								
Albacore Tuna	700	30	39%	na	67	1655	32	78
Avocado & Turkey	675	28	37%	na	35	1605	27	80
Avocado, Cucumber & Alfalfa Sprout	635	28	40%	na	6	1150	16	85
BBQ Beef	725	22	27%	na	88	2120	39	94
BBQ Chicken	560	8	13%	na	95	1540	48	74
California Roasted Chicken	510	15	26%	na	65	1770	36	73
Egg Salad w. Cheese	730	35	43%	na	456	1765	29	76
Ham & Cheese	660	26	35%	na	68	2900	33	76
Hot Pastrami	705	26	33%	na	72	2260	34	85
Meatballs w. Pizza Sauce	710	28	36%	na	97	1605	36	78
Mort., Provolone & Dry Salami/Cotto	785	39	45%	na	84	2300	36	74
Roast Beef (Hot or Cold)	550	11	18%	na	84	1535	42	75
Roasted Bell Pepper & Provolone	580	22	34%	na	33	1755	21	79
Seafood Salad	610	21	31%	na	105	2010	31	74
Smoked Turkey	725	19	24%	na	96	2545	46	94
Spicy Chkn w. Jamaican seasoning	560	14	22%	na	85	1190	32	78
Turkey & Bacon Club	665	26	35%	na	80	2110	37	73
Turkey & Cranberry	625	13	19%	na	50	1905	30	96
Turkey, Ham, Salami & Cheese	700	26	34%	na	88	2975	40	77

Weinerschnitzel®

na - figures not available	Cal	Fat	%Fc	S.Fat	Chol	Sod	Pro	Carb
Breakfast Burrito	570	37	58%	13	530	1105	na	na
Chicken Sandwich	540	32	53%	9	48	960	na	na
Chili Burger	625	40	58%	12	96	1350	na	na
Deluxe: Hamburger	580	37	57%	12	90	1145	na	na
Cheeseburger	635	42	60%	14	103	1350	na	na
Bacon Cheeseburger	690	46	60%	16	110	1520	na	na
Patty Melt	580	35	54%	16	108	1330	na	na
Dogs: Chili Dog	295	16	49%	5	28	935	na	na
Chili Cheese Dog	350	21	54%	8	41	1140	na	na
Corn Dog	290	23	71%	8	26	460	na	na
Deluxe Dog; Kraut Dog	275	14	46%	5	21	1620	na	na
Mustard Dog	260	14	48%	5	21	795	na	na
Relish Dog	280	14	45%	5	21	900	na	na
Western Dog	380	23	54%	9	43	985	na	na
Fries: Small	175	13	67%	8	19	345	na	na
Chili Fries	470	36	69%	19	64	1000	na	na

Wendy's®

	Cal	Fat	%Fc	S.Fat	Chol	Sod	Pro	Car
Sandwiches: Big Bacon Classic	580	30	46%	12	100	1460	34	46
Chicken Club	470	20	38%	4.5	65	940	30	47
Classic Single with Everything	410	19	43%	7	70	920	25	37
Grilled Chicken	300	7	23%	1.5	55	740	24	36
Kids' Meal: Jr. Hamburger	270	9	33%	3	30	620	14	33
Jr. Cheeseburger	310	12	37%	6	45	800	17	33
Deluxe	350	16	42%	6	50	860	18	36
Jr. Bacon Cheeseburger	380	19	45%	7	55	870	20	34
Spicy Chicken	410	14	33%	2.5	65	1280	28	43
French Fries: Medium	420	20	44%	3	0	130	6	55
Biggie	470	23	44%	3.5	0	150	7	61
Great Biggie	570	27	43%	4	0	180	8	73
Fresh Salads-To-Go: No Dressing								
Caesar Side	110	5	41%	2.5	15	380	9	6
Deluxe Garden	110	6	49%	1	0	320	7	10
Grilled Chicken	200	7	36%	1.5	55	780	27	10
Side Salad	60	3	45%	0.5	0	160	4	5
Soft Breadsticks	130	3	21%	0.5	5	250	4	23
Taco Salad	380	19	45%	10	65	1040	26	28
Taco Chips, 15 chips	210	9	47%	1.5	0	160	3	28
Tomato, wedged, 1 piece	5	0	0%	0	0	0	0	1
Dressings & Sauce: Per Packet								
Barbeque Sauce	45	0	0%	0	0	160	1	10
Blue Cheese	360	38	100%	7	30	350	2	1
French	250	21	75%	3	0	670	0	13
French Fat Free	70	0	0%	0	0	300	0	18
Hidden Valley Ranch	200	20	100%	3	25	410	1	3
Reduced Fat	120	11	75%	2	20	470	1	4
Honey Mustard	130	12	83%	2	10	220	0	6
Italian Caesar	230	24	96%	4	25	350	1	1
Italian Reduced Fat	80	7	67%	1	0	340	0	6
Sweet & Sour Sauce	50	0	0%	0	0	120	0	12
Thousand Island	260	25	80%	4	20	380	1	7
Baked Potato: Plain	310	0	0%	0	0	25	7	72
Bacon & Cheese	530	17	30%	4	25	820	16	78
Broccoli & Cheese	470	14	27%	3	5	470	9	80
Sour Cream & Chives	370	5	14%	4	15	75	7	72
Whipped Margarine	70	7	100%	1.5	0	115	0	0
Chili: Small	210	7	30%	2.5	30	800	15	21
Large	310	10	29%	3.5	45	1190	23	32
Cheddar Cheese, shredded, 2 Tbsp	70	6	77%	3.5	15	110	4	1
Saltine Crackers, 2	25	0.5	18%	0	0	80	1	4
Chicken Nuggets: 5 Piece	230	16	63%	3	30	470	11	11
4 Piece Kid's Meal	190	13	62%	2.5	25	380	9	9
Frosty Dairy Dessert: Junior, 6 oz	170	4	21%	2.5	200	100	4	26
Small, 12 oz	330	8	22%	5	35	200	8	56
Medium, 16 oz	440	11	22%	7	50	260	11	73

Whataburger®

Burgers/Sandwiches:	Cal	Fat	%Fc	S.Fat	Chol	Sod	Pro	Carb
Justaburger®	295	12	39%	5	35	80	16	27
Whataburger®	605	29	39%	9	75	1165	31	53
Small bun no oil	425	21	42%	7	75	875	27	31
Double Meat Whataburger®	835	46	50%	20	150	1305	51	53
Whataburger Jr.®	305	15	36%	6	35	90	17	29
Grilled Chicken Fajita Taco	335	9	19%	2	75	1080	28	37
Beef Fajita Taco	325	13	33%	3	42	1150	21	30
Grilled Chicken Sandwich: w. dressing	455	18	28%	3	84	1165	31	49
No dressing	395	12	20%	2	75	1075	31	47
No bun oil or dressing	370	9	14%	2	75	1075	31	47
Small bun, mustard (no dressing)	335	8	9%	1	75	1125	29	30
Whatacatch®	460	33	48%	4	32	860	18	44
Whatachick'n®	500	23	41%	4	40	1120	27	51
Salads: Garden Salad	55	0.5	8%	0	0	30	3	11
Grilled Chicken Salad	215	5	7%	1	75	630	25	19
Shakes: Chocolate (Jr. Size)	615	17	24%	5	60	325	13	100
French Fries: Junior	240	4	49%	7	0	205	3	37
Regular	420	21	49%	11	0	310	5	51
Large	560	29	49%	14	0	410	7	69
Breakfast: Biscuit w. Bacon, Egg, Chse	490	29	58%	14	245	1370	21	35
Breakfast-On-A-Bun™: w. Sausage	460	30	55%	13	255	840	23	29
Egg Omelet Sandwich	290	15	40%	7	225	725	15	28

Winchell's®

Baked Products	Cal	Fat	%Fc	S.Fat	Chol	Sod	Pro	Carb
Bagel	310	1	3%	na	na	320	8.6	22
Banana Nut Muffin	535	28	47%	na	na	480	13	63
Blueberry Muffin	440	25	51%	na	na	470	10	54
Blueberry Muffin, Low Fat	410	3	7%	na	na	470	6	42
Bran Muffin, Low Fat	405	3	7%	na	na	270	7	44
Chocolate Chip Muffin	480	22	41%	na	na	475	9	54
Croissant	260	17	59%	na	na	280	5	28
Cake Donuts: Glazed Old Fashion	250	18	65%	na	na	210	4	28
Iced Donut Holes (4)	230	15	59%	na	na	220	2	28
Plain Donut Holes (4)	215	14	59%	na	na	215	1.5	26
Raised Donuts: Apple Fritter	670	41	55%	na	na	220	6	55
Bear Claw	560	30	48%	na	na	220	6	47
Chocolate Bavarian	325	18	50%	na	na	195	6	36
Chocolate Rounds	240	16	60%	na	na	125	4	29
Chocolate Twist	240	16	60%	na	na	125	4	29
Glazed Cinnamon Roll	430	24	50%	na	na	195	6	12
Glazed Rounds	230	15	59%	na	na	120	1.5	27
Glazed Twist	230	15	59%	na	na	120	1.5	27
Sugar Jelly	315	17	49%	na	na	190	6	36
Sugar Rounds	225	15	60%	na	na	120	1.5	27
Sugar Twist	225	15	60%	na	na	120	1.5	27

White Castle®

	Cal	Fat	%Fc	S.Fat	Chol	Sod	Pro	Carb
Hamburgers: Hamburger	135	7	47%	3	10	135	6	11
Cheeseburger	160	9	51%	4	15	250	7	11
Sandwiches: Chicken	190	8	38%	2	20	360	8	21
Fish (w/out Tartar), 1 serving	160	6	34%	1	15	220	8	18
Breakfast Sandwich	340	25	66%	10	130	900	14	17
Bacon Cheeseburger	200	13	59%	6	25	400	10	12
French Fries: Small	115	6	47%	1	15	15	2	15
Onion Chips, small	180	9	45%	2	0	580	3	25
Onion Rings, 8 piece	540	26	45%	na	0	1300	8	69

Yoshinoya®

	Cal	Fat	%Fc	S.Fat	Chol	Sod	Pro	Carb
Bowls								
Beef Bowl: Regular, 15 oz	840	30	32%	13	75	1120	32	109
Large, 21 oz	1160	41	32%	18	105	1530	44	153
Kids, 9 oz	340	11	29%	5	30	690	13	48
Chicken Bowl: Regular,19 oz	760	15	18%	4.5	80	1280	33	125
Large, 30 oz	1110	22	18%	7	120	2120	49	180
Kids, 10 oz	370	9	22%	3	55	720	20	53
Combo Bowl: Regular, 17 oz	750	19	23%	7	70	1120	29	117
Large, 27 oz	1220	36	27%	14	135	2080	54	171
Vegetable Beef Bowl: Regular,18 oz	770	23	27%	10	55	1240	26	114
Large, 28 oz	1090	32	26%	13	75	1970	37	163
Vegetable Bowl: Regular 19 oz	530	3.5	6%	0.5	0	870	9	116
Large, 32 oz	780	5	6%	1	0	1710	14	169
Tempura: Fish Tempura, 22 oz	990	24	22%	6	80	1720	26	168
Fish & Beef Tempura, 30 oz	1450	45	28%	15	135	2520	47	214
Fish & Chicken Tempura, 31 oz	1450	37	23%	10	160	2560	53	225
Shrimp Tempura, 20 oz	890	19	19%	4.5	55	1540	20	160
Shrimp & Beef Tempura, 28 oz	1350	40	27%	14	110	2450	41	206
Shrimp & Chicken Tempura, 29 oz	1340	32	22%	8	135	2480	48	217
Extras: Beef, 5¹/2 oz	370	28	68%	12	75	1090	25	6
Chicken & Vegetables, 9¹/2 oz	300	12	36%	4	80	1250	26	21
Rice, 10 oz	460	2.5	5%	0.5	0	30	7	104
Vegetable, 9 oz	60	0.5	8%	0	0	840	2	12

Note: Yoshinoya Beef Bowl Restaurants are based in California.

Zantiago®

	Cal	Fat	%Fc	S.Fat	Chol	Sod	Pro	Carb
Burrito								
Hot Cheese, Chilito	330	15	41%	7	35	466	14	35
Mild Cheese, Chilito	335	15	41%	7	35	505	14	36
Enchilada: Beef	315	15	43%	5	30	904	18	26
Cheese	390	23	53%	11	40	759	20	26
Taco: Burrito	415	19	41%	8	40	815	21	41
Regular	200	12	55%	4	20	318	10	13

Notes on Cholesterol

- **Cholesterol** is a white waxy substance produced mainly by our liver. It is also found in animal food products. Plant foods have no cholesterol.

- **Cholesterol is essential to life.** It is a structural part of every body cell wall and is the building block for vitamin D, sex hormones, and bile acids which help in the digestion of dietary fats.

- **The body makes sufficient cholesterol** for its needs and does not rely on cholesterol in the diet. Dietary fats have a major influence on blood cholesterol levels - more so than dietary cholesterol.

- **A high blood cholesterol increases** the risk of atherosclerosis - the thickening of arteries that can reduce or block blood flow to the heart muscle, brain, eyes, kidneys, sex organs and other body parts.

  This in turn increases the risk of heart attack, stroke, blindness, kidney failure, impotence and other blood circulatory problems.

  Other risk factors which increase the risk of atherosclerosis include high blood pressure, tobacco smoking, obesity and diabetes (uncontrolled).

HEART ATTACK WARNING SIGNALS

Many victims die before reaching hospital by ignoring warning signals and delaying medical help.

Symptoms vary and commonly include:

- **Chest pain,** vice-like squeezing or burning sensation in centre of chest or between shoulder blades, or feeling of severe indigestion.

- **Pain** may spread to shoulders, neck, jaw or arms.

- **Sweating,** nausea, dizziness, shortness of breath, irregular pulse.

If you experience any of the above symptoms seek IMMEDIATE medical attention!

Every minute counts.

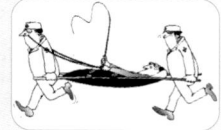

BLOOD CHOLESTEROL

Check Your Risk!

Cholesterol Level (mg/dL)	Risk of Heart Attack
240 and above	~ High Risk
200 - 239	~ Borderline/High
Below 200	~ Desirable

❤ Know your cholesterol level, particularly if there is a family history of heart disease or stroke. If high, see your doctor.

❤ All adults should have their cholesterol, HDL and triglycerides tested at least every 5 years.

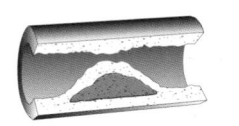

▲ Atherosclerosis can clog arteries and impede blood flow to the heart muscle or other body organs.

▼ A thrombus (blood clot) can form on unstable, festering atherosclerotic plaque and rapidly block blood flow.

A heart attack or stroke can result.

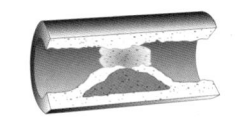

Fats & Cholesterol Guide

The amount and type of dietary fat has the greatest influence on blood cholesterol levels.

Fats in food are a mixture of 3 basic types: saturated, monounsaturated, and polyunsaturated. Animal fats are mainly saturated while plant oils and fish oils are mainly mono- and polyunsaturated.

Saturated fats have subgroups known as long chain, medium chain, and short chain fats. Most of the long chain fats raise blood cholesterol; and increase the risk of blood clots and thrombosis leading to artery blockage.

Long chain saturated fats are found mainly in full cream milk, cheese, butter, cream, fatty meats and sausages, and processed foods.

Monounsaturated fats tend to more selectively lower 'bad' LDL-cholesterol and maintain the protective 'good' HDL-cholesterol in the bloodstream - but only if they replace saturated fats in the diet.

Foods rich in monounsaturates include canola and olive oils, canola margarine, peanuts, and avocados.

Polyunsaturated fats consist of two main classes. **Omega-6** polyunsaturates tend to lower blood cholesterol. Rich sources include safflower, sunflower and corn oils.

Omega-3 polyunsaturated fats can lower blood cholesterol, and also confer extra benefits by lowering blood triglycerides, and reducing the risk of thrombosis, heart arrhythmias, and artery spasm.

Best practical omega-3 sources include canola oil and margarine, soybean oil and fish. (See adjoining chart)

A balanced intake of the two omega classes is important for optimal health. Increasing slightly omega-3 intake by Americans would help to attain a more ideal balance. Adequate vitamin E intake is also important.

All fats are high in calories and need to be limited for weight control.

DIETARY FATS COMPARISON

- ■ Saturated Fat
- ■ Monounsaturated Fat
- ■ Linoleic (Omega-6)
- ■ Alpha-Linolenic (Omega-3)

OILS — PERCENTAGE CONTENT

OIL	Saturated Fat	Monounsaturated Fat	Linoleic (Omega-6)	Alpha-Linolenic (Omega-3)
CANOLA OIL	7	63	20	10
LINSEED/FLAX OIL	9	19	17	55
SAFFLOWER OIL	9	14	77	
GRAPESEED OIL	10	22	68	
SUNFLOWER OIL	11	23	66	
CORN OIL	14	32	52	2
OLIVE OIL	14	76	10	
SOYBEAN OIL	15	23	54	8
PEANUT OIL	19	45	34	2
COTTONSEED OIL	26	16	58	
PALM OIL	51	39	10	

SPREADS & FATS
Saturated Fat includes 'Trans Fats' ❑ WATER CONTENT

	Saturated	Mono	Omega-6	Omega-3	Water
LIGHT MARGARINE	14	14	21		51
CANOLA MARGARINE	18	45	12	6	19
POLYUNSATURATED MARG.	24	20	36		20
BUTTER	57	18	2	4	
LARD	41	47	12		
BEEF FAT	44	37	4	15	

GOOD SOURCES OF OMEGA-3 FATS

Plant Sources	Omega-3 Fats (Grams)
Canola Oil, 1 Tbsp, 1/2 fl.oz	1.5g
Flaxseed Oil, 1 Tbsp	8g
Soybean Oil, 1 Tbsp	1.2g
Canola Margarine, 1 Tbsp, 1/2 oz	1g
Soybeans, cooked, 1/2 cup, 4 oz	0.5g
Walnuts, 1/2 oz	0.5g

FISH - Per 4 oz Serving
High Content: Salmon (Chinook), Tuna, 3g
Trout (Lake), Sardines, Herring, Mackerel 3g
Medium Content:
Salmon (Pink/Red/Coho), 4 oz 2g
Fair Content: Per 4 oz Serving
Bass, Catfish, Cod, Grouper, Hake, Halibut, Kingfish, Perch, Pollock, Shark, Trout (Rainbow), Tuna (Skipjack), Crab, Oysters, Blue Mussel, Shrimp, Squid } 0.5-1g

How Much is Needed?
As little as 1-2 grams daily of omega-3 fats may benefit general health. High doses of fish oil supplements should only be taken as directed by your doctor.

Dietary Cholesterol

Cholesterol in food varies in its effect on blood cholesterol level (BCL) from person to person. Much depends on the amount and type of fat, and fiber eaten at the same meal.

Any elevating effect of dietary cholesterol on BCL is more likely to occur when the diet is high in saturated fat. Little elevation, if any, generally occurs when dietary fats are balanced in favour of mono- and polyunsaturated fats (including omega-3 fats).

For example, while fish does contain cholesterol, the omega-3 fats can prevent any increase in BCL. Conversely, a meal containing no cholesterol but rich in saturated fat, may see a significant increase in BCL.

Consequently, the need to be overly concerned about dietary cholesterol is being de-emphasised in favour of a stricter approach to limiting total fats, and saturated fat in particular.

The liver usually cuts back its own cholesterol production in response to cholesterol in the diet. Many people can consume normal amounts of high cholesterol foods without concern.

However, it is difficult to identify just who is at risk - the so-called 'hyper-responders' - and because over 50% of Americans have a BCL above ideal levels, the **American Heart Association** advises all Americans to be prudent and limit their cholesterol intake to less than 300mg daily.

This limitation still allows the inclusion of most foods regularly eaten - even the overly maligned egg.

Note: Eggs contain a modest 5 grams of fat per large egg of which barely 2 grams are saturated, the rest being mono- and polyunsaturated.

By comparison, a cup of whole milk has almost 10g fat of which 6g are saturated.

CHOLESTEROL COUNTER

Cholesterol is found only in foods of animal origin. Plant foods contain no cholesterol. AHA recommends limiting dietary cholesterol to less than 300mg/day.

	Chol mg
Meat - Average all types:	
Lean Meat, cooked, 4 oz	70
Fatty Meat, cooked, 4 oz	105
Fat, thick strip, 2 oz	35
(Note: While lean meat and fat have similar amounts of cholesterol, choose lean meat to limit fat intake.)	
Chicken/Turkey, average, 4 oz	90
Organ Meats: Liver, fried, 4 oz	500
Brains, beef, pan fried, 3 oz	1700
Sausages: Frankfurter, 1.5 oz	25
Salami, 2 slices, 2 oz	40
Bacon: 3 slices, cooked, 1 oz	20
Fish: Fish fillets, average, ckd, 4 oz	70
Tuna/Salmon, canned, 3 oz	30
Scallops, 9 medium, 3 oz	30
Shrimp, 12 large, raw, 3 oz	130
Oysters, raw, 6 medium, 3 oz	45
Lobster, Crab, raw, 3 oz	80
Eggs (Chicken), 1 large	210
1 medium	180
Egg White, *Egg Beaters*	0
Milk/Yogurt: Whole, 1 cup, 8 fl.oz	35
1% Milk, 1 cup	10
Skim/Non-fat, 1 cup	5
Soy Milk	0
Cheese: Natural/Hard/Cream 1 oz	30
Cottage, lowfat, 4 oz	5
Ricotta, part skim, 4 oz	25
Fats: Butter, 2 Tbsp, 1 oz	60
Margarine, Oils (vegetable)	0
Mayonnaise, 1 Tbsp	10
Cream: Heavy, whipping, 2 T, 1 oz	40
Half & Half/Sour, 2 Tbsp, 1 oz	10
Icecream: Regular, $1/3$ cup, 4 fl.oz	30
Fruit, Vegetables, Avocados	0
Nuts, Seeds, Grains	0
Coffee, Tea, Soda, Beer, Wine	0

Fast-Foods ~ See Pages 167 - 250

Blood Cholesterol ~ Diet Hints

DIETARY HINTS TO LOWER BLOOD CHOLESTEROL

1. **Maintain a healthy weight.**
   If overweight, lose weight with lowfat eating and daily exercise.

2. **Reduce saturated fat intake by:**
   (a) eating less dairy fat. Choose lowfat or fat-reduced varieties of milk, yogurt, cheese, and icecream. Enjoy soy drinks.

   (b) replacing saturated fats with fats and oils rich in mono- and polyunsaturated fats; and carbohydrate-rich foods. Choose vegetable oils such as canola, olive, sunflower and soybean. Avoid solid frying fats. *Take Control* and *Benecol* (spreads) contain plant stanol esters which can lower total and LDL cholesterol.

   (c) eating less fat from meat and poultry. Choose lean cuts of meat and skinless chicken. Go easy on luncheon meats, salamis and fatty sausages. Enjoy fish.

   (d) eating less saturated fats from baked and fried fast-foods. Avoid deep-fried foods. Avoid donuts, cakes, pastries and cookies unless made with healthier fats and oils.

3. **Increase your 'soluble' fiber intake.**
   Foods rich in 'soluble' fiber include dried beans, baked beans, lentils, chick peas, hummus, nuts, seeds, psyllium seed husks and psyllium fiber supplements.
   Oat bran, rice bran and barley are also useful, as are fruit, veges and avocados.

4. **Eat more soya bean products** such as: soy drinks, tofu, tempeh (cultured soya beans), soy flour and soy vegetarian foods.
   Soy protein in place of animal protein can significantly decrease high blood cholesterol levels - as well as 'bad' LDL-cholesterol and blood triglycerides. Good' HDL-cholesterol is maintained. For best results, eat at least 25g of soy protein per day (from 3-4 servings)

5. **Eat more fruit and vegetables in place of high-fat foods.**
   Aim for 2 fruits and 5 servings of vegetables per day. They also contain valuable antioxidants.
   The fat of avocados (and most nuts and seeds) is mainly unsaturated and lowers blood cholesterol levels.

6. **Limit cholesterol to 300mg per day**
   (Extra Notes ~ See Previous Page)

7. **Avoid brewed unfiltered coffee** (espresso; plunger-style). It contains oily compounds (diterpenes) which can raise blood cholesterol. American style filtered coffee is fine.

8. **Spread your food intake over the day**
   Have 5-6 small meals per day rather than just 2-3 large meals. Nibbling, versus gorging, favors lower blood cholesterol.

ALCOHOL - WINE

Alcohol is a mixed bag. Moderate amounts of 1-2 drinks daily appear to reduce the risk of heart attack and ischaemic stroke in older persons.

However, larger amounts increase the risk of high blood pressure, obesity, heart failure and hemorrhagic stroke; and can aggravate hypertriglyceridemia - in addition to many other health hazards.
(See Alcohol Guide - p.155)

The over-riding harmful effects of excess alcohol do not allow its recommendation for any aspects of health promotion.

Notes On Wine:

Red wine (more so than white) contains antioxidants which may help protect cholesterol in the blood from becoming oxidized.

Many fruits, vegetables and tea also contain protective antioxidants.

...ts in the diet not only affect blood cholesterol levels. ...ney can also strongly influence blood clot formation ...d thrombosis, as well as blood flow and ultimate ...xygen delivery to body parts and organs.

...hile advanced atherosclerosis can impede blood flow ... the heart and other organs, it is thrombosis ...omplete blockage by blood clots) or arterial spasm ...hich commonly result in a heart attack or stroke.

...ant and fish oils rich in omega-3 fats lessen the ...sk of blood clots, thrombus formation and artery ...asm by reducing platelet stickiness and adhesion to ...tery walls. This reduces the risk of atherosclerotic ...aque becoming unstable and reactive.

...mega-3 fats also improve blood flow by reducing ...ood viscosity; and increasing the flexibility of red ...ood cells (RBC) that need to flex and twist on ...emselves in order to squeeze through tiny narrow ...pillaries often half their diameter.

...diet high in saturated fats has the opposite effect ...y stiffening RBC membranes and increasing blood ...scosity thereby hindering blood flow. The stiffening ...the RBC membrane also reduces its ability to release ...tal oxygen to body cells and take up carbon dioxide.

...iff red blood cells may also form aggregates like coin ...acks. In narrow blood vessels, this further impedes ...ood flow and impairs oxygen release through the ...uch lessened surface area of red blood cell ...embranes exposed to blood. (Smoking, lack of exercise, ...d stress can have similar adverse effects on thrombosis, ...d blood cell flexibility and blood flow.)

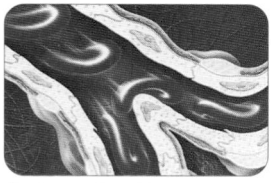

▲ Picture of Healthy Blood Flow

Flexible red blood cells twist and slide through tiny capillaries - often half the diameter of red blood cells.

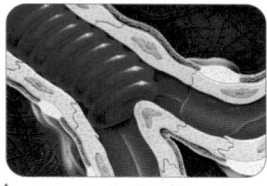

▲ A Not-So-Healthy Picture!

Red blood cells have lost their flexibility and ability to twist and slip through capillaries. They are stacked up thereby impeding blood flow.

A diet high in saturated fats can contribute to this picture - as can smoking, lack of exercise and stress.

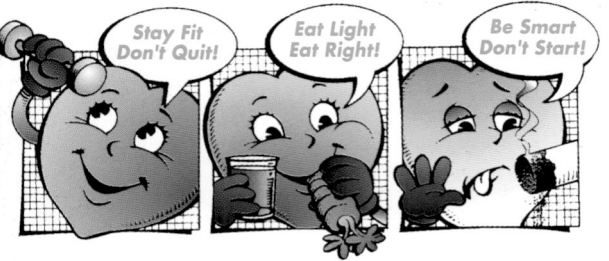

Calcium's Role in the Body

Calcium plays a vital role in nerve and muscle function, clotting of blood, enzyme regulation, insulin secretion and overall bone strength. Bones and teeth store 99% of the body's calcium.

The calcium level in blood is kept at a steady level by the continual exchange of calcium between blood and bone. When insufficient calcium is obtained from food the body draws calcium out of the bones.

This bone loss over a period of years may lead to **osteoporosis** - thinning of the bones (*porous bones*).

The bones become weak, brittle and easy to fracture, particularly the bones of the wrist, hips and spine. Loss of height and curvature of the spine may also result, as may periodontal disease - the deterioration of the jaw bones that support the teeth.

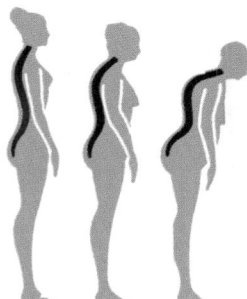

As osteoporosis progresses after menopause, vertebrae may collapse causing the spine to curve and shoulders to hunch.

Osteoporosis - Common in Women

While osteoporosis also occurs in men, women are particularly vulnerable (1 in 4 by age 60). They have about 30% less bone than men, and a greater bone loss at menopause when estrogen levels drop. Slender framed women are at greater risk. (A woman in her eighties can have lost up to two thirds of her skeleton.)

Insufficient dietary calcium during pregnancy and breastfeeding will see bone reserves drawn upon, increasing the risk of osteoporosis.

Causes of Osteoporosis

The major factors associated with the bone loss of osteoporosis appear to be:

- **Hormone changes of menopause.**
- **Insufficient calcium in the diet. (Absorption decreases with age.)**
- **Insufficient exercise (weight bearing - such as walking, cycling.)**
- **Family history of osteoporosis.**
- **Other contributing factors may include:** excess amounts of alcohol, protein and phosphorus (from meats and soft drinks); insufficient vitamin D and magnesium; and cigarette smoking.

RECOMMENDED DAILY INTAKE OF CALCIUM

		Calcium
Infants:		
	0-6 mths ~	360mg
	6-12 mths ~	540mg
Children:		
	1-10 yrs ~	800mg
	10-12 yrs ~	1200mg
Teenagers:		
	13-18 yrs ~	1200mg
	16-18 yrs ~	800mg
Adults:	19+ yrs ~	800mg
Women:		
Pre-menopausal	~	1000mg
Menopausal(beginning)	~	1200mg
Post-menopausal	~	1500mg
Pregnancy/breastfeeding:		
	10-18 yrs ~	1600mg
	19+ yrs ~	1200mg

Early Prevention Important

Gradual loss of bone begins in the thirties after maximum bone mass is reached. The stronger the bones at that time, the less trouble is likely to occur later. The earlier that prevention or treatment begins the greater the benefit. **The key to prevention** is to build strong, dense bones early in life. **By age 16,** some 80% of peak bone mass is reached.

Young women may lessen the risk by eating high-calcium foods, not engaging in excessive dieting that results in period cessation (less estrogen), taking regular exercise and not smoking.

In menopausal women, hormone therapy as well as calcium supplements and exercise, can help retard osteoporosis. Your doctor can advise you.

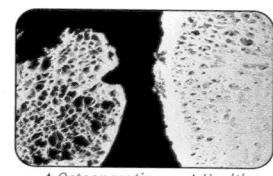

▲ Osteoporotic Fragile Bone   ▲ Healthy Dense Bone

Dietary Sources of Calcium

Milk, yogurt, calcium-enriched soy drinks and cheese are the richest sources of calcium. (Lowfat and nonfat varieties contain similar calcium.)

Canned fish with edible bones (salmon/sardines) are high in calcium. Tofu (soybean curd), tempeh, broccoli and dried beans are also good sources.

- Soy drinks (calcium-enriched) may be preferable to cow's milk. Body calcium losses are much greater with animal protein. Soy protein is relatively 'bone-sparing'.

- Phytoestrogens in soy foods may also lessen calcium losses at menopause. Soy drinks are suitable for persons with lactose intolerance.

Extra Notes on Calcium

Persons who have difficulty eating sufficient calcium-rich foods should consider a **calcium supplement.** Prescribed high doses of calcium (1500-2000mg/day) may benefit persons with osteoporosis - as well as vitamins D and K, and magnesium.

Daily calcium above 2000mg is unlikely to provide any additional benefit.

Calcium in food reduces iron absorption by up to 60% when eaten with iron-containing foods. Consume calcium-rich foods/supplements at smaller meals and mid-meal snacks.

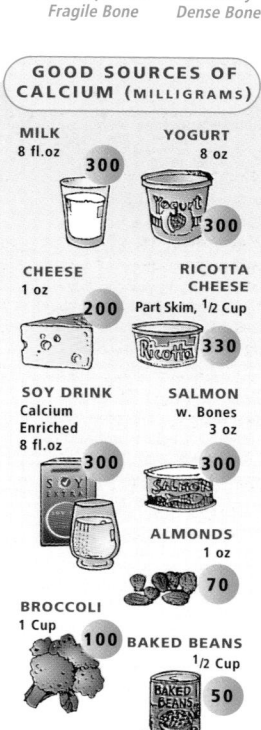

GOOD SOURCES OF CALCIUM (MILLIGRAMS)

MILK 8 fl.oz — 300

YOGURT 8 oz — 300

CHEESE 1 oz — 200

RICOTTA CHEESE Part Skim, 1/2 Cup — 330

SOY DRINK Calcium Enriched 8 fl.oz — 300

SALMON w. Bones 3 oz — 300

ALMONDS 1 oz — 70

BROCCOLI 1 Cup — 100

BAKED BEANS 1/2 Cup — 50

Milk & Milk Drinks

	Calcium (mg)
Milk Fluid:	
Whole: 1 cup, 8 fl.oz	300
1 small glass, 6 fl.oz	220
1% or 2%: 1 cup, 8 fl.oz	300
Lowfat/Skim: 1 cup, 8 fl.oz	300
Hi-Calcium *(Borden)*, 1 cup	1000
Viva, w. extra Calcium, 1 cup	500
Condensed Milk, sweet, 1 fl.oz	110
Evaporated Milk: Skim, 1 fl.oz	90
Whole/Lowfat	80
Dry/Powder: Whole, 1/4 cup	290
Skim/Nonfat, 1/4 cup	380
Other Milks & Milk Drinks	
Buttermilk, average, 1 cup	300
Chocolate Milk, average, 1 cup	300
Goats Milk, 1 cup	320
Malted Milk, 1 cup	350
Milkshakes: Medium, 15 fl.oz	450
Café Latte, 1 cup, 8 fl.oz	220
Cappuccino, 1 cup, 8 fl.oz	150
Milk Drink Powders:	
Malted Milk, dry powder, 1 oz	80
Chocolate, Instant, 3 Tbsp	10
Cocoa Powder: Regular, 1 Tbsp	10
Cocoa Mix: *Hershey*, 1/3 cup	40
Alba High Calcium, 1 envelope	320

Soy & Grain Drinks

Soy: Regular, non-fortified, 1 cup	60
Enriched/Calcium-fortified, 1 cup	300
Dry Powder, 1 oz	80
Rice/Oat Drinks: Average, 1 cup	10

Yogurt

Average All Brands, **1 cup, 8 oz**	350
Fruit-flavored, 1 cup, 8 oz	250
Small cup, 6 oz	230
4 1/2 oz cup	350
Plain: Average, 1 cup, 8 oz	430
Dannon, Nonfat/Lowfat, 8 oz	200
Custard-style, 6 oz	100
Frozen Yogurt, average, 1/2 cup	150

Fats/Oils

Butter, Margarine, Spreads, Oils	0
I Can't Believe It's Not Butter	0
w. Sweet Cream and Calcium, 1 Tbsp	100

Cream

	Calcium (mg)
Average: Unwhipped, 1 Tbsp	15
Whipped, 1 heaping Tbsp	15
Half & Half, 1 Tbsp	15
Non-dairy Creamers, 1 tsp	0

Ice Cream & Ices

Ice Cream: Regular, 1 scoop	65
1/2 cup	90
Premium *(Ben & Jerry's)*, 1/2 cup, 4 oz	150
Soft Serve, 1/2 cup	120
Lowfat, 1/2 cup, 4 oz	150
Ice Milk, average, 1/2 cup	100
Sherbet, average, 1/2 cup	50
Fruit Sorbet	0
Sundae, regular, 6 fl.oz	200
Soy/Tofu Ices, average, 1/2 cup	10

Cheese: Per 1 oz (1 1/2" cube)

Natural, Hard: Average, 1 oz	200
Processed Cheese: Average, 1 oz	150
Single-wrapped, 3/4 oz	120
Cheese Substitutes: Average, 1 oz	200
Specific Cheeses:	
Blue, 1 oz	150
Brie	50
Camembert	110
Cheddar	200
Cottage Cheese: 1 round Tbsp, 1 oz	20
1/2 cup, 4 oz	80
Cream Cheese	20
Dorman's Light, average 1 oz	200
Edam, Gouda	200
Feta	140
Goat, semi-soft	85
Gruyere	290
Kraft Light Naturals, average	250
Light-Line *(Borden)*, singles	200
Monterey Jack	210
Mozzarella, average	170
Parmesan, grated, 1 Tbsp	70
Processed	160
Provolone	210
Ricotta, part skim, 1/2 cup, 4 1/2 oz	330
Swiss	270
Cheese Dishes: Souffle, 4 oz	240
Macaroni & Cheese, 1 cup, 8 oz	150
Ham & Cheese Crepes, 8 oz	350
Quiche, 1 serve, 6 oz	200

Eggs	Calcium (mg)
1 large Egg	30
Scrambled, with Milk	50
Omelet w. Cheese (1/2 oz)	260

Fish & Seafood	
Canned Fish: Tuna, canned, 3 oz	10
Salmon: with bones, 3 oz	190
without bones, 3 oz	10
Sardines, with bones, 3 oz	90
Fresh Fish: cooked, average, 4 oz	35
Seafood: Lobster, cooked, 4 oz	60
Mussels/Oysters (10), 4 oz	95
Crabmeat, cooked, 4 oz	50

Meats & Poultry	
Average all types, cooked, 4 oz	20
Vegetarian Soy Burgers:	
Example: *BocaBurger*, 1 pattie, 2 1/2 oz	100

Soups: *Average all types*	
No Milk or Cheese added, 1 serve	30
with Milk, 1/2 cup, 1 serve	180
Sauces: Non-Dairy, average, 2 Tbsp	10
Cheese/White Sauce, 2 Tbsp	40
Spices: Average all types, 1 tsp	5

Bread, Bagels	
Bread: White, 1 slice, 1 oz	30
Wholewheat, Rye, 1 slice, 1 oz	30
Bagels, average	30
Buns/Rolls: Small	40
Large	90
English Muffins, 2 oz	90
Pita, 6 1/2 " diameter, 2 oz	50
Tortillas, Corn, 1 oz	40

Breakfast Cereals	
Ready To Eat: Average all types, 1 oz	20
with 3/4 cup Milk/Soy (enriched)	250
All-Bran, 1/2 cup, 1 oz	150
Harmony (General Mills), 1 1/4 c., 2 oz	600
Life (Quaker), 1 cup, 1 oz	100
Special K Red Berries, 1 cup	150
Total (General Mills), all types, 1 oz	1000
Wheaties (General Mills), 1 cup, 2 oz	350
Hot Type, cooked: Corn Grits, 1 cup	5
Cream of Wheat, 1 cup	50
Oatmeal/Rolled Oats: Regular, ckd, 1 cup	20
Instant, fortified, 1 pkt	100

Note: Breakfast cereals are a good medium for calcium-rich milk or soy drinks (150mg per 1/2 cup).

Flours, Grains	Calcium (mg)
Wheat Flour: All-purpose, 1 cup	20
Self-rising, 1 cup	330
Whole-wheat, 1 cup	50
Carob Flour, 1 cup, 3 1/2 oz	360
Corn meal, 1 cup, 4 oz	20
Soybean Flour, 1 cup, 3 oz	170
Grains, Barley, Rice: Cooked, 1 cup	15

Pasta, Spaghetti	
Average all types, cooked, 1 cup	15
Lasagne, average, 1 serve	300
Macaroni & Cheese, aver., 1 cup	150
Spaghetti w. Meat Sce, 1 serve	20
with 1 Tbsp Parmesan	90

Sugar & Syrups, Honey	
Sugar: White	0
Brown, 1 Tbsp	10
Syrups: Table Syrup, 2 Tbsp	0
Choc., Thin type, 2 Tbsp	5
Fudge type, 2 Tbsp	40
Molasses: Light, 2 Tbsp	70
Blackstrap, average, 1 Tbsp, 3/4 oz	270
Honey, Jam, Jelly	0

Cookies & Cakes, Desserts	
Cookies: Average all types, 1 cookie	5
Crackers, average, 1 only	5
Cake: Plain, average, 2 oz	40
Carrot Cake with Icing	45
Cheesecake, 1 piece	80
Fruitcake, 1 piece	40
Croissants, average, 2 oz	20
Custard, average, 1/2 cup	150
Danish pastry, average, 2 oz	60
Donuts, average, 2 oz	20
Gelatin, plain w. water, 1/2 cup	2
Muffins: Regular, average, 1 1/2 oz	40
English Muffins, 2 oz	90
Pancakes, 4" diameter, average, 1 oz	40
Pies: Apple/Fruit, average, 5 oz	20
Custard Pie, average, 5 oz	140
Pecan Pie, 1 piece, 5 oz	70
Pumpkin Pie, 1 piece, 5 oz	80
w. Icecream, 1 scoop: Add	70
Puddings: Canned, aver., 5 oz	80
Dry Mix, made w. milk, 1/2 cup	150
Rice Pudding, 1/2 cup	120
Waffles, 7" diameter average	160

Candy, Chocolate

	Calcium
Chocolate: Milk Chocolate, 1 oz	50
Plain/Fruit, 1 oz	65
with Almonds, 1 oz	80
Kit Kat Wafer (1^{1}/$_{2}$oz); Mars Bar (1.8 oz)	80
Milky Way Bar, 2 oz	60
Carob Bar, average, 2 oz	220
Sugar Candy, Jelly Beans, M'mallow, 1 oz	0

Snacks & Nutrition Bars

Breakfast Bars *(Carnation)*	20
Corn Chips; Tortilla Chips, 1 oz	40
Granola Bars, average	30
Popcorn, 1 cup	5
Potato Chips, 1 oz	10
Nutrition Bars: *Balance Oasis* Bars	350
Dr Soy Bars	350
GeniSoy 'Soy Nutty' Bar	250
Jenny Craig; Power Bars	300
MetRx, After Fx, Pure Protein Bars	500
Nature's Plus Calcium Almond Blitz	1200
Slim-Fast 'Meal On The Go'	300
SoBeBars; Vita-Trim Bars (Market America)	350
TwinLab Protein Fuel Bars	350
Viactiv Bar	300
Wholefoods Everyday Bars	300

Nuts & Seeds (Shelled)

Almonds, 12-15 nuts, ^{1}/$_{2}$oz	40
Brazil Nuts, 4 medium, ^{1}/$_{2}$oz	30
Cashews, 6-8 nuts, ^{1}/$_{2}$oz	5
Coconut, fresh, ^{1}/$_{2}$oz	5
Filberts (Hazelnuts), ^{1}/$_{2}$oz	40
Macadamias, 6 medium, ^{1}/$_{2}$oz	10
Peanuts, raw, 1 oz	25
Walnuts, 1 oz	20
Seeds: Pumpkin, 1 oz	15
Sesame, 1 Tbsp	10
Sunflower, 1 oz	30
Tahini, 1 Tbsp, ^{1}/$_{2}$oz	20

Drinks - Alcohol, Soda, Water

Beer, Cider, Wine, 1 glass	5
Spirits, Liqueurs	0
Coffee, Tea, Soda, Fruit Drinks	5
Water: Tap, average, 1 cup	5
Mineral Water *(Perrier)*, 1 glass, 6 oz	20

Fruit & Fruit Juice

	Calcium (mg)
Fresh Fruit: Average all types, 1 serve	20
Apple, 1 medium	10
Avocado, 1 medium	20
Banana, 1 medium	10
Orange, 1 medium	50
Pear, 1 medium	20
Rhubarb, cooked, ^{1}/$_{2}$ cup	170
(calcium largely not available to body)	
Dried Fruit: Average, 1 oz	20
Figs, 3 medium, 1^{1}/$_{2}$oz	55
Fruit Juice: Average, 1 cup, 8 fl.oz	25
Orange Juice, calcium fortified:	
Citrus Hill Plus Calcium, Hi-C	300
Minute Maid (Premium Calcium)	300
Jui2ce, 8 fl.oz	200
Tropicana Grapefruit & Calcium	300
Welch's Healthy Sensation, 1 cup	350

Vegetables

Average all types, 1 cup	40
Higher Calcium Content:	
Beans, dried: cooked,^{1}/$_{2}$ cup	50
Baked/Refried Beans, ^{1}/$_{2}$ cup	60
Broccoli, chopped, 1 cup	100
Chickpeas, boiled, ^{1}/$_{2}$ cup	40
Collards, cooked, 1 cup	150
Dandelion Greens, cooked, 1 cup	150
Kale, 1 cup	130
Mustard Greens, 1 cup	100
Soybeans, cooked, ^{1}/$_{2}$ cup, 3 oz	60
Spinach, cooked, ^{1}/$_{2}$ cup	120
Potato: Plain, 1 large	20
Au Gratin, 1 cup	200
Mashed w. Milk, 1 cup	60
Tofu: *Mori Nu:* Silken, 4 oz	90
Azumaya: Silken, 3 oz	20
Firm/Extra Firm, 3 oz	150
Hinoichi: Regular, 1" slice, 3 oz	100
Firm/Extra Firm, 3 oz	150
Soft, 1" slice, 3 oz	60
Nasoya: Firm, Soft, 3 oz	120
Extra Firm, 3 oz	150
Silken, 3 oz	60
Tree of Life: Firm, 3 oz	150
Miso: ^{1}/$_{2}$ cup, 5 oz	100
Tempeh: 4 oz serving	100

Frozen Entrees/Meals

	Calcium (mg)
Budget Gourmet Light	
Chicken Parmigiana; Ziti Parmesano	160
Three Cheese Lasagne	360
Lean Cuisine: Cheese Ravioli, 2.5 oz	150
Cheese Lasagna, 10 oz	200
Chicken Fettucine, 9.25 oz	150
French Bread Pizza, Deluxe, 6 1/8 oz	360
Stouffer's: Cheese Manicotti	320
Chicken Enchilada; Fettucini Alfredo	200
Extra Cheese Pizza	280
Five Cheese Lasagna	400
Weight Watchers	
Bowtie Pasta & Mushroom Marsala	160
Lasagna w. Meat Sauce	320
Tuna Noodle Casserole	160

Frozen Pizzas

	Calcium (mg)
Average All Brands: Cheese, 1/4 pizza	350
Meats (Sausage/Pepperoni), 1/4 pizza	250

Calcium Supplements

	Calcium (mg)
Caltrate 600, 1 tablet	600
Citracal, 1 tablet	200
Ethical Nutrients 'Bone Builder', 1	200
IDN LifePak: Reg./Prime, 2 pkts	500
Women, 2 pkts	1000
Isotonix Calcium (Mkt Amer.), 2 capfuls	750
Nature's Life 'Super Cal-Mag', 1	500
Os-cal; 1 tablet	500
Posture Calcium, 1 tablet	600
Tums: Regular, 1 tablet	200
Extra Strength, 1 tablet	300
Viativ Soft Calcium Chews, 1 chew	500

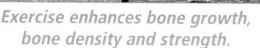

*Exercise enhances bone growth,
bone density and strength.*

Fast-Foods, Restaurants

	Calcium (mg)
Chicken: Grilled/BBQ, 1/4 chicken	20
Battered & Fried, 2 pieces	80
Nuggets, 6 pack	20
Crispy Chicken Deluxe Sandwich	50
Croissant Sandwich: Plain	40
with Cheese, 1 oz	240
Fish Sandwich: no Cheese	60
with Cheese	140
Fish Filet Deluxe	70
Fish, fried, 2 pieces	20
French Fries: Small Serving	10
Hamburgers: Average all outlets,	
Regular, no Cheese	120
Cheeseburger, regular	120
McDonald's: Big Mac	160
Quarter Pounder w. Cheese	120
Egg McMuffin	120
Hot Dog: Plain	60
with Cheese	150
Mexican: Burrito	120
Enchilada	300
Nachos, regular	200
Taco, regular	140
Taco Bell Salad	400
Pizza: Average all types,	
Medium (12"), 2 slices	250
Double Cheese, 2 slices	350
Large (16"), 2 slices	350
Double Cheese, 2 slices	500
Pizza Hut:	
Cheese, medium, 2 slices	290
Pepperoni, medium, 2 slices	300
Potato: Plain, baked, 8 oz	20
Stuffed w. Cheese Topping	100
with Cheese Filling	300
Sandwiches: no Cheese	60
with 1 oz Cheese (regular)	260
with Cream Cheese	80
Subway: 6" Sandwich, average	100
Cheese & Egg Bkfst Sandwich	150
Steak & Cheese Wrap	150
Cheese (extra fixin'), 3 triangles	150
Pocket Sandwich, CheeseLess	150
Salads (Classic), average	100
Salads: Chef, regular	300
Coleslaw, small	20
Shakes, average	330

Fiber Guide

Introduction

Fiber is the general term for those parts of **plant** food that we cannot digest (although bacteria in the large bowel partly digests fiber through fermentation). It is not found in foods of animal origin (meats, dairy products).

Fiber promotes intestinal health, bowel regularity, can benefit diabetes and blood cholesterol levels, and may help prevent colon cancer. High fiber foods also assist weight control.

Most Americans don't eat enough fiber - less than 20 grams/day - instead of a **healthier 25 to 35 grams/day.**

Types of Fiber

Plant foods contain a mixture of different fibers in varying proportions. Insoluble and soluble fiber categories are based on their solubility in water. All types of fiber are beneficial to the body.

◆ **Insoluble fibers** (cellulose, hemi-celluloses, lignin) make up the structural parts of plant cell walls. The **best sources** are wheat bran, corn bran, rice bran, wholegrain cereals and breads, dried beans and peas, nuts, seeds and the skins of fruits and vegetables.

These fibers absorb many times their own weight in water. They create a soft bulk and hasten the passage of waste products through the intestines.

They promote bowel regularity, and aid in the prevention and treatment of uncomplicated forms of **constipation, diverticulosis and haemorrhoids.**

The risk of colon cancer may also be reduced by fiber's diluting effect of potentially harmful substances.

◆ **Soluble fibers** (pectin, gums, mucilages) are found mainly within plant cells, soy milk (whole bean) and products.

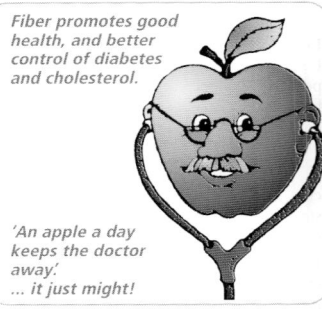

Fiber promotes good health, and better control of diabetes and cholesterol.

'An apple a day keeps the doctor away.'
... it just might!

Types of Fiber (Cont)

Best Sources of Soluble Fiber:
Fruits and vegetables, oat bran, barley, dried beans and peas, psyllium and flax seed.

These fibers form a gel which slows both stomach emptying and the absorption of sugars from the intestines. This helps to control **blood sugar** levels.

Weight control is also aided by the slower emptying of the stomach and the feeling of **fullness provided by soluble fiber.**

Some soluble fibers can lower **blood cholesterol** by binding bile acids and excreting them. More body cholesterol must then be broken down to supply bile acids for emulsification of dietary fats. **Rice bran, while not high in soluble fiber can also lower blood cholesterol.**

◆ **Resistant starch** is that part of starchy foods (approx. 10%) which is tightly bound by fiber and resists normal digestion. Friendly bacteria in the large bowel ferment and change the resistant starch into short-chain fatty acids which are important to bowel health and may protect against colon cancer.

Starchy foods include bread, cereals, rice, pasta, potatoes and legumes.

Fiber & Weight Control

Fiber can assist weight control in several ways. Fiber-rich foods such as fresh fruit and vegetables, potatoes and whole-grain bread contain few calories for their large volume (due to their lowfat, high water content).

Their bulk fills the stomach and satisfies appetite much earlier than fiber-depleted foods. The extra chewing time also contributes to satiety, and gives the stomach time to register a feeling of fullness. Excessive calories are less likely to be consumed.

Fiber-depleted foods and drinks are more concentrated in calories; e.g. fats, sugar, candy, soft drinks, fruit juices, alcohol. They require little or no chewing. Large amounts with excessive calories can be consumed before appetite is satisfied.

Example: Whereas one fresh apple might satisfy our appetite, an apple juice drink with the equivalent sugars and calories of 2-3 apples does little to satisfy appetite. (See illustration below.)

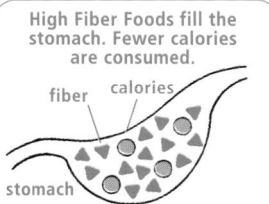

High Fiber Foods fill the stomach. Fewer calories are consumed.

fiber   calories

stomach

Low Fiber Foods are more concentrated in calories. More food must be eaten to fill the stomach.

calories

fiber

stomach

EFFECTS OF REMOVING FIBER FROM FOOD

2-3 pieces of fresh fruit produces 1 glass of fruit juice.
The removal of fiber concentrates the sugar and calories.

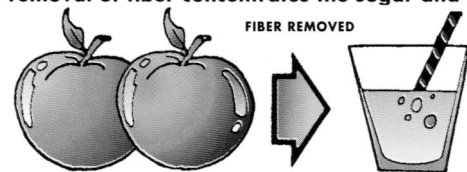

FIBER REMOVED

Fresh Fruit		Fruit Juice
High Fiber	←	Negligible Fiber
Low Calorie Density	←	High Calorie Density
Long Eating Time	←	No Eating Time (Drink)
Satisfies Hunger	←	Does Not Satisfy Hunger
Sugar Slowly Absorbed	←	Sugar More Quickly Absorbed
Less Insulin Required	←	More Insulin Required

Constipation

Constipation can reasonably be defined as a failure to have a bowel movement at least every second day - and just as importantly, without straining or pain.

Typically, stools are too hard, too narrow, and too small . . . *sinkers* rather than *floaters*.

The **main cause** is simply a lack of dietary fiber. Other contributing factors include insufficient fluids, too little exercise, emotional stress, gastro-intestinal disease, lack of proper dentition to chew high-fiber foods, and some medications (e.g. some antacids, antidepressants, tranquilizers).

Note: Check with your doctor to rule out any underlying medical problem – especially if you notice a change in bowel habits in middle-age or later years.

DESIRABLE FIBER INTAKE

Adults: 25-35gm per day
Children (under 18): Age + 5gm
Example: 6-year old (6 + 5)= 11gm

SAMPLE FOOD QUANTITIES

For 35 Grams of Fiber/Day **Fiber**

Breakfast Cereal (higher-fiber)	5g
plus 4 slices whole wheat Bread	6g
plus 3 servings fresh Fruit	9g
plus 1 medium Potato (w. skin) **or** 1 cup Brown Rice **or** $^1/_2$ cup whole-wheat Pasta	4g
plus 3-4 servings Veges/Salad	6g
plus 1 cup Bean Soup **or** $^1/_4$ cup Baked/Soy Beans **or** $^1/_2$ cup Corn/Peas/Lentils **or** 1$^1/_4$ oz Almonds (natural) **or** 3 medium Figs	5g

---

HINTS TO INCREASE FIBER AND AVOID CONSTIPATION

1. Breakfast is an important contributor to daily fiber intake. Eat high-fiber breakfast cereals (bran-based cereals, oatmeal etc.). Add 1-2 tablespoons of unprocessed bran (wheat/ barley/ rice) and wheat germ if required.

Dried fruits, chopped nuts, soy grits, and seeds are also excellent additions to cereals.

Note: A gradual increase in fiber will prevent bloating, gas or pain. Persons intolerant to bran may benefit from psyllium-based fiber supplements and cereals.

2. Drink 6-8 glasses of water daily. Fiber works by absorbing many times its own weight of water.

3. Eat wholegrain breads, or fiber-enriched breads. One slice of whole-wheat bread has over double the fiber of regular white bread.

4. Enjoy fruit as fresh fruit with skins rather than as fruit juice. Enjoy whole-wheat pasta, barley, brown rice, nuts and seeds.

5. Eat more vegetables, salads and legumes - especially dried beans, baked beans, lentils, potatoes with skins, avocado, broccoli, brussel sprouts, cabbage, carrots, celery, and peas.

6. Add bran (barley/rice/wheat) or soy grits to soups, casseroles, yogurt, desserts, biscuits, cakes. Also use wholemeal flour or soy flour in place of white flour. Use nuts and seeds.

7. Snack on fresh or dried fruits, carrot or celery sticks, popcorn, nuts or seeds, wholegrain crackers, high-fiber bars (low-fat). Limit amounts if overweight.

8. Exercise regularly to strengthen abdominal muscles and stimulate the gut. Keep up fluids, especially in warm weather.

9. Avoid indiscriminate and regular use of harsh laxatives. They can overstimulate the intestinal muscles and may make normal bowel activity impossible. It may take several weeks to restore normal bowel function.

FOODS WITH ZERO FIBER
- Dairy Products (Milk, Cheese, etc)
- Meats, Poultry, Fish, Eggs
- Fats/Oils, Sugar/Syrups

(Only foods of plant origin contain fiber.)

Breakfast Cereals	Fiber
General Mills: Basic 4, 1 cup, 2 oz	3
Cheerios (Wholegrain/Heart Healthy), 1 cup	3
Team Cheerios, 3/4 cup, 1 oz	1
Crispy Wheaties, 1 cup, 1 oz	3
Fiber One, 1/2 cup, 1 oz	13
Multi-Bran Chex, 1 cup, 2 oz	8
Oatmeal Crisp, 1 cup, 2 oz	4
Raisin Nut Bran, 3/4 cup, 2 oz	5
Total, average all types, 1 oz	3
Wheat Chex; Wheaties Raisin Bran, 1 cup	5
Wheaties Energy Crunch, 1 cup, 2 oz	4
Health Valley: 10 Bran O's, 3/4 cup	4
Amaranth Flakes, 3/4 cup	4
Corn Bran Flakes, 3/4 cup	4
Fiber 7 Flakes, 3/4 cup	4
Golden Flax, 1/4 cup	6
Granola (Fat Free), 2/3 cup	6
Healthy Crunches & Flakes, 3/4 cup	4
Healthy Fiber Flakes, 3/4 cup	4
Oat Bran Flakes, all types, 3/4 cup	4
Real Oat Bran, 1/2 cup	5
Kellogg's: All-Bran, 1/2 cup, 1 oz	10
All-Bran w. Extra Fiber, 1/2 cup, 1 oz	13
Bran Buds, 3/4 cup, 2 oz	12
Bran Flakes, 3/4cup, 1 oz	5
Corn Flakes, Fruit Loops, Smacks, 3/4 cup	1
Cracklin' Oat Bran, 3/4 cup, 2 oz	6
Cocoa/Rice Krispies, 1 cup	0
Complete Wheatbran Flakes, 3/4 c., 1 oz	5
Frosted Mini Wheats, 1 cup	6
Healthy Choice, all types, 1 cup	5
Nutri-Grain (Almond Raisin), 1 1/4 cup	4
Cereal Bars, 1 bar	4
Mueslix (Almond. Raisin Date), 2/3 cup	4
Raisin Bran, 2.2 oz	8
Smart Start, 1 cup	2
Special K; Product 19, 1 cup	1
Special K Red Berries, 1 cup	4
Nabisco: 100% Bran, 1/2 cup, 1 oz	8
Shredded Wheat, 2 biscuits	5
Shredded Wheat & Bran, 1 1/4 cup, 2 oz	8

Fiber ~ Fiber (grams)	
Breakfast Cereals (Cont)	**Fiber**
Kashi: GoLEAN Cereal, 3/4 cup	10
GoLEAN Crunch!, 1 cup	8
GoLEAN Bars	6
Breakfast Pilaf, 1/2 cup, cooked	6
'From Kashi to Good Friends', 3/4 cup	8
Heart to Heart, 3/4 cup	5
Kashi 'Go', all varieties, 1/2 cup	6
Puffed Kashi, 1 cup, 0.8 oz	2
Quaker: Per 1 oz	
100% Natural Cereals, average,1/2 cup	3
Cap'n Crunch; Cr. Nut Oh's, 3/4 cup	1
Crunchy Bran, 3/4 cup	5
Life Cereal (3/4 cup), Oat Squares (1/2 c.)	2
Oat Bran, 1/3 cup	6
Oatmeal, average, 1 packet	3
Puffed Rice, 1 cup	1
Puffed Wheat, 1 cup	2
Quisp, 3/4 cup, 1 oz	1
Toasted Oatmeal; Honey Nut, 1 cup	3
Post: 100% Bran, 1/2 cup	8
Blueberry Morning, 1 1/4 cup, 2 oz	2
Cocoa/Fruity Pebbles, 3/4 cup	0
Cranberry Almond Crunch, 1 cup, 2 oz	3
Frosted Alpha Bits, 1 cup	1
Fruit & Fibre, 1 cup, 1 3/4 oz	5
Grape-Nuts, 1/2 cup, 2 oz	5
Great Grains, 2/3 cup, 2 oz	4
Honey Bunches of Oats, 3/4 cup, 1 oz	1

Brans & Supplements	
Oat Bran: 1 Tbsp (level)	0.8
1/3 cup, (5 1/3 Tbsp), 1 oz	4.2
Rice Bran: 1/3 cup, 1 oz	6
Wheat Bran: unprocessed: 1 Tbsp	1.6
2 Tbsp (level), 1/4 oz	3.2
1/4 cup, (4Tbsp), 1/2 oz	6.4
1/2 cup, 1 oz	13
Corn Germ: 1/4 cup, 1 oz	5
Wheat Germ: 1/4 cup, 1 oz	3
Psyllium Seed Husks, 2 Tbsp	8
Metamucil, 1 dose	3.4

Hot Cereals, Oatmeal	
Bulgur (cracked Wheat), ckd, 1 cup	8
Cream of Wheat, ckd, 2/3 cup	1
Hominy Grits, dry, 3 Tbsp, 1 oz	1.2
Oatmeal (uncooked 1/3 cup), ckd, 2/3 cup	2.7

Breads & Crackers	Fiber
Bread: White, 1 slice, 1 oz	0.7
Whole-wheat, 1 slice, 1 oz	1.5
Whole-grain, 1 slice, 1 oz	2
Rye, Pumpernickel, 1 oz	1.5
Bagel/Roll/Bun, 1 medium, 2 oz	1.5
Pita, whole wheat, 5" pocket	4.5
Crackers: Graham, average, 2	1.4
Saltine, 4 crackers	0.3
Crispbreads (Rye), average, 2	4
Matzo 1 board, 1 oz	1
Rice Cakes: Average, 1 cake	0.3
Tortilla: Regular, 6"	0.5
Whole-wheat, 6"	1.3

Barley, Pasta, Rice & Flours	
Barley, pearled, raw, 1/4 cup, 1.7 oz	5
Rice: White, cooked, 1 cup, 7 oz	1.6
Brown, cooked, 1 cup	3.2
Rice-A-Roni, average, 1 cup	1.5
Spaghetti/Noodles: cooked, 1 cup	2
Whole-wheat, cooked, 1 cup	7
Amaranth *(Health Valley),* 1 cup	9
Flour: Wheat, All-purpose, 1 cup, 4 1/2 oz	3.5
Whole-wheat, 1 cup, 4 1/2 oz	15
Cornmeal, stone ground, 1 cup, 4 1/2 oz	13
Carob Flour, 1 cup, 3 1/2 oz	13
Rye Flour, 1 cup, 3 1/2 oz	15
Soy Flour: Defatted, 1 cup, 3 1/2 oz	17
Full-fat, raw, 1 cup, 3 oz	8
Soy Meal, defatted, 1 cup, 4 1/2 oz	14

Frozen Entrees & Dinners	
***Average All Brands:** Per Serving*	
Beans/Chili base, average	6-10
Potato/Pasta base, average	4-6
Vegetable base, average	3
Meat/Chicken base, average	2-3
Pizzas, 1/4 large, average	3
Vegetarian Soy Burgers, 1 pattie	5

Soups	
Chicken Noodle, 1 cup	<0.5
Tomato Soup, average, 1 cup	<1
Vegetable Soup, average, 1 cup	3
Health Valley: Per 1 Cup Serving	
Black Bean; Minestrone	10
Tomato	4
5-Bean Vegetable; Lentil & Carrots	13
Mushroom & Barley; Split Pea; Vegetable	7
Chili: w. Beans, average, 1 cup, 8.8 oz	7
without Beans, average, 1 cup, 8.3 oz	3

Fast Foods & Restaurants	Fiber
Hamburgers: Small, average	1.5
Large/Whopper, average	2.5
Hot Dog, Regular	1.5
French Fries: Small serving, 2 1/2 oz	2.5
Regular/Medium, 3 1/2 oz	3.5
Chicken Nuggets, 6 pack	<0.5
Chicken Sandwich, average	2
Taco, average	4
Sundaes, Shakes, Soft Drinks	0
Arby's: Baked Potato w. Broccoli	9
Roast Beef Sandwich, regular	3
Denny's: Oriental Chicken Salad	7
Dennyburger w. fries	3
Club Sandwich	3
Grilled Chicken Sandwich	1
Domino's (Pizza): Veggie, 2 sl. (12")	4
Pepperoni, 2 slices (12")	2.5
Cheese., Saus/Mushr., 2 slices, (12")	3
McDonald's: Crispy Chicken	4
Big Mac	3
Egg McMuffin	1
Salads: Garden; Grilled Chicken	2
Pizza Hut: Per 2 slices, Medium	
Pan Pizza: Cheese, Pepperoni	2
Supreme	4
Thin 'n Crispy: Supreme	4
Hand-Tossed, average	3
Personal Pan Pizza, 1 whole	5
Subway: Sandwich, white roll	2.5
w. Honey Wheat Roll	3.2
Footlong, w. Wheat Roll	6.4
Salads, average	2

Cakes, Cookies, Snack Bars	
Apple/Fruit Pie, 1 serving	2
Cake: w. plain flour, 1 serving	1
w. whole-wheat flour, 1 serving	3
Carrot Cake, 1 serving	2
Cookies, oatmeal, (3 small/1 large)	3
Donuts	0
Fruit Cake, 1 serving	3
Fig Bars, 2	1.3
Muffins, Oat Bran (2 small, 1 large), 4 oz	4
Granola Bars, average, 1 bar	1
Fi-Bar (Natural Nectar), 1 bar	4
Health Valley: Fat-Free Fruit Bars	4
Oat Bran Jumbo Fruit Bars	7
IDN Fiberry Snack Bar	3
SoBeBars (Mkt America), Peanut	3
Vita-Trim Bars (Mkt America)	5

Chocolate, Chips, Popcorn · Fiber

Cheese Balls/Curls/Twists	0
Chocolate, Hard Candy, Cheese Balls	0
Chocolate with nuts/fruit, 2 oz bar	1
Mars Bar	1
Potato Chips, corn chips, 1 oz	1
Popcorn, 3 cups	2
Pretzels, Twists, 6	1

Nuts, Seeds

Almonds: Natural, 25 kernels, 1 oz	4
Blanched (skins removed), 1 oz	3
Cashews, Filberts, Pecans, 1 oz	1.7
Peanuts, Mixed Nuts, Coconut, 1 oz	2.5
Peanut Butter, 2 Tbsp, 1 oz	1.8
Pistachio Nuts, dried, shelled, 1 oz	3
Walnuts, Black/dried, dried, 1 oz	1.5
Seeds: Amaranth, 2¹/₂ Tbsp, 1 oz	3.5
Flax Seeds, 3 Tbsp, 1 oz	7
Psyllium Seed Husks, 5 Tbsp, 1 oz	20
Quinoa Seeds, 3 Tbsp, 1 oz	2.7
Sesame Seeds, whole, 1 oz	3
Sesame Butter/Tahini, 2 Tbsp, 1.1 oz	3
Sunflower kernels, ¹/₄ cup, 1 oz	4.4
Teff Seeds, 1 oz	3.8

Fruit – Fresh

Apples: 1 medium, 6 oz (whole)	
with skin + core	5.5
with skin, no core	4.5
without skin, no core	3.7
Apricots, 2 medium, 4 oz	2
Avocado, average, ¹/₂ medium	3
Banana, 1 medium, 6 oz (w. skin)	2
Blueberries, raw, ¹/₂ cup, 5 oz	4.4
Cherries, sweet, raw, 10 fruits, 2¹/₂ oz	1.5
Grapefruit, average, ¹/₂ fruit, 8¹/₂ oz	1
Grapes, 1 medium bunch, seedless, 7 oz	3
Kiwifruit, 1 medium, 3 oz	3
Mango, 1 medium, 11 oz (whole)	1.6
Melons, cantaloup, 4 oz (edible)	1
Nectarine, 1 medium, 4 oz	1.8
Olives, average all types, 7 jumbo, 2 oz	1.5
Oranges, 1 medium (7-8 oz w. skin)	
5¹/₂ oz (peeled)	3.8
Passionfruit, 2 medium, 2¹/₂ oz	5
Peaches, 1 large, 6 oz	2
Pears, raw, 1 medium, 6 oz	4.5
Pineapple, 1 slice, 3 oz	1.8
Plums, 2 medium, 6 oz	2.8
Strawberries, 6 medium/3 large, 2 oz	1.5
Watermelon, 4 oz (edible)	0.5

Fruit – Dried, Juice · Fiber

Dried Fruit: Apricots, 8 halves, 1 oz	2.2
Dates (3 med); Raisins (2 Tbsp), 1 oz	1.5
Figs, 3 medium,1¹/₂ oz	5
Prunes, 4 medium, 1 oz	2
Fruit Juice: Orange/Apple etc, 1 glass	<0.5
Prune Juice, 5 oz	1.4
Carrot Juice, 8 oz	1.8

Vegetables

Asparagus, 4 spears	2
Bean Sprouts, ¹/₂ cup, 2¹/₄ oz	1.5
Beans: Snap/Green, ¹/₂ cup, 2¹/₂ oz	2
Baked Beans in Tom Sce, ¹/₂ c, 4¹/₂ oz	10
Dried Beans, ckd, average, ¹/₂ cup	7
Beets, ckd, slices, ¹/₂ cup, 3 oz	1.5
Broccoli, cooked, ¹/₂ cup, 3 oz	2.2
Brussels Sprouts, ckd, ¹/₂ cup, 3 oz	3.5
Cabbage: White, ckd, ¹/₂ cup, 2¹/₂ oz	1
Red, ckd, ¹/₂ cup, 2¹/₂ oz	2
Carrots, 1 medium (7¹/₂"), ¹/₂ cup, 3 oz	2.7
Cauliflower, cooked, ¹/₂ cup, 3 oz	2.8
Celery, raw, diced, ¹/₂ cup, 2¹/₂ oz	1
Chick Peas (Garbanzos), ckd, ¹/₂ c., 3¹/₂ oz	6
Corn, kernels, ckd, ¹/₂ cup, 2¹/₂ oz	2.5
Cream-style, ¹/₂ cup, 4¹/₂ oz	1.5
Cucumber/Lettuce/Mushrooms, 2 oz	0.5
Eggplant, raw, sliced, ¹/₂ cup	2.5
Lentils, cooked, ¹/₂ cup, 3¹/₂ oz	4
Onions, 1 medium, 4 oz	2
Spring Onions, chop., ¹/₄ cup, 1 oz	1.5
Peas: Green, ¹/₂ cup, 3 oz	3
Cowpeas (Black-eyed), ckd, ¹/₂ cup	10
Split Peas, ckd, ¹/₂ cup, 4¹/₂ oz	6.5
Peppers, sweet, raw, 1 large, 3¹/₂ oz	1.5
Potatoes: 1 medium, with skin, 5 oz	4
without skin	2
¹/₂ cup mashed, 3¹/₂ oz	1.5
French Fries, 3 oz serving	3
Spinach, cooked, ¹/₂ cup, 3 oz	2
Squash: Summer, cookd, 3 oz	1.2
Winter, cooked, 3 oz	2.4
Tomatoes: 1 medium, 5 oz	2
Tomato Sauce, 1 cup	0.3
Frozen: Mixed Vegetables, ckd, ¹/₂ cup	3
Soybean Products: Miso, ¹/₂ c., 5 oz	7.7
Tempeh, 1 piece, 3 oz	2
Tofu, 4 oz	1.4

Salads: Side Salad, average

Bean Salad, ¹/₂ cup	5
Coleslaw, ¹/₂ cup	1
Potato Salad, ¹/₂ cup	2

General Notes

- **Protein has many important body functions.** It builds and repairs muscle, and is the basis of our body's organs, hormones, enzymes, and antibodies to fight infection.

- **Protein is also an emergency fuel** in the absence of sufficient carbohydrate and fats. For this reason, weight loss should be gradual so as to preserve protein levels in muscle, the heart and other body organs.

- **It is easy to obtain sufficient protein,** even if vegetarian. **Plant proteins are not inferior to animal proteins.** In fact, eating more soy and other plant proteins, and less animal protein, may help to build stronger bones and prevent osteoporosis; and may help to control blood cholesterol levels.

- **When changing to a vegetarian diet,** include soybeans, and other dried beans, soy milk drinks (calcium-enriched), lentils, tofu, tempeh, nuts, and wholegrain breads and cereals. Milk, yogurt, cheese and eggs may enhance nutrient intake.

Protein & Muscle

- Although muscles are built of protein, protein is not a special fuel for working muscle cells - carbohydrates and fats are.

- In fact, a diet high in protein (and fat) and low in carbohydrate, can significantly reduce the performance of endurance sports athletes. **Carbohydrate** is the best fuel for muscles exercised for long periods.

- Any **extra protein** required by athletes and body-builders, can easily be obtained from the extra food eaten to satisfy hunger and energy needs - even allowing an excessive 120g protein daily for a 170 lb athlete (0.7g/lb body wt; twice the RDI).

- Remember, **excess protein** in food will not build bigger muscles. Any excess is converted and stored as fat. Excess protein can also strain the kidneys which excrete the waste products of protein metabolism.

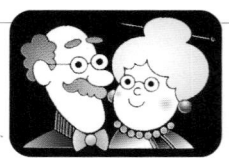

Elderly people (and dieters) must eat sufficient food to ensure adequate protein intake.

Inadequate protein leads to a drop in immune response with greater susceptibility to illness and infections. Muscle strength and muscle mass also drop.

Protein needs are easily met with sensible eating. Athletes who eat enough food for their energy needs, can obtain sufficient protein.

PROTEIN
RECOMMENDED DAILY INTAKE (Grams)

(Figure in brackets - Recommended amount of protein per lb of ideal body weight.)

Pro

Infants:	0-6 mths	13g	(1g/lb)
	6-12 mths	14g	(0.7g/lb)
Children:	1-3 yrs	16g	(0.6g/lb)
	4-6 yrs	24g	(0.5g/lb)
	7-10	28g	(0.5g/lb)
Males:	11-14 yrs	45g	(0.45g/lb)
	15-18	59g	(0.4g/lb)
	19-24	58g	(0.36g/lb)
	25+	50g	(0.4g/lb)
Females:	11-14 yrs	46g	(0.45g/lb)
	15-18	44g	(0.37g/lb)
	19-24	46g	(0.36g/lb
	25+	50g	(0.36g/lb)
Pregnancy:		60g	
Breastfeeding:		65g	

Note: Above figures allow for a large safety margin for most persons.

Iron & Anemia Guide

- **Iron deficiency** is one of the most common nutritional deficiencies in women. The risk is increased in dieters who do not eat well-balanced meals. Chronic shortage of iron leads to **anemia**.

- **Women** between 11 and 50 years of age are at greater risk because of the monthly loss of menstrual blood. Pregnancy, growth, and endurance sports also demand extra iron.

- **In red blood cells**, iron combines with protein to form **hemoglobin** - the red pigment which carries oxygen in the blood. A lack of iron limits the production of hemoglobin and hence the amount of vital oxygen delivered to body cells.

Note: A blood test will tell you if your Hb and Iron stores (ferritin) are adequate. (Iron stores can be low even when Hb is normal.)

- **Vitamin C** (in fruits/veges/salads) enhances absorption of 'non-heme' iron in bread, cereals, milk, vegetables, nuts, eggs and iron supplements. Small amounts of meat, fish or poultry also help. (They contain 'heme' iron).

- **Iron absorption is lessened** by up to 60% when high calcium foods are consumed with iron-rich main meals. Tea, coffee, phytates (in bran) and oxalates lessen absorption of non-heme iron.

- **For infants to 1 year**, use iron-fortified milk/soy formula if not breast-feeding. Introduce iron-fortified baby cereals at 4-6 mths.

Note: Iron deficiency in children (even without anemia), can result in lethargy, irritability, repeated infections, and developmental problems.

Iron Supplements

- **Most people** can obtain adequate iron from their diet. **A wide variety** of animal and plant foods contain iron. (See Iron Counter)

- **Iron supplements** are only recommended for women with heavy menstrual blood losses, during pregnancy (if tests show a low-iron status), endurance athletes with low blood ferritin (iron stores) and for persons with diagnosed anemia. Check with your doctor.

- While the 5 mg of iron in multi-vitamin/mineral supplements is safe for most people, large amounts can be toxic, (especially in persons with hemochromatosis iron-overload condition).

ANEMIA SYMPTOMS

Anemia reduces the amount of oxygen carried in the blood. The body tissues become starved of oxygen. Symptoms include:

- **Pale skin; brittle finger nails (may turn up into spoon shape).**

- **Excessive tiredness or fatigue**

- **Breathlessness**

- **Feeling of malaise and irritability.**

- **Always feel cold.**

- **Decrease in attention span.**

Note: Other medical conditions may also cause similar symptoms. Check with your doctor.

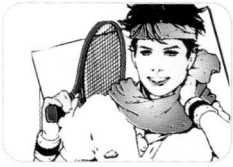

A nutritious diet with adequate iron is important - particularly for women and athletes.

RECOMMENDED DAILY IRON INTAKE (mg)

			Iron
Infants (0-6 mths):			
	Breastfed	~	0.5mg
	Bottlefed	~	3mg
	6-12 mths	~	9mg
Children:	1-11 yrs	~	6-8mg
Males:	12-18 yrs	~	10-13mg
	19+ yrs	~	7mg
Females:	12-50yrs	~	12-16mg
	51+ yrs	~	5-7mg
	Pregnancy	~	22-36mg
	Breastfeeding	~	12-16mg

Pro ~ Protein (grams)   **Iron** ~ Iron (mg)

Meat

	Pro	Iron
Steak: Average all cuts, lean (no fat)		
Small (4 oz raw/3 oz ckd)	23	2.3
Medium (6 oz raw/4^1/4 oz ckd)	34	3.4
Large (10 oz raw/7^1/4 oz ckd)	57	5.7
Roast Beef: lean, 2 slices, 3 oz	24	2.5
Ground Beef patty, lean, ckd, 3 oz	21	2
Lamb chop, broiled, 3 oz	22	1.5
Liver, cooked, 3 oz	23	5.5
Veal cutlet, 1 medium	23	1
Pork, cooked, lean, 3 oz	24	1
Bacon, 3 medium slices	6	0.3
Ham, roasted, 2 pieces, 3 oz	18	1
Ham, luncheon, 2 slices, 1^1/2 oz	7	0.3
Pastrami *(Oscar Mayer),* 3 sl., 1^3/4 oz	10	1.3
Sausages: Bologna, 2 sl., 2 oz	7	1
Braunschweiger, 2 sl., 2 oz	8	5.3
Pork link, thick, 2 oz	6	0.4
Frankfurter, 1^1/3 oz	5	0.5
Salami, hard 3 slices, 1 oz	7	0.5
Vegetarian *(BocaBurger),* 1 pattie	13	2

Chicken/Turkey

	Pro	Iron
Chicken, ckd; Breast portion, 3 oz	27	1
Leg/Thigh, lean, 3 oz	24	1
^{1}/2 Whole Chicken	60	2.5
Drumstick, 1 medium, 3 oz	12	0.6
Turkey, cooked: Light meat, 3 oz	24	2
Dark meat, lean, 3 oz	24	2

Fish

	Pro	Iron
Finfish: *Per 4 oz, cooked*		
Cod, Flounder/Sole, Pollock	28	0.5
Catfish, Haddock, Halibut, M/Mahi	28	1.3
Ocean Perch, Swordf., Orange Roughy	28	1.3
Canned Fish: Tuna, Light, 3 oz	25	1.5
White, 3 oz	23	0.5
Salmon, pink, 3 oz	17	0.7
Salmon, red, 3 oz	17	1
Sardines, 3 whole (3"), 1^1/4 oz	9	1
Anchovies, 1 can, 1^1/2 oz	13	2
Shellfish: Crabmeat, 3 oz	17.5	0.7
Clams, raw, 4 large/9 sml, 3 oz	11	12
Crayfish, cooked, 3 oz	20	2.7
Lobster, cooked, 3 oz	17	0.5
Oysters, raw, 6 medium, 3 oz	7	5
Scallops, 2 lge/5 small, 1 oz	5	0.1
Shrimp, raw, 6 large, 1^1/2 oz	8.5	1
Fish Products: Fish Sticks, 4 sticks	10	0.5
Fish Portions, in batter, 4 oz	13	0.6
Gefilte Fish, 1 medium ball, 2 oz	8	1

Eggs

	Pro	Iron
1 Large Egg, whole	6	0.7
Egg Yolk	3	0.7
Egg White	3	0
Omelet: Plain, 2 eggs	13	1.7
Ham & Cheese	17	3
Egg Substitutes (liquid):		
Eggbeaters, 1 egg equiv.	4.5	1
Scramblers, ^{1}/4 cup, 2 oz	6	0.7

Milk, Yogurt, Icecream

	Pro	Iron
Milk: Whole/Lowfat/Skim, 8 fl.oz cup	8	0.1
Protein Enriched, 1 cup	10	0.1
Chocolate Milk, 1 cup	8	0.6
Thick Shake, Chocolate, 10 oz	9	1
Vanilla, 10 oz	11	0.3
Soymilk (fortified), average, 1 cup	7	1
Yogurt: Plain, 6 oz	10	0.1
Fruit flavors: 6 oz	8	0.3
8 oz	11	0.5
Ice-Cream: Rich, ^{1}/2 cup	2	0
Regular, Vanilla, ^{1}/2 cup	2.5	0
Sherbet, ^{1}/2 cup	1	0
Custard, baked, ^{1}/2 cup	7	0.5

Cheese

	Pro	Iron
Hard Cheeses, average, 1 oz	7	0.2
4 oz piece	28	0.8
Cottage Cheese, ^{1}/2 cup	13	0.3
Ricotta, part skim, ^{1}/2 cup	14	1

Bread, Bagels, Biscuits

	Pro	Iron
Bread (w. enriched flour): 1 slice, 1 oz	2	1
4 slices, about 4 oz	8	4
4 thick slices, 6 oz	1.2	6
Bagel, plain 2 oz	6	1.5
Biscuits, 1 oz	2	0.7
Pita Bread, 1 pita, 1^1/2 oz	4	1
Pumpernickel, 1 slice, 1 oz	3	1

Infant/Baby Foods

	Pro	Iron
Infant Formula Milk:		
Enfamil/Gerber/Similac, 5 fl.oz		
Regular/Low Iron	2.2	0.2
With Iron	2.2	1.8
Isomil/Nursoy/ProSobee	3	1.8
Baby Cereals: *Average All Brands*		
Dry, 4 Tbsp, ^{1}/2 oz	1	7
Jars (w. fruit), 4^1/2 oz	1	7

Breakfast Cereals | Pro | Iron

Hot Type, cooked:

	Pro	Iron
Bulgur, cooked, 1 cup, 5 oz	9	2
Oatmeal: Reg., non-fortified, 1 cup	6	1.5
Instant, fortified, average, 1 pkt	4	8
Quaker Extra, all flavors	4	18
Total, all types, 1 pkt	4	18
Corn/Hominy Grits: Reg., 1 cup	3	1.5
Quaker: Reg., 3 Tbsp, 1 oz	2	0.8
Instant White, 1 packet	2	8
Cream of Wheat, 1 cup	4	10

Ready-To-Eat: Per 1 oz serving

	Pro	Iron
Arrowhead: Average, all varieties	3	1
General Mills: Basic 4, 1 cup, 2 oz	4	3.8
Cheerios, regular, 1 cup, 1 oz	3	6.8
Cocoa Puffs, 1 cup, 1 oz	1	3.8
Corn Flakes, 1 cup	2	6.8
Fiber One, 1/2 cup	2	3.8
Kix, 1 1/3 cups; Kaboom, 1 1/4 cup	2	6.8
Multi-Bran Chex, 1 cup, 2 oz	4	16
Total, average all types, 1 cup, 2 oz	4	18
Wheaties Energy Crunch, 1 cup, 2 oz	6	18
Health Valley: 10 Bran O's, 3/4 cup	3	0.9
Amaranth Flakes, 3/4 cup	3	0.6
Bran Cereal w. Raisins, 3/4 cup	5	1.5
98% Fat Free Granola, 2/3 cup	5	1.2
Real Oat Bran, 1 cup	6	1.2
Golden Flax, 1/4 cup	6	1.2
Kellogg's: All Bran, 1/2 cup	4	4.5
Bran Flakes, 3/4 cup	3	8.5
Cocoa Krispies, 3/4 cup	1	1.8
Corn Flakes, 1 cup	2	8.4
Just Right, 1 cup	4	16
Nutrigrain Almond Raisin, 1 1/4 cup	4	1.4
Product 19, 1 cup, 2 oz	2	18
Raisin Bran, 1 cup, 2 oz	6	4.5
Raisin Squares, 3/4 cup	4	16
Rice Krispies, 1 1/4 cup	2	1.8
Special K, 1 cup	6	8
Nature Valley: All varieties, 1/3 cup	2	0.7
Post: Raisin Bran, 1 oz	3	4.5
Grape Nuts, 1 oz	3	1
Quaker: Crunchy Bran, 2/3 cup	2	8
Oat Squares, 1/2 cup, 1 oz	4	6
100% Natural Cereal, 1/4 cup	3	1
Life, 1/4 cup, 1 oz	3	4.5
Puffed Rice/Wheat, 1 cup, 1/2 oz	1	0.5
Shreaded Wheat, 2 biscuits	4	1

Brans & Wheatgerm | Pro | Iron

	Pro	Iron
Oat Bran, raw, 1 Tbsp	2	0.5
Rice Bran, raw, 2 Tbsp	1	1
Wheat Bran, unprocessed, 2 Tbsp	1	1
Wheat Germ, 2 Tbsp, 1/2 oz	4	1.3

Grains & Flours

	Pro	Iron
Amaranth, 1 cup, 1/2 oz	10	3
Barley, 1/2 cup, 3 1/2 oz	8	2
Buckwheat Flour, dark, 1 cup	11.5	2.7
light, 1 cup	6	1
Carob Flour, 1 cup	5	3
Corn Flour, 1 cup, 4 oz	9	2
Corn Meal, enriched, 1 cup	11	3.5
Flour: White, enriched, 1 cup, 4 1/2 oz	13	6
Wholegrain, 1 cup, 4 1/4 oz	16	5
Millet, wholegrain, 1 cup, 3 1/2 oz	10	7
Rye Flour, dark, 1 cup, 4 1/2 oz	21	6
light, 1 cup, 3 1/2 oz	10	1
Soy Flour, full fat, 1 cup, 3 oz	32	5.5
Yeast: Brewer's, dry, 1 Tbsp	3	1.5

Rice, Spaghetti

	Pro	Iron
Rice: Brown/White, average 1 cup cooked, 6 1/2 oz	5	1
Spaghetti/Macaroni/Noodles (enriched):		
Cooked, 1 cup, 4 1/2 oz	7	2
Canned: in Tomato Sauce, 1/2 cup	2	0.5
w. Meatballs, 1 cup, 8 oz	9	2

Soups

	Pro	Iron
With Noodles/Vegetables, 1 cup	3	0.5
With Meat/Beans/Peas, 1 cup	8	1.5

Fruit

Fresh/Canned: Average, all types, 1 serving

	Pro	Iron
1 medium/2 small fruit	1	0.5
Avocado, 1/2 medium	2	1
Dried Fruit: Apricots, 8 halves, 1 oz	1	1.3
Dates, 6 dates, 2 oz	1.5	0.7
Figs, 4 medium figs, 2 oz	2	1.7
Prunes, 5 medium, 1 1/2 oz	1	1
Raisins, 1 oz	1	0.7
Fruit Juice: Average, 1 cup	0.5	0.5
Prune Juice, 6 fl.oz	1	2.5
Tomato Juice, 6 fl.oz	0.5	1

King Kong was a vegetarian!

Protein & Iron Counter

Vegetables

	Pro	Iron
Beans: Snap/green, 1/2 cup	1	0.8
Dried: Average all types, cooked, 1/2 cup	7	2.5
Baked Beans, 1/2 cup 4 1/2 oz	5	2
Bean Sprouts, mung, 1 cup	3	1
Broccoli, 3/4 cup pieces, 4 oz	4	1.4
Cabbage; Cauliflower, 1 cup	1	0.6
Corn, 1/2 cup kernels, 3 oz	2.5	0.3
1 ear trimmed to 3 1/2"	2	0.4
Lentils, cooked, 1/2 cup, 3 1/2 oz	9	3.3
Mushrooms, raw, 1/2 cup, sliced	0.5	0.5
Peas: green, 1/2 cup, 3 oz	4	1.2
Split Peas, cooked, 1 cup	16	2.5
Potatoes, cooked,		
1 medium, with skin, 5 oz	3.3	2
without skin, 4 oz	2.3	1
French Fries, 3 oz	3	1
Potato Salad, 1/2 cup	3.5	2.5
Pumpkin, 1/2 cup mashed	1	2.5
Seaweed, kelp, 1 oz	<1	2.5
Spinach, cooked, 1/2 cup, 3 oz	2.7	2.5
Squash, ckd, all types, 1/2 cup	1	0.3
Tomatoes, 1 medium, 4 1/2 oz	1	0.6
Vegetables, mixed, ckd, 1 cup	2.5	0.7
Soybeans, cooked, 1/2 cup, 3 oz	14	4.4

Tofu, Tempeh, Miso

Tofu, raw, firm, 1/2 cup, 4 1/2 oz	10	1.5
Tempeh, 1/2 cup, 3 oz	16	2
Miso, 1/2 cup, 5 oz	16	4
Soybean Protein (TVP), 1 oz	18	3

Cakes, Pastries, Pies

(Made with enriched flour)

Carrot w. cream cheese frosting, 4 oz	4	1.3
Cheesecake, 1 piece, 3 1/2 oz	5	0.5
Chocolate, 1 piece, 2 oz	2	2
Fruitcake, 1 piece, 1 1/2 oz	2	1.2
Plain, 1 piece, 3 oz	4	1.2
Croissant, plain, 2 oz	5	2
Danish Pastry, 1 pastry, 2 1/4 oz	4	1.3
Donuts, average, 2 oz	4	1.2
Muffins, average, 1 medium, 1 1/2 oz	3	1
Pancakes, 4" diam., two, 2 oz	4	1
Pies: Fruit, 1 piece, 5 1/2 oz	4	1.5
Pecan, 1 piece, 5 oz	7	4.5
Puddings, average, 1/2 cup, 4 1/2 oz	4	0.3
Waffles, 1 large, 2 1/2 oz	7	1.5

Sugar, Honey, Jam

	Pro	Iron
Sugar: White	0	0
Brown, 1 Tbsp	0	0.3
Molasses: Light/Medium, 1 Tbsp	0	1
Blackstrap, 1 Tbsp, 3/4 oz	0	3
Corn Syrup, 1 Tbsp, 3/4 oz	0	1
Honey, Jams, Jelly	0	0.2

Candy, Chocolate, Carob

Candy, sugar-based	0	0
Chocolate: Plain, 2 oz bar	4	0.8
with nuts, 2 oz bar	6	0.8
Carob, plain, 2 oz	6	0.5

Cookies, Crackers, Chips

Cookies, average, 4 cookies	2	1
Crackers: Graham, 2 1/2" sq., 2	1	0
Rice Cakes, average, one	1	0
Corn/Potato Chips, 1 oz	2	0.3
Nuts: Almonds, shelled, 20-25 nuts	6	1
Brazil Nuts, 7-8 medium nuts, 1 oz	4	1
Cashews, 12-16 nuts, 1 oz	5	1.5
Macadamias, 1 oz	2	0.5
Peanuts, dry roasted, 40 nuts, 1 oz	6	0.5
Pecans, 24 halves, 1 oz	2	0.5
Walnuts, 15 halves, 1 oz	4	0.7
Peanut Butter, 1 Tbsp	1	0.5
Seeds: Sesame Seeds, dry, 1 Tbsp	2	0.6
Pumpkin Kernels, dry, hulled, 1 oz	7	4.2
Sunflower Seeds, dried, hulled, 1 oz	6	1.9
Tahini, 1 Tbsp, 1/2 oz	2.5	1.4

Granola & Food/Protein Bars

Granola Bars, average, 1 bar, 2 oz	2	0.5
Balance Oasis Bars, 1.7 oz	9	6.3
Bariatrix: Nutra Bars, 1	11	3.6
Choice dm Bar, 35g	6	3.6
Dr Soy Soy Protein Bars	11	18
Gatorade Bars, Chocolate, 2.3 oz	7	3.5
Genisoy Protein Bar, 2.2 oz	14	4.5
IDN: proGram-16, 65g	16	3.6
Jenny Craig Bars, 2 oz	10	3.6
Met-Rx Bar, 100g	27	7.2
Optifast Nutra Recipes Bars	8	5
Planters Peanut Bar, 1 1/2 oz	7	0.7
Power Bar, 1 oz	10	6.3
Slim-Fast Bar, 34g	6	4.5
SoBeBars (Mkt America), Peanut	18	6.3
Source One Bar, 2.2 oz	15	4.5
Sweet Success Bar, 33g	2	2.7
Twin Lab Protein Fuel, 3 oz	35	4.5
High Energy Bars, 3 oz	15	1.5
Vita-Trim (Market America)	14	6.3

Nutritional & High Protein Drinks	Pro	Iron
Bariatrix Shakes, dry, 1 oz	15	3.6
Fruit Drinks, mix, 20g	15	0
Proti-Max Meal Replacement, 67g	35	6.3
Boost Nutrition Energy Drink, 8 oz	10	3.6
Carnation Instant Breakfast, 10 oz	12	4.5
Diet Center Meal Repl. Powder, 1 pkt	12	6.3
Ensure, all flavors, 8 oz	9	2.3
Ensure Plus, 8 oz	13	3
GatorPro, 11 oz	17	5.5
GeniSoy Shake: Pro-Cal 100, 1 pkt	14	3.6
JDN Appeal, 1 pkg, 1 cup	16	2.7
Met-Rx, Drink Mix, 72g	38	9
Nature's Best, Protein Shake, 11 oz	20	3.6
Nutra Start, 11 oz	10	3.6
Optifast 800, made-up, 8 oz	14	3.6
Resource (Novartis) Standard, 8 fl.oz	9	4.5
SoBeShakes (Mkt America), 1 pkt	22	6.3
Slim Fast Shakes 325 ml can	10	2.7
Sustacal/Plus, 8 oz	15	4
Sweet Success (Nestle), 10 fl.oz can	10	4.5
Ultra Slim Fast, powder, 3 Tbsp, 33g	5	6.3
Usana Nutrimeal Mix, 2 scoops, 1½ oz	12	6
VitaTrim Shakes (Mkt America), 2 oz pkt	22	6.3
Walgreens Nutritional Suppl.: Plus, 8 oz	9	4.5
Advanced, 8 oz can	13	2.7
Lite, 8 oz can	10	4.5
Weider: Muscle Builder, 2 scoops	18	9
90% Plus Protein, 3 Tbsp	24	2.7

Coffee, Tea, Soda

	Pro	Iron
Coffee, Coffee Substitutes, 1 cup	0	0.1
Tea (all types); Soft Drinks/Soda	0	0
Hot Chocolate, 6 fl.oz	2	2.2

Beer, Wine, Spirits

	Pro	Iron
Beer, 12 fl.oz	1	0
Wines, red/white, 1 glass	0	0.4
Spirits/Liquor	0	0

Fast-Foods/Burgers

Note: See Fast-Foods Section for comprehensive protein counts.

	Pro	Iron
Arby's: Roast Beef Sandwich, reg.	21	4
Giant Roast Beef S/wich	32	6
Italian Sub	29	2
Roast Chicken Club	29	3
Burger King: Whopper S/wich	29	2.5
Hamburger	19	1.5
Double Bacon Cheeseburger	41	2.5
Chicken Sandwich; Big Fish Sandwich	25	2
Carl's Jr: Famous Star Hamburger	24	2

Fast Foods/Burgers (Cont)	Pro	Iron
Carl's Jr (Cont): Ranch Crispy Chicken	24	2
Super Star Hamburger	41	3
Charbroiled Chicken Club Sandwich	35	2
Domino's Pizza: Deep Dish (12"), 2 sl.		
Cheese, 2 slices	42	4
Pepperoni, Sausage, Ham	41	4
X-tra Cheese & Pepperoni	50	4.5
KFC: Original, Wing & Breast	35	0.4
3-Pce. Dinner, Original	51	0.4
Crispy Strips, 3	26	0.4
Colonel's Chicken Sandwich	29	1.5
McDonald's: Big Mac	24	2.5
Cheeseburger	15	1.5
Chicken McNuggets (6)	15	0.6
Filet-O-Fish	15	1.5
Grilled Chicken Caesar Salad	17	1
Grilled Crispy Chicken Deluxe	23	1.5
Hamburger	12	1.5
Sourdough Supreme Burger	21	2.5
Quarter Pounder	23	2.5
French Fries: Small, 2½ oz	3	0.2
Large, 5 oz	8	0.6
Breakfast: Egg McMuffin	17	1.5
Hotcakes w. Marg/Syrup	9	1.5
Sausage McMuffin w. Egg	19	1.5
Muffin, Lowfat, Apple Bran	6	1
Pancakes: 3 Pancakes	8	2
Pizza Hut: Per Medium, 2 slices		
Pan Pizzas, average	26	4
Thin 'n Crispy: Supreme	24	2
Hand Tossed: Pepperoni	26	3
Personal Pan Pizza: Beef	26	4
Shakes, Chocolate	12	0.4
Subway: 6" Subs, average	20	2
Rst Chicken Breast	25	3.5
Steak & Cheese, 6"	23	6
Steak & Cheese Wrap	22	7
Subway Club	22	3.5
Sundaes: Average all outlets	7	0.3
Taco Bell: Bean Burrito	13	3.5
Beef Burrito	17	3.5
Tostado	10	1.5
Enchirito; Chicken; Steak	22	3
Taco Supreme	10	2
Gordita Baja Beef	13	2.5
Chicken Quesadilla	25	3
Wendy's: Single w. Everything	25	3
Big Bacon Classic	34	3
Jr Hamburger Kid's Meal	14	2
Grilled Chicken Sandwich	24	1.5

High Blood Pressure Guide

High Blood Pressure

Many American adults have hypertension (high blood pressure), and are unaware of it. It is generally symptomless, so **have your blood pressure checked annually** - particularly if there is a family history of hypertension.

Untreated hypertension overworks the heart, damages arteries and promotes atherosclerosis. This in turn greatly increases the risk of heart disease, stroke, blindness, kidney disease and impotence. The earlier hypertension is detected, the sooner it can be brought under control.

Treating Hypertension

If your blood pressure is high, consult your doctor about diet and medication. You may be referred to a dietitian for more detailed dietary advice and meal planning.

High-Normal and Stage 1 hypertension can often be treated by reducing sodium intake, losing weight if overweight, limiting alcohol to 2 drinks or less daily, exercising regularly, and dealing with stress.

Stages 2, 3 and 4 hypertension usually require drug therapy. However, salt restriction, abstaining from alcohol and the above lifestyle changes will improve the success of drug therapy, and enable smaller drug doses to be prescribed.

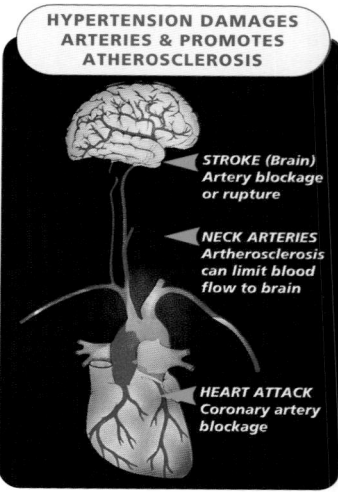

HYPERTENSION DAMAGES ARTERIES & PROMOTES ATHEROSCLEROSIS

STROKE (Brain) Artery blockage or rupture

NECK ARTERIES Artherosclerosis can limit blood flow to brain

HEART ATTACK Coronary artery blockage

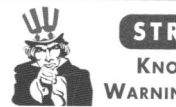

STROKE
KNOW THE WARNING SIGNS!

If you notice one or more of these signs, **call your doctor immediately.** They may be signalling a possible stroke or transient ischemic attack:

- **Sudden weakness** or numbness in your face, arm or leg on one side of your body.
- **Sudden dimness,** blurring or loss of vision, particularly in one eye.
- **Loss of speech,** or trouble talking or understanding speech.
- **Sudden severe headache** - 'a bolt out of the blue' - with no apparent cause.
- **Unexplained dizziness,** unsteadiness or a sudden fall, especially if accompanied by any of the other symptoms.

BLOOD PRESSURE CLASSIFICATIONS
National High Blood Pressure Educ. Prog. (1993)

	DIASTOLIC	SYSTOLIC
Normal ►	80-84	120-129
High-Normal ►	85-89	130-139
Stage 1 ►	90-99	140-159
Stage 2 ►	100-109	160-179
Stage 3 ►	110-119	180-209
Stage 4 ►	120 or over	210 or over

Salt & Sodium

Sodium is a mineral element most commonly found in salt (sodium chloride). It also occurs naturally in much smaller amounts in animal and plant foods, and water is normally sufficient for our needs without having to add salt.

Sodium is required for nerve and muscle function as well as to balance the amount of fluid in our tissues and blood.

Sodium acts like a sponge to attract and hold fluids in body tissues.

Excess sodium can cause water retention, and increase the risk of developing hypertension. Very high salt intake may also increase the risk of stomach cancer.

Too little sodium may cause low blood pressure (hypotension), and decrease blood flow to the heart, brain and kidneys - especially during exercise. (A certain blood volume is required to sustain the blood pressure needed for adequate blood flow in the capillaries.)

Salt - Sensitive Persons

Normally, our kidneys excrete excess dietary sodium. The thirst we feel after a salty meal is the body calling for water to dilute the sodium, and enable the kidneys to flush out excess sodium.

However, 'salt sensitive' persons (perhaps 1 in 2-3 adults) tend to retain excess sodium (above approximately 3000mg daily) instead of excreting it. Such persons are more likely to develop hypertension and would most benefit from sodium restriction. Assume you are susceptible if there is a family history of hypertension.

Although not everyone will benefit, all Americans are being asked to moderate their salt and sodium intake as a public health measure - particularly that so many do not know whether or not they have hypertension; and also because we do not know just who is salt-sensitive.

SAFE SODIUM LEVELS

The American Heart Association recommends a maximum sodium intake of 2400mg per day for adults with normal blood pressure. Many Americans have double this amount.

Persons with hypertension and kidney ailments are usually restricted to as little as 1000mg sodium per day. Your doctor will discuss the correct sodium level for you.

Persons engaged in prolonged strenuous work or exercise may lose sodium through heavy sweating - especially in hot, humid weather. Adequate salt (and fluids) is necessary to avoid dehydration. A little extra salt at mealtimes is usually sufficient to satisfy any extra need. Do not take salt tablets.

FINDING HIDDEN SODIUM

On average, only one third of our sodium intake comes from the salt shaker. The rest is hidden in processed foods that have salt added during manufacture.

Sodium compounds added to food or medicinals can also contribute significant sodium.

Sodium bicarbonate in particular is widely used in antacid tablets and powders, and saline drink powders (such as *Alka Seltzer*). Sodium bicarbonate contains 27% sodium by weight. Each gram contributes 270mg sodium. Large amounts of sodium can be unwittingly consumed.

Other sodium compounds include monosodium glutamate (MSG), sodium ascorbate, sodium nitrite, and sodium citrate.

ALCOHOL

Excess alcohol causes up to 20% of hypertension in America.

Susceptible persons should abstain to normalize their blood pressure.

Salt-Sodium Guide

Sodium accounts for only 40% of the weight of salt (sodium chloride). Examples:
1 gram (1000mg) Salt has 400mg Sodium

1 teasp. (5g) Salt has 2000mg Sodium

Hints to Reduce Sodium

● **Watch the salt shaker.** Start with an easy 50% cut in sodium by using Lite Salt (*Morton*). Then gradually cut back until you can leave the salt shaker off the table.

● **Taste your food before salting.** Use the pepper shaker (small holes) for more controlled sprinkling of salt.

● **Choose low sodium,** sodium free, and reduced sodium products in place of regular salted products.

● **Check labels for sodium levels.** The following sodium descriptors may appear on labels:

　Reduced Sodium: At least 75% less sodium than the original product.
　Low Sodium: 140 mg or less/serving.
　Very Low Sodium: 35mg or less/serving.
　Sodium Free: Less than 5mg per serving.

● **Use reduced-sodium breads,** butter and margarine. Regular varieties contain up to 2% salt. This is considered high in view of their significant contribution to our diet.

● **Go easy on condiments and sauces** such as tomato ketchup, mustard, soy sauce and spaghetti sauces, plus salad dressings. Use low sodium varieties.

● **Limit pizzas and salty fast-foods.** Check the *Fast-Food Restaurant* Section.

● **Avoid salty snack foods** such as potato chips, corn chips, salted nuts, pretzels and cheesy-flavoured snacks. **Choose unsalted** popcorn, nuts or seeds. Eat more fruit.

● **Don't salt children's food** to your taste.

● **Limit or avoid antacids and saline powders** with sodium bicarbonate (such as *Alka-Seltzer*). They are high in sodium.

FOODS HIGH IN SODIUM

● Cheese, Butter, Margarine
● Pickles, Sauerkraut, Olives
● Condiments, Sauces
● Salad Dressings
● Canned vegetables/salads/beans
● Deli Salads (with dressing)
● Frozen/Packaged Meals/Entrees
● Soups: Canned/dry; bouillon cubes
● Meats: Ham, bacon, sausage, luncheon meats, smoked meats
● Canned Fish (in brine)
● Seasoning Salts (e.g. garlic, celery)
● Snack Foods (potato chips, pretzels)
● Tomato Jce (Canned), V8 Vegetable Juice
● Fast Foods: Pizza, Burgers, Chicken
● *Alka-Seltzer* Antacid

MODERATE SODIUM

● Bread (Reduced Salt)
● Meat, Fish, Poultry - Unprocessed
● Milk, Yogurt, Soy Drinks, Eggs
● Peanut Butter
● Breakfast Cereals (<200mg/serving)
● Chocolate Candy, Fruit/Nut Bars
● *Reduced & Low-Sodium* Products

FOODS LOW IN SODIUM

● Products labelled *Very Low Sodium,* or *Sodium Free*
● Fresh fruits and vegetables
● Canned and Dried Fruits
● Potatoes, Rice, Pasta
● Dried Beans & Lentils, Tofu
● Nuts & Seeds (unsalted)
● Corn & Popcorn (unsalted)
● Pepper, Spices, Herbs
● Jam, Honey, Syrup
● Candy, Gum
● Hard & Jelly Candy
● Coffee, Tea, Alcohol
● Fresh Fruit Juices, Water

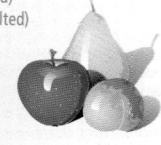

The American Heart Association recommends a sodium intake of **less than 2400mg/day**

Sod ~ Sodium (mg)

Milk & Dairy Products | **Sod**

Milk: Whole/lowfat/skim, average	
1 cup, 8 fl.oz	120
Whole, low sodium, 1 cup	5
Choc Milk (*Hershey's*), 1 cup	130
Human Milk, 8 fl.oz	40
Soy Milk, 8 fl.oz	30
Buttermilk, cultured, 8 fl.oz	250
Dry/Powder, skim, 1/4 cup, 1 oz	110
Yogurt: with fruit aver., 8 oz	130
Cheese:	
Blue, 1 oz	330
Parmesan, 1 oz	450
Kraft: Cheddar, 1 oz	180
Philadelphia Brand Cream Cheese	85
Process Cheese., average,1 oz	430
Swiss, 1 oz	40
Cottage Cheese, 1/2 cup, 4 oz	450
Ricotta Cheese, 1/2 cup, 4 oz	150

Icecream, Frozen Yogurt

Icecream, average, 1/2 cup	50
Frozen Yogurt, 1/2 cup	50

Fats/Oils

Butter/Margarine:	
Regular, 2 Tbsp, 1 oz	230
Unsalted, reg., 2 Tbsp, 1 oz	5
Mayonnaise, aver., 2 Tbsp, 1 oz	160
Molly McButter, 1 tsp	120
Oils/Lard/Dripping	0
Cream, average, 1 Tbsp	6
Coffee-Mate: Powdered, 1 tsp	2
Liquid, 1 Tbsp	5

Eggs

Whole, 1 large	70
Omelet, 2 egg, plain	220
w. cheese	400
Egg Beaters (*Fleischmann's*), 1/4 cup	80

Meats

Meat, average all types, cooked	
(Beef/Lamb/Veal/Pork), 4 oz	80
Corned Beef, cooked, 3 oz	800
Bacon, cooked, 2 slices, 1/2 oz	270
Ham, 3 oz	1100

Chicken & Turkey

Chicken/Turkey, cooked, unsalted, 4 oz	80
Stuffing Mixes, average., 1/2 cup	500

Sausages & Meats | **Sod**

Bologna, 1 oz	280
Frankfurter, 2 oz	640
Ham, chopped, 3/4 oz slice	290
Liverwurst (Braunschweiger), 1 oz	320
Pepperoni, 5 slices, 1 oz	570
Salami, cooked, 1 oz	350
dry/hard, 1 oz	600
Sausage, 1 oz link	220
Pork, 2 oz patty	260
Turkey Roll, 1 oz	160

Fish: Fresh Fish, average, plain

Cooked, 4 oz (no bone)	60
Broiled w. butter, 4 oz	150
Breaded & fried, 4 oz	320
Fish fillets, bat.-dipped 3 oz	350
Fish sticks, 1 oz stick	160
Gefilte Fish (w. broth), 1 pce, 1 1/2 oz	220
Herring, pickled, 2 pces, 1 oz	260
Lobster, meat only, 4 oz	180
Oysters, fresh, 6 med., 3 oz	95
Salmon, canned, 3 oz	460
No Salt Added, 3 oz	65
Smoked fish, average, 3 oz	650
Tuna, canned, 3 oz	330
No Added Salt, 3 oz	40

Entrees & Meals

Frozen Meals, average	600-900
Lean Cuisine, average	700
Stouffer's, average	580
Dinners, average	900-1200
Side Dishes, average	400-600
Pizza, frozen, 1/4 large, 6 oz	800-1200
Microwave Cup Meals	900-1200
Cup O'Noodles, average	1500

Fast-Foods & Restaurants

(Comprehensive listings in **Fast-Foods Section**)

Cheeseburger	750
Chicken Dinner (3 piece)	2200
Chicken Nuggets w. Sauce	800
Fish/Chicken Sandwich	1000
French Fries, small, 2 1/2 oz	150
Hamburger: Regular	500
Large with cheese	1100
Hot Dog (Frankfurter)	800
Pizza, 2 medium slices	1200
Shake, chocolate	250
Taco	400

Sodium Counter

Sod ~ Sodium (mg)   **Sod**

Soups: Condensed, 1 c., 8 oz	800-1000
Low Sodium	70
Chicken Noodle, 1 cup	900
Bouillon Cube, average	950
Cup-A-Soup, average	850
Lite, average	450
Soup Mixes, average, 1 cup	900

Condiments, Sauces, Dressings

A-1 Sauce, 1 Tbsp	270
Barbecue Sauce, 1 Tbsp	130
Bragg Liquid Aminos, 1 tsp	220
Chili Sauce, 1 Tbsp	230
Ketchup: tomato, 1 Tbsp	180
Low Sodium, 1 Tbsp	20
Mayonnaise, 1 Tbsp	80
Mustard, 1 tsp	70
Pizza Sauce, 1/2 cup	700
Salad Dressings, 2 Tbsp, 1 oz	160-400
Spaghetti Sauce, 1/2 cup	500
Soy Sauce, 1 Tbsp	900
Lite (Kikkoman), 1 Tbsp	600
Sweet & Sour, 1/2 cup	250
Tabasco, 1 tsp	25
Vinegar, Lemon Juice	0
Worcestershire, 1 Tbsp	200
Tomato: Sauce, 1 cup	1200
Paste/Puree (salted), 1/2 cup	1000
No Salt Added, 1/2 cup	25

Salt & Salt Substitutes

Table Salt: 1 tsp, 6g	2400
Single Serve packet, 1 g	400
Lite Salt (Morton), 1 tsp, 6g	1200
No Salt Alternative, 1 tsp	5
Garlic/Seasoned Salt 1 tsp, 4g	1300
Sea Salt, 1 tsp, 5g	2250

Seasonings, Herbs & Spices

Baking Powder, 1 tsp, 3g	340
Baking Soda (Sodium bicarb), 1 tsp, 3g	810
Accent (Flavor Enhancer), 1 tsp	600
Chili Powder, 1 tsp, 3g	25
Herbs/Spices: Curry Powder	0
Lemon Pepper (Lawry's), 1 tsp	340
Meat Tenderizer, 1 tsp, 5g	1750
MSG (Monosodium glutamate), 5g	500
Mrs Dash (Herb/Spice Blend), 1 tsp	0
Pepper, Mustard (dry), 1 tsp	1
Yeast, Nutritional, 1 Tbsp	10

Breakfast Cereals

Kellogg's: All-Bran, 1/3 cup, 1 oz	260
Bran Flakes, 2/3 cup, 1 oz	220
Corn Flakes, 1 cup, 1 oz	290
Just Right, 2/3 cup, 1 oz	200
Shredded Wheat Squares, 1/2 cup, 1 oz	5
Health Valley Cereals, 1 serving	5
Quaker: Crunchy Bran, 1 oz	320
100% Natural, 1 oz	15
Puffed Rice/Wheat, 1 oz	1
Total, 1 cup, 1 oz	140
Nature Valley: Average, 1 oz	90
Oatmeal: Regular, 3/4 cup	1
Instant (Quaker), 2/3 cup (1 pkt)	270

Breads, Bagels, Crackers

Bread: Average all types, 1 oz	140
Low Sodium, 1 oz	10
Bagels, plain, 2 oz	200
Sara Lee, 3 oz	500
Biscuits, average, 1 oz	180
Bun/Roll, 1 medium, 1 1/2 oz	200
Crackers: Saltine, 2 crackers	70
Low Salt (Premium), 2	45
Graham, 2 regular	50
Croissant, average, 2 oz	280
Rice Cakes, average	25
RyKrisp Crispbread, Sesame, 2	100

Cookies, Cakes, Desserts

Cookies, average, 2-3 cookies, 1 oz	100
Mrs Fields', average, 2 1/2 oz	180
Baked Custard, 1/2 cup	100
Brownie, 1/4 oz piece	75
Cake, average, 3 oz piece	250
Cinnamon Sweet Roll, 2 oz	250
Danish, Apple	250
Donut, average	150
Muffins, 1 medium, 2 oz	150
Sara Lee, average, 2 1/2 oz	300
Pancakes, 3 x 4"	360
Pie, average 1/6 of 9" pie	300
Pudding, average, 1/2 cup	160
Jell-O (Mix), Instant, 1/2 cup	400
Waffles:	
Home-made, 7", 2 1/2 oz	350
Frozen, average, 1 1/4 oz	260
Aunt Jemima, aver., 2 1/2 oz	630

Fruit & Juices

	Sod
Fresh Fruit, average all types, 1 serving	1
Dried/Canned Fruit, 1/2 cup	1
Fruit Juice: Fresh, sqz'd, 6 fl.oz	1
Commercial, aver., 6 fl.oz	20
Carrot Juice (*Ferraro's*), 8 fl.oz	230
Tomato Juice (*Campbell's*), 6 fl.oz	570
Low Sodium (No Salt Added)	20
V8 Vegetable (*Campbell's*), 6 fl.oz	600
(No Salt Added), 6 fl.oz	45

Vegetables

Fresh/Frozen (No Salt Added), 1/2 cup

Asparagus, Bean Sprouts, Corn	3
Beets, Carrots, Celery, 1/2 cup	40
Broccoli, Cabbage, Cauliflower	10
Cucumber, Green Beans, Mushroom, Okra	3
Onions, Peas, Potato, Pumpkin, Squash	3
Peppers, Hot Chili, raw, each	3
Spinach, Turnips, 1/2 cup, ckd	40
Tomato, 1 medium, 5 oz	10
Canned: Asparagus, 4 spears	300
Beans, baked in tomato sauce	450
Beets, 1/2 cup, 3 oz	240
Corn Kernels, 1/2 cup, 3 oz	190
Creamed, 1/2 cup, 41/2 oz	330
Mushrooms w. butter sce, 2oz	550
Peas, 1/2 cup, 3 oz	250
Sauerkraut, 1/2 cup, 4 oz	750

Pickles, Olives

Olives, pickled: Green, 1 large	90
Ripe/black, 1 large	40
Pickles: Bread & Butter, 4 sl., 1 oz	200
Dill, 1 pickle, 21/2 oz	900
Sweet, 1 gherkin, 1/2 oz	130

Soybean Products

Miso (Soy Paste), 1/4 c., 21/2 oz	2500
Soybean Protein Isolate, 1 oz	280
Tempeh, 1/2 cup, 3 oz	5
Tofu, average, 1/2 cup, 4 oz	5

Jam, Honey, Syrups

Jam/Jelly, 1 Tbsp	2
Honey/Maple Syrup, 1 Tbsp	1
Log Cabin Syrup, 1 fl.oz	35
Lite, 1 fl.oz	90

Peanut Butter

Peanut Butter, regular, 1 Tbsp	70
Unsalted, 1 Tbsp	1

Snacks, Nuts

	Sod
Cheese Balls/Curls, 1 oz	280
Corn/Tortilla Chips, aver., 1 oz	220
Granola bars, aver., 1 bar	80
Nuts: Plain, unsalted, 1 oz	1
Lightly salted, 1 oz	80
Salted or Honey Roasted, 1 oz	160
Popcorn: Plain (unsalted), 1 cup	1
Flavored, average, 1 cup	60
Salt added, 1 cup	180
Potato Chips, plain, 1 oz	160
Flavored, average, 1 oz	250
Pretzels, regular, 3, 1 oz	450

Candy, Chocolate

Chocolate, milk, 1 oz	30
Carob Milk Bar, 1 oz	55
Fudge, chocolate, 1 oz	55
Candy Bars, average, 11/2 oz	60
Hard Candy, Jelly Beans, 1 oz	10
Licorice, 1 oz	30

Beverages, Alcohol

Coffee (& Substitutes), Tea, 1 cup	1
Cocoa, dry, plain, 1 Tbsp	0
Mix, average, 1 envelope	120
Quik (*Nestle*), 2 tsp	35
Soft Drinks, average, 8 fl.oz	20
Mineral Water, Perrier, 8 fl.oz	5
Gatorade Thirst Quencher, 8 fl.oz	110
Water, average, 1 cup, 8 fl.oz	5
Drier regions, 1 cup	20+
Alcohol: Beer, average, 12 fl.oz	15
Wines, average, 4 fl.oz	10
Spirits (distilled), 11/2 fl.oz	1

Antacids – Alka-Seltzer

	Sod
Alka-Seltzer (Per Tablet):	
Alka-Seltzer P.M., 1 tablet	500
Original (Light Blue Box)	570
Extra Strength (Dark Blue Box)	590
Flavored Lemon/Lime & Cherry	500
Antacid (yellow Box)	310
Gelatine Capsule, 1	0
Alka-Mints, chewable	0
Bromo Seltzer, 3/4 capful	760
Rolaids: All types	0
Tums: Regular/Extra Strength	0
Sodium Bicarbonate (27% sodium), 1g	270

279

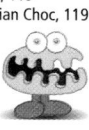

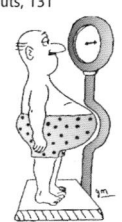

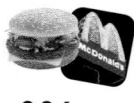

FAST-FOOD RESTAURANTS INDEX
~ SEE PAGE 167 ~

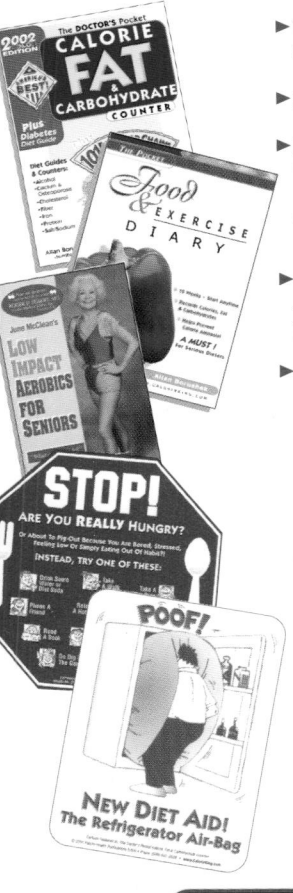
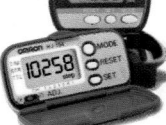

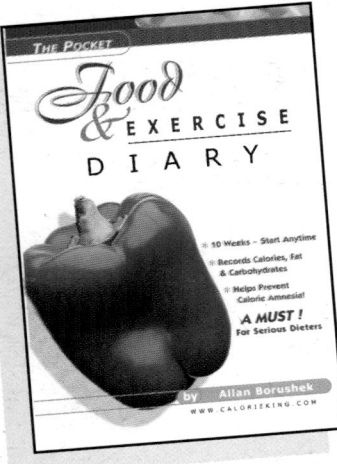
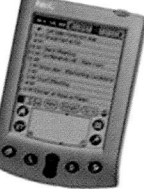